CLINICAL
IMMUNO-ONCOLOGY

CLINICAL IMMUNO-ONCOLOGY

JOHN E. NIEDERHUBER, MD

Adjunct Professor
Department of Surgery and
Department of Oncology;
Deputy Director
Johns Hopkins Clinical Research Network
Johns Hopkins University School of Medicine
Baltimore, Maryland
United States

ELSEVIER

Elsevier
1600 John F. Kennedy Blvd.
Ste 1800
Philadelphia, PA 19103-2899

CLINICAL IMMUNO-ONCOLOGY

ISBN: 978-0-323-87763-3

Executive Content Strategist: Nancy Anastasi Duffy
Senior Content Development Specialist: Malvika Shah
Publishing Services Manager: Shereen Jameel
Project Manager: Gayathri S
Design Direction: Bridget Hoette

Printed in India

Last digit is the print number: 9 8 7 6 5 4 3 2 1

Working together
to grow libraries in
developing countries

www.elsevier.com • www.bookaid.org

Parul Agarwal, MD
Assistant Professor
Department of Medicine
Abramson Cancer Center, Perelman School
    of Medicine
University of Pennsylvania
Philadelphia, Pennsylvania
United States

Vinod P. Balachandran, MD
Assistant Attending
Hepatopancreatobiliary Service
Department of Surgery
Memorial Sloan Kettering Cancer Center;

Assistant Member
Immuno-Oncology Service, Human
Oncology and Pathogenesis Program
Memorial Sloan Kettering Cancer Center
New York, New York
United States

Challice L. Bonifant, MD, PhD
Assistant Professor
Department of Oncology
Sidney Kimmel Comprehensive Cancer
    Center
Johns Hopkins University School of
    Medicine
Baltimore, Maryland
United States

Timothy N. J. Bullock, PhD
Professor
Department of Pathology
University of Virginia
Charlottesville, Virginia
United States

William R. Burns, MD
Assistant Professor
Department of Surgery
Johns Hopkins University School of Medicine
Baltimore, Maryland
United States

Sophia Y. Chen, MD, MPH
Resident Physician
Department of Surgery
Johns Hopkins University School of
    Medicine
Baltimore, Maryland
United States

Daniel Delitto, MD, PhD
Assistant Professor
Department of Surgery
Stanford University
Stanford, California
United States

Stephen Desiderio, MD, PhD
Professor Emeritus
Department of Molecular Biology and
    Genetics
Department of Medicine
Johns Hopkins University School of
    Medicine
Baltimore, Maryland
United States

Jad Farouqa, BSc, MSc
Graduate Student
Australian Institute for Bioengineering and
    Nanotechnology
University of Queensland
Brisbane, Queensland
Australia

Maria J. Gutierrez, MD, MHS
Assistant Professor
Division of Pediatric Allergy, Immunology
    and Rheumatology
Johns Hopkins University School of
    Medicine
Baltimore, Maryland
United States

Thatcher R. Heumann, MD
Assistant Professor
Division of Hematology and Oncology
Vanderbilt Ingram Cancer Center
Nashville, Tennessee
United States

Hyun Min Jung, MS, PhD
Assistant Professor
Department of Pharmacology and
    Regenerative Medicine
University of Illinois at Chicago
Chicago, Illinois
United States

Silvia Manzanero, PhD
Associate Professor
Jamieson Trauma Institute
Metro North Health
Herston, Queensland;
Australian Institute for Bioengineering and
    Nanotechnology
The University of Queensland
Brisbane, Queensland
Australia

Jamileh Nabizadeh, B Biotech, PhD
Research Scientist
Australian Institute for Bioengineering and
    Nanotechnology
The University of Queensland
Brisbane, Queensland
Australia

John E. Niederhuber, MD
Adjunct Professor
Department of Surgery and Department of
    Oncology;
Deputy Director
Johns Hopkins Clinical Research Network
Johns Hopkins University School of Medicine
Baltimore, Maryland
United States

Olamide Olayinka, DVM, MVSc, MS
Graduate Research Assistant
Department of Pharmacology and
    Regenerative Medicine
University of Illinois at Chicago
Chicago, Illinois
United States

Nadya Panagides, PhD, BSc (Honours)
Research Scientist
Australian Institute for Bioengineering
    and Nanotechnology
Brisbane, Queensland
Australia

Luis A. Rojas, PhD
Research Associate
Immuno-Oncology Service
Human Oncology and Pathogenesis Program
Memorial Sloan Kettering Cancer Center;
Hepatopancreatobiliary Service
Department of Surgery
Memorial Sloan Kettering Cancer Center
New York, New York
United States

Barbara E. Rolfe, BSc, PhD
Associate Professor
Principal Research Fellow and Group Leader
Australian Institute for Bioengineering and
    Nanotechnology
The University of Queensland
Brisbane, Queensland
Australia

Melanie Rutkowski, PhD
Assistant Professor
Department of Microbiology, Immunology,
    and Cancer Biology
University of Virginia
Charlottesville, Virginia
United States

Stefan E. Sonderegger, Mag, Dr
Research Scientist
Australian Institute for Bioengineering and
    Nanotechnology
University of Queensland
Brisbane, Queensland
Australia

Brant M. Weinstein, PhD
Associate Scientific Director
Division of Developmental Biology
Eunice Kennedy Shriver National
    Institute of Child Health and Human
    Development
National Institutes of Health
Bethesda, Maryland
United States

Trent M. Woodruff, BSc, PhD
Professor of Pharmacology
School of Biomedical Sciences
The University of Queensland
Brisbane, Queensland
Australia

Lei Zheng, MD, PhD
Professor
Department of Oncology
Johns Hopkins University School of Medicine
Baltimore, Maryland
United States

In 2013, the journal *Science* recognized the scientific accomplishments that enabled the new era of cancer immunotherapy as the scientific breakthrough of the year.[1] This recognition represented more than six decades of study by immunologists to show that the immune system has an important role in the recognition of abnormal cell growth. These early tumor experiments in mammals and the clinical experience with immunology brought about by the advent of organ transplantation began to define the cellular components of the immune response, immune cell interdependence, and active proteins of the complex immune system. These research efforts, over time, confirmed the potential of the immune system as a potent tool to suppress or even reject the malignant cells of cancer. Though our understanding of the complexity of the immune system continues to expand as immunologists define the rules and principles of the system, clinical applications designed to empower the patient's own immune system against their cancer are demonstrating the exciting therapeutic potential of "clinical immuno-oncology."

Recognizing the excitement of today's successes in cancer immunotherapy, and as I worked to put this text together, I could not help reflecting on memories of those early days of my training at the Karolinska Institute and in the formation of my first laboratory in the Department of Microbiology at the University of Michigan. At that time, in the early 1970s, little was known regarding the actual origins and functions of the T- and B-lymphocyte subpopulations of the immune system and the process of antigen presentation. It was in the Möller laboratory at the Karolinska Institute that I learned the valuable *in vitro* culture techniques of the time, the "Mishell-Dutton" methods for culturing mouse spleen cells to measure antibody responses to sheep red blood cells (SRBC).[2] I remember well the hours of counting hemolytic plaques (Jerne and Nordin) to enumerate the anti-SRBC antibody–producing B cells.[3] I have learned so much working with Professor Erna Möller, producing and using antisera that were specific at that time for the two major lymphocyte immune cell populations, T-dependent and B-dependent lymphocytes. Alloantisera against the theta antigen was used with complement to eliminate T lymphocytes from the spleen-derived mixed lymphoid cell populations. A rabbit antimouse B-lymphocyte serum (anti-MBLA) was used in a similar fashion to eliminate the B lymphocytes.

Using these antisera enabled studies to determine T cell–B cell interactions in response to antigens, or the ability of these cell populations to generate immune response "help" and immune "memory." Following my time in the Möller lab, I was able to bring these *in vitro* culture methods to my new laboratory in the Department of Microbiology at the University of Michigan. There, we used these same *in vitro* models to study the adaptive immune response and the role played by the murine I (immune response) region's Ia genes of the *H-2* major histocompatibility complex in the immune response to antigen stimulation.

From those early days dissecting the functions of cells involved in the immune response and the identification of a number of cytokines critical to the adaptive immune response, the science of immunology soon progressed to the advent and application of the technologies brought about by the exciting era of "molecular biology." Soon thereafter, the introduction of massively parallel DNA sequencing enabled the Human Genome Project, which later empowered the whole genome sequencing of many cancers (The Cancer Genome Atlas [TCGA]). TCGA-acquired data continue to have tremendous effects on cancer immunology. The introduction of immune checkpoint inhibition into the treatment of cancer was recognized in 2018 by the awarding of the Nobel Prize in Physiology or Medicine to cancer immunologists James P. Allison and Tasuku Honji. Already, checkpoint inhibition is beginning to be integrated with other immunotherapies such as adaptive T-cell transfer therapy (ATC) and chimeric antigen receptor (CAR) T-cell therapy, further expanding anticancer immunotherapy.

In addition to the advances in immune therapy, there is remarkable progress in the development of new computational pipeline tools that continue to expand our ability to characterize even more precisely functionally specific subclasses of cells that are members of major immune system cell populations; for example, the development of single-cell mRNA sequencing and specific cell characterization not based on morphologic markers but instead defined by the cell's gene transcription profile and secretion of specific functioning proteins. As an example, this approach has identified several functionally distinct fibroblast subpopulations such as inflammatory cancer-activated fibroblasts (CAFs), myofibroblast CAFs, and antigen-presenting CAFs expressing major histocompatibility complex class II antigen presentation complexes, as well as subpopulations within other cell phenotypes comprising the tumor microenvironment.

There is no other more rapidly advancing and therefore promising field in cancer treatment than immuno-oncology. Today, we have a much greater and, in fact, continually expanding understanding of the complex relationships existing between the host's tissues, the host immune system, the tumor, and the tumor microenvironment as these entities relate to the process of tumor initiation and tumor progression. The goal of this book is to enable its readers—those caring for patients with cancer no matter their specialty—to achieve a greater in-depth understanding of these relationships and how they can be engineered to drive the immune system to effectively treat the cancer. It is hoped that this text will enable the trainee and the practicing oncologist to acquire the language of immunology and, in so doing, facilitate the more purposeful reading of the rapidly evolving clinical immuno-oncology literature. Empowered by this knowledge, it is hoped that practitioners will be optimally prepared to discuss and apply immunotherapies in translational research and in the actual care of their patients.

John E. Niederhuber, MD

1. Couzin-Frankel J. Cancer Immunotherapy. *Science*, Dec. 20, 1913; 342:1432-1433.
2. Mishell RJ and Dutton RW. Immunization of dissociated spleen cell cultures from mice. *J. Exp. Med.* 1967; 126:423-442.
3. Jerne NK and Nordin AA. Plaque formation in agar by single antibody producing cells. *Science* 1963; 140: 405-408.

ACKNOWLEDGMENTS

I am indebted to the numerous teachers, clinical mentors, faculty colleagues, and especially my patients with cancer, from whom I have learned a great deal over the years about the challenges of caring for the patient with this devastating disease. I owe special mention to Professors Erna and Göran Möller, who welcomed me to their laboratory at the Karolinska Institute, Stockholm, Sweden, and were responsible for launching my career in immunology. I am, of course, especially grateful for the support and understanding of my family, especially my wife Kathy, during this project. Kathy generously spent many hours proofreading text and critiquing figures. A special mention goes to my son Matthew, whose own interest in science was a major factor in encouraging me to undertake this project and the writing of certain chapters.

My gratitude goes out to the many contributing authors for their dedication to this project and for their willingness to share their subject-matter expertise. Their generosity of time and their efforts to make the content easy to understand and nicely integrated across the individual chapters is greatly appreciated.

I very much appreciate the ongoing support and special opportunity afforded me by my Johns Hopkins colleagues. They have generously welcomed my continued participation in the mentoring of surgical oncology trainees and in cancer research. Special mention goes to Dr. Andrew Cameron, director, Johns Hopkins Department of Surgery, and Drs. Lei Zhang and William R. Burns, leaders of the NCI T32 Training Program in Surgical Oncology. These individuals and many others at Hopkins make life very fulfilling. Finally, I am in debt to Robin Carter, senior content strategist at Elsevier, whose gentle persuasion convinced me to undertake this project. I am extremely grateful for the expert assistance provided by Malvika Shah of Elsevier Development and Production for her constant availability and support as we put these chapters together.

This text is dedicated, as it should be, to the many students, postdoctoral fellows, and surgery residents who worked with me in my laboratories at University of Michigan, Johns Hopkins, Stanford, and the National Cancer Institute. Their presence in my life and the many special friendships remain a daily reminder of the importance of science to the ultimate goal of improving the care of the patient with cancer.

CONTENTS

CHAPTER 1

Development and Structure of the Lymphoid System

Olamide Olayinka ■ Brant M. Weinstein ■ Hyun Min Jung

SUMMARY OF KEY FACTS

- The lymphatic system is a complex, blind-ended vascular tree distinct and separate from the blood circulatory system.
- Lymphatics facilitate tissue fluid homeostasis, nutrient uptake, and immune functions.
- Lymphatic vessels and lymphatic endothelial cells have unique features promoting uptake and transport back to the blood circulation.
- Lymphatic endothelial cell specification and differentiation are promoted by specific molecular programs.
- Heterogeneity and plasticity of lymphatic endothelial cells help create specialized tissue- and organ-specific lymphatic vascular beds.
- Lymph nodes are complex structures with unique layers of endothelial cells that function as key immune surveillance centers.
- Lymphatic vessels are present in the tumor microenvironment where they are active in tumor metastasis.
- Tumor-associated lymphatic vessels have distinct molecular profiles compared with normal lymphatic vessels.
- Crosstalk between the lymphatic system and tumors is important for cancer progression and metastasis.
- For example, VEGFC and VEGFD are major growth factors attracting VEGFR3-expressing lymphatic endothelial cells and accelerating tumor lymph angiogenesis.
- Most of our current knowledge regarding the function of lymphatics in cancers is limited to a few cancer types such as melanoma, breast cancer, and glioblastomas, so there is much still to be explored.

Introduction

The vascular system in our body is essential for supplying nutrients, macromolecules, and cells to tissues and organs but also critical for efficiently removing waste products. The blood and lymphatic vascular systems are responsible for these roles. The lymphatic system is a blind-ended network of vessels that runs parallel to the blood vessels and collects fluid from interstitial spaces to return it back to the bloodstream.[1,2] Although the first description of lymph nodes and glands is found in the Hippocratic treatise "On glands" from around 400 BC,[3,4] the 17th century was the golden age for the investigation of the lymphatics with several key discoveries: gut lacteals, cloacal bursa, reservoir of the chyle, extraintestinal lymphatic vessels, and hepatic lymph

1

circulation.[5,6] In the early 20th century, Florence Sabin and other classical anatomists character-ized the lymphatic system in detail using dye injection and histology to characterize fluid uptake.[7-13] In addition to its important function in tissue and systemic fluid homeostasis, the lymphatic system plays a vital role in immune surveillance by regulating production and transportation of immune cells in response to immunogenic stimuli.[14] Moreover, certain organs contain specialized lymphatic networks that support their function. For example, lacteal lymphat-ics absorb fatty acids in the intestine and meningeal lymphatics regulate cerebral spinal fluid homeostasis.[15-17] Therefore lymphatics play numerous important physiologic roles in human health, and lymphatic research is a rapidly emerging field in cardiovascular medicine.

In this chapter, we review structural, molecular, and functional aspects of lymphatic system development and further discuss the importance of understanding this system in oncology.

Overview of the Lymphatic System

The lymphatic system consists of an extensive network of vessels that transport lymph (called lymphatic vessels) and nodal centers that filter the lymph (called lymph nodes). Unlike the blood circulation, the lymphatic network is a unidirectional, low-pressure system that drains excess in-terstitial fluid from tissues and returns it back to the blood circulation (Fig. 1.1). Interstitial fluid is collected by lymphatic capillaries (also called initial lymphatics), composed of a single layer of loosely connected lymphatic endothelial cells (LECs) that lack a continuous basement mem-brane, a surrounding smooth muscle cell layer, or pericytes.[18,19] Unlike endothelial cells in blood vessels joined by continuous junctions creating a tight barrier to passage of fluid and macromol-ecule, LECs in initial lymphatics are connected by button-like junctions that permit free passage of fluid (see Fig. 1.1). In addition, anchoring filaments connect the LECs of initial lymphatics to the surrounding collagenous extracellular matrix and nearby tissues. Tissue swelling from inter-stitial fluid buildup causes these filaments to stretch and pull on the LECs, increasing the size of the gaps between LECs, promoting increased fluid uptake and decreased interstitial pressure. Lymph contains water, macromolecules (protein and lipids), white blood cells, cell debris, and foreign antigens that are absorbed by initial lymphatics and then transported to lymph nodes via larger caliber collecting lymphatic vessels. Unlike initial lymphatics, collecting lymphatic vessels have elongated LECs that are tightly connected by zipper-like junctions as well as specialized smooth muscle cells, pericytes, and valves that facilitate unidirectional lymph flow.[20] Protein-rich lymph is filtered in lymph nodes to prevent reentry of noxious stimuli into the circulation. Filtered lymph empties into the left (thoracic) duct and right lymphatic ducts, which then empty into subclavian veins where lymph returns to the bloodstream (see Fig. 1.1). Returning lymph to the circulation is critical for regulating tissue fluid homeostasis and normal blood volume and pressure. Failure of the lymphatic system to maintain fluid homeostasis results in excessive buildup of fluid in tissues (lymphedema) a disease afflicting up to 200 million individuals globally.[21] In addition to being disfiguring and interfering with limb function and mobility, long-term accumulation of protein-rich lymph leads to further pathologic changes in tissues and skin, making this a significant cause of morbidity. Lymphedema is classified as primary lymphedema (genetic) or secondary lymphedema (acquired). Primary lymphedema is a congenital condition that causes defects and malformation of the lymphatic system. Although the causes of primary lymphedema are not fully understood, it is frequently associated with genetic mutations and developmental anomalies that disrupt lymphangiogenesis or lymphatic valve development and function.[22,23] Secondary lymphedema is an acquired disorder resulting primarily from underlying conditions that cause lymphatic obstruction. Although the most common cause of secondary lymphedema worldwide is filariasis (e.g., infection by *Wuchereria bancrofti*), in developed coun-tries lymphedema occurs most commonly as sequelae to cancer and cancer treatment. This includes surgical resection of lymph nodes and lymphatic defects caused by chemotherapy and

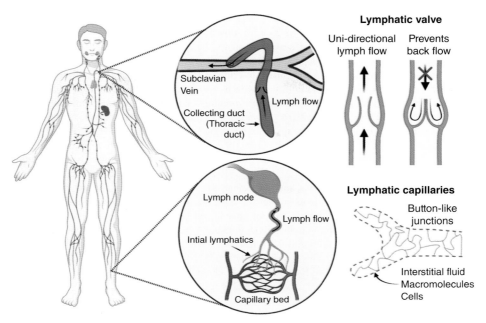

Fig. 1.1 Overview of lymphatic vascular function. Lymphatic capillaries take up fluid from the interstitial spaces of tissues after it has leaked from the blood capillary bed and then transport this lymph fluid to lymph nodes. Lymphatic capillaries are composed of endothelial cells with button-like junctions that enable easy uptake of interstitial fluid containing macromolecules and cells into the vessels. Lymph drains from lymphatic capillaries through collecting lymphatics to collecting ducts (e.g., thoracic duct), where it is returned to circulation via the subclavian vein. Lymph valves are critical components of collecting lymphatics, helping to promote unidirectional flow. (Created with BioRender.com.)

radiotherapy.[22,24-26] Indeed, 1 in 5 women surviving breast cancer develops lymphedema,[27] and over 90% of patients with head and neck cancer experience some form of lymphedema in the first 18 months posttreatment,[28] making lymphedema one of the most common long-term comorbidities of cancer and cancer treatment.

Embryonic Development of the Lymphatic System

Lymphatic vessels begin to develop during midgestation, shortly after blood circulation is established. Studies using *in vivo* imaging in zebrafish and lineage tracing in mice have confirmed that the majority of initial lymphatics originate from the cardinal vein and other primitive veins,[29-31] as originally proposed by Florence Sabin over a century ago.[7] LECs also emerge from alternative nonvenous sources[32-35] via organ-specific mechanisms that appear to be conserved in mammals. Hemogenic endothelium contributes to mesenteric lymphatics,[36] nonvenous cells derived from blood capillaries supplement dorsal skin lymphatics,[37,38] hematopoietic cell and second heart field-derived cells give rise to cardiac lymphatics,[39-41] bone marrow–derived cells play a role in forming corneal lymphatics,[42] and inflammation-associated macrophages incorporate into renal lymphatics.[43] Lymphatic endothelial progenitors coalesce and expand to form a primitive lymphatic plexus that further develops and elaborates to form a defined, tree-like network of capillaries and collecting lymphatic vessels.[30,44,45] Extensive postnatal lymphangiogenesis also occurs through sprouting of preexisting lymphatic vessels and by proliferation and migration of fully differentiated lymphatic ECs, as shown in both mice and zebrafish.[31,45,46]

Several important molecular pathways critical for lymphatic vessel development have been identified. The transcription factor, prospero homeobox 1 (PROX1), is required for lymphatic commitment and maintenance.[47-49] Additional transcription factors including SRY-box transcription factor 18 (SOX18), Chicken ovalbumin upstream promoter transcription factor II (NR2F2 (also known as COUP-TFII)), and GATA binding protein 2 (GATA2) act upstream of and promote expression of PROX1.[50-52] Prox1-positive progenitor cells bud from the endothelium of the cardinal vein and other primitive veins and begin to express vascular endothelial growth factor receptor 3 (FLT4 (also known as VEGFR3)), which allows the lymphatic progenitors to respond to vascular endothelial growth factor C (VEGFC) signals to migrate and form the primitive lymph sacs that gives rise to the lymphatic network.[53-57] Several different cell types such as fibroblasts, neurons, endothelial cells, smooth muscle cells, and macrophages express VEGFC and can attract LECs and help guide their migration.[53,58-60] Loss of Vegfc or Vegfr3 results in lymphatic malformation, edema, and lethality, confirming the critical role of this ligand–receptor pair in lymphatic development.[53,57,61] Collagen and calcium binding EGF domains 1 (CCBE1) and a disintegrin and metalloproteinase with thrombospondin motifs 3 (ADAMTS3) are required for proteolytic activation of VEGFC, and their loss also causes lymphatic defects.[62-64] Chemokine signals such as the CXC motif chemokine receptor 4 (CXCR4) - CXC motif chemokine ligand 12 (CXCL12) axis provide critical guidance cues for lymphatic network assembly and patterning (Fig. 1.2).[65,66] Notably, mutations in VEGFR3, VEGFC, CCBE1, and ADAMTS3 are found in human congenital lymphatic diseases including congenital lymphedema, Milroy disease, and Hennekam syndrome,[67-70] reinforcing the importance of understanding more about the molecular mechanisms of lymphangiogenesis.

Animal models have been critical to our understanding of the development of the lymphatic system. The lymphatic vasculature is highly conserved throughout the vertebrates, including in aquatic animals.[71] The zebrafish is a superb genetically and experimentally accessible vascular model organism that has already yielded many important discoveries regarding lymphatic vessel development.[29,30,45,46,57,65,72-77] Studies in the fish have shown that a subset of venous endothelial cells bud from the posterior cardinal vein and form secondary sprouts that give rise to lymphatic progenitor cells on the horizontal myoseptum region, called *parachordal lines* or *parachordal lymphangioblasts*.[30,45,46] This subset could be angioblasts from the ventral side of the posterior cardinal vein that migrates toward the dorsal side of the vein and gives rise to lymphatic sprouts.[78] The venous cells committed to lymphatic fate acquire Vegfc-promoted Prox1 expression that regulates asymmetric cell division and helps direct their differentiation and migration to become lymphatic progenitors.[79] As in mammals, Vegfc/Vegfr3 and cxcr4/cxcl12 signaling pathways are critical to guide migration and patterning of these progenitor cells in fish,[57,65] and zebrafish ccbe1 and adamts3 genes are essential for cleavage of precursor Vegfc, and their loss impairs lymphatic vessel development.[60,64] The extensive conservation of mechanisms of lymphatic development among the vertebrates permits genetically and experimentally accessible animal models such as the zebrafish to be used to experimentally probe molecular mechanisms and biologic processes required for lymphatic development and their links to human lymphatic diseases.

The primitive lymphatic vascular network further matures and remodels to develop a functional system. A hierarchical structure consisting of capillaries and precollecting and collecting lymphatics forms to ensure efficient unidirectional lymph transport.[2] Blind-ended lymphatic capillaries are composed of oak-shaped LECs that overlap and connect via discontinuous button-like junctions. This unique shape and structure allow interstitial fluid to easily drain from the interstitial spaces of tissues into the lymphatic vessels and inhibits backflow out of lymphatic capillaries (Fig. 1.3A).[12,19] The downstream collecting lymphatics are more complex vessels that consist of continuous zipper-like junctions that prevent fluid leakage, and they are covered with basement membrane and a contractile smooth muscle layer that promotes transport of fluid

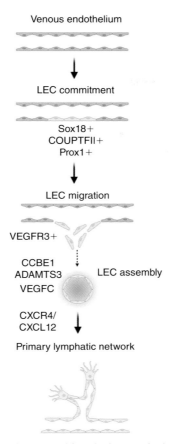

Fig. 1.2 Stepwise embryonic development of lymphatic vessels. Lymphatic vessels start to develop after the primary blood vasculature forms. A subset of venous endothelial cells acquires Prox1 expression, promoted by Sox18 and COUPTFII, committing them to a lymphatic identity. These progenitors express VEGFR3 and migrate toward cells expressing VEGFC. Proteolytic activity of CCBE1 and ADAMTS3 is required to process the precursor form of VEGFC. Lymphatic progenitors cluster and assemble into lymph sacs that give rise to the initial lymphatic plexus. The Vegf pathway and CXCL12 signaling guides patterning of the lymphatic network. (Created with BioRender.com.)

toward the lymph node and eventually back to blood circulation.[80] The presence of valves is an important additional feature of collecting lymphatics that helps prevent backflow (see Fig. 1.3B). Strong expression of the forkhead box C2 (FOXC2) and nuclear factor of activated T cells 1 (NFATC1) transcription factors in a subset of LECs helps regulate lymphatic maturation and valve formation.[81,82] Animals with defective FOXC2 or NFATC1 display abnormal lymphatic vessel patterning, failed remodeling of lymph sacs, and deficient valve formation.[81,83] Lymph flow causing oscillatory shear stress is one of the factors that regulates FOXC2,[84] whereas as discussed later, microRNA-204 (miR-204) posttranscriptionally regulates nfatc1.[85] Interestingly, suppression of either FOXC2 or NFATC1 leads to lymphatic hyperplasia, suggesting that these factors also regulate LEC proliferation.[85,86] Another transcription factor important for lymphatic development is GATA2. Knockdown of Gata2 leads to overgrowth of lymphatics and defective lymphatic valve in mice and zebrafish.[52,87] Gata2 promotes Vegfr3 expression required for LEC

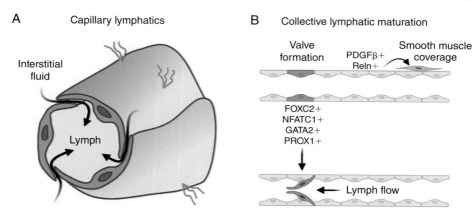

Fig. 1.3 **Key characteristics of capillary and collecting lymphatic vessels.** (A) Lymphatic capillaries are blind-ended tubes with LECs that overlap each other to form a flap-like structures. These structures serve a valve function, promoting directional flow from the interstitium to the lymphatic lumen and preventing backflow. (B) Collecting lymphatics form intraluminal valves by remodeling mediated by transcription factors FOXC2, NFATC1, GATA2, and PROX1. These valves regulate unidirectional lymph flow. LECs on collecting lymphatics also express factors such as PDGFB and RELN that promote recruitment of smooth muscle cells. (Created with BioRender.com.)

migration and vessel patterning.[88] LECs contributing to collecting lymphatic vessels also express secreted signals such as platelet derived growth factor subunit B (PDGFB) and reelin (RELN) that recruit smooth muscle cells to support these vessels.[89,90] Smooth muscle coverage of collecting lymphatic vessels is critical for lymphatic contractility.[20,80]

    Research on the role of microRNAs in lymphatic biology has begun to uncover important functions for these factors in regulating lymphatic vessel development. Small RNA profiling of human blood and LECs led to identification of lymphatic microRNAs.[85,91] The expression of miR-204 is highly enriched in human and zebrafish LECs compared with blood vessel endothelial cells (BECs) and the miR-204-deficient animals fail to form lymphatic progenitors and the lymphatic vessel network.[85] miR-204 targets NFATC1, and the lymphatic defects in miR-204-deficient animals can be reversed by manipulating nfatc1, suggesting that this regulatory axis is important for developmental lymphangiogenesis.[85] In primary cultured rat mesenteric LECs, tumor necrosis factor (TNF) treatment induces miR-9 to regulate Nuclear factor kappa-light-chain-enhancer of activated B cells (NF-κB) level and suppress inflammation.[92] MicroRNAs miR-181a and miR-31 bind to the 3′ untranslated region of PROX1 and negatively regulate LEC genes such as VEGFR3 and FOXC2 in blood endothelial cells to maintain their BEC identity.[91,93] Expression of some of these microRNAs is regulated by bone morphogenic protein (BMP) activity to help direct the lymphatic fate decision.[94] MicroRNA-466 has also been shown to suppress Prox1, inhibiting lymphangiogenesis in a rat corneal model.[95] The pan-endothelial miR-126 targets cxcl12a and vegfr3 signaling and directs LEC sprouting and extension.[96,97]

Heterogeneity of Lymphatic Endothelial Cells and Organ-Specific Lymphatic Vessels

Although LECs in diverse lymphatic vessels share many similarities, they are remarkably heterogeneous and plastic in different organs and in different physiologic and pathologic states. Although lymphatic capillaries and collecting lymphatics have distinct morphologic and functional characteristics (discussed in **Embryonic development of the lymphatic system**), LECs on both vessels express PROX1, the master transcription factor of lymphatic differentiation and identity.[47-49] They also both express other important lymphatic regulators such as podoplanin (PDPN),[98-100] VEGFR3,[54,55] and neuropilin 2 (NRP2).[101,102] Although the organization of their cell–cell junctions varies, all lymphatic vessels also express similar sets of junctional proteins like VE-cadherin, claudin-5, and platelet and endothelial cell adhesion molecule 1 (PECAM-1).[19] Although the LECs of lymphatic capillaries and collecting vessels have many similarities, they are also clearly distinguishable by molecular profiling. Notably, lymphatic capillaries express high levels of the lymphatic vessel endothelial hyaluronan receptor 1 (LYVE1)[103] and the chemokine, C-C motif chemokine ligand 21 (CCL21).[104] LYVE1 is used as a common lymphatic marker, although its molecular function is not well understood. LYVE1 is expressed in LEC progenitors and in primitive blood vessels during embryonic development,[45,46,105] but mice deficient in Lyve1 are viable and develop macroscopically normal lymphatic vessels.[106,107] However, lymphatic capillaries with limited distensibility in organs such as the liver and intestine undergo morphologic changes that alter fluid uptake.[108,109] Lyve1 also plays a critical role in docking dentric cells to the basolateral surface of lymphatic vessels.[110] CCL21 is a strong chemoattractant for C-C motif chemokine receptor 7 (CCR7)-positive immune cells, guiding their migration toward lymphatic vessels.[104,111,112] Unlike lymphatic capillaries, collecting lymphatics express low levels of LYVE1 and CCL21 and, as a result, migration of immune cells to and through these vessels is thought to be passive.[113-115] In contrast to capillary vessels that are specialized for fluid uptake and immune cell recruitment, collecting vessels are designed for transport (see Fig. 1.3). Collecting vessels also have luminal valves that are critical for unidirectional flow (see Fig. 1.1). These valves express high levels of transcription factors FOXC2, NFATC1, GATA2, and integrin subunit alpha 9 (ITGA9), which are required for their formation (see Fig. 1.3B).[52,81,87,116]

LECs respond to inflammatory stimuli and show remarkable plasticity in pathologic conditions. Inflamed peripheral lymphatics suppress migration of leukocytes by atypical chemokine receptor 2 (ACKR2)[117] and inhibit dendritic cell maturation via altered expression of intercellular adhesion molecule 1 (ICAM1).[118] Interestingly, LECs respond differently to some inflammatory stimuli and can influence dendritic cell migration in CCL21-, ICAM1-, and CCR7-independent fashion, suggesting that LECs are highly plastic and respond in a stimulus-specific manner as shown in the case of skin inflammation.[119] The molecular profile changes observed in tumor-associated lymphatics further support the idea that LECs are highly plastic.[120] These new findings add layers of complexity to understanding the plasticity of LECs in health and disease state including infection, inflammation, and cancer. Lymphatic vessels also acquire unique features and contribute to specialized functions according to the functional demands of each organ, guided by organ-specific cues.[1,2] We discuss a few well-characterized organ-specific lymphatic vascular beds later.

Intestinal lymphatic vessels play vital roles in lipid absorption, preservation of gut immunity and intestinal homeostasis.[15] The intestinal lymphatics are composed of two unique vascular networks that connect to form the largest lymphatic bed in the human body. Lacteals are blind-ended lymphatic capillaries that drain excess fluid from the vascular bed within the intestinal villi. These lacteal lymphatic capillaries link back to the submucosal lymphatics and the muscular lymphatic network that drains the smooth muscle layer of the intestine. Both vascular networks connect to larger collecting vessels in the mesentery to transport fluid to mesenteric lymph nodes.[121] Lacteals have distinct specialized functions in absorption of dietary fats (chylomicrons) and fat-soluble vitamins from the villi to be delivered directly to the circulation via the cisterna chyli and thoracic duct. Nevertheless, it is unclear exactly how chylomicron uptake occurs; it may involve paracellular transport across LEC junctions as well as transcellular transport in vesicles.[122] Like dermal lymphatic capillaries, lacteals have high expression of LYVE1 and CCL21, and they provide an entry point for dendritic cells in the villi to access draining mesenteric lymph nodes. This serves as an essential mechanism of gut immunosurveillance and oral tolerance.[121,122] However, unlike most lymphatic capillaries, lacteals have a mixture of both discontinuous button-like and continuous zipper-like cell–cell junctions. In addition, lacteal LECs continuously proliferate at a slow rate under homeostasis.[123] Postnatal deletion of VEGFC resulted in lacteal regression and diminished lipid uptake with no effects on the integrity of quiescent adult dermal lymphatics.[124] This regenerative mechanism may be important in lacteals to manage the constant cellular stress from exposure to dietary products. Although lacteals play a primary role in uptake of dietary fat, lymphatic vessels outside the gastrointestinal tract can also affect fat metabolism. This is evident in patients suffering from chronic lymphedema, who frequently present with accumulation of adipose tissue in affected body parts.[125] Dysfunction in lymph transport can also result in chylous effusions in the abdominal cavity (ascites) and thoracic cavity (chylothorax) and may contribute to cholesterol-associated conditions like atherosclerosis.[126,127]

In the brain, fluid homeostasis and clearance of waste and cellular debris are maintained by the glymphatic system named after its dependence on glial cells and comparable draining functions to lymphatics.[128,129,130] The lymphatic vascular network in the dural meningeal layers surrounding the brain has led to a new understanding of central nervous system (CNS) lymphatics.[6,7,128,131] Meningeal lymphatics function as drainage channels for clearance of cerebrospinal and interstitial fluid macromolecules. They also provide paths for lymphocytes and dendritic cell trafficking from the cerebrospinal fluid (CSF), through deep cervical lymph nodes, to the peripheral lymphatic system. Ligation of the meningeal lymphatic vessels results in accumulation of immune cells within the meninges.[16,132] Phenotypically, meningeal lymphatic vessels express classic LEC markers like PROX1, VEGFR3, LYVE1, and CCL21. Unlike lymphatic vessels in other organs, meningeal lymphatic vessels develop postnatally in response to VEGFC signaling in the blood vasculature. In mice, inhibition of VEGFC signaling hinders meningeal lymphatic vessel development and overexpression of VEGFC promotes excess meningeal lymphangiogenesis, highlighting the remarkable plasticity and regenerative potential of the meningeal lymphatics.[133] Meningeal lymphatic vessels (mLVs) consist of dorsal mLVs and basal mLVs.[134] Interestingly, although dorsal mLVs have similar features as capillary LVs, dorsal mLVs have continuously sealed zipper-like junctions, whereas basal mLVs have discontinuous sealed loss button-like junctions.[134] Interestingly, basal mLVs display a precollecting vessel phenotype characterized by lymphatic valves but no smooth muscle cells (SMC). These distinct features promote CSF and interstitial fluid (ISF) uptake and maintenance of unidirectional lymph flow.[16,133,134] In addition, the close anatomic proximity of the basal mLVs to the subarachnoid space suggests that basal mLVs are hotspots for fluid drainage into the lymphatic system.[134] Meningeal lymphatics are highly conserved including in lower vertebrates such as the zebrafish, where high-resolution optical imaging of lymphatics in living animals can be used to understand its function in brain homeostasis.[75] A better understanding of mechanisms regulating the meningeal lymphatic system may have clinical implications in neurodegenerative diseases (e.g., Alzheimer disease), autoimmune neuroinflammatory conditions (e.g., multiple sclerosis), and cancer.

There are also some hybrid vascular beds that share lymphatic and blood vessel properties. The Schlemm canal (SC) is an endothelium-lined channel that creates a vascular route for the drainage of the aqueous humor within the anterior eye chamber.[135,136] This structure is regarded as an intermediate vessel type between lymphatic and blood vessels (hybrid) but has functional and molecular similarities closer to those of lymph vessels.[137,138] SC endothelial cells express typical lymphatic markers like PROX1, VEGFR3, CCL21 and are responsive to VEGFC-induced angiogenesis, although they lack expression of LYVE1 and podoplanin. In addition, they express TEK receptor tyrosine kinase (also known as TIE2) and endomucin, which are generally blood endothelial cell markers.[135,137,138] During postnatal development, the SC sprouts from the choroidal veins in a manner analogous to the formation of primitive embryonic lymph sacs from Prox1 + endothelial cells in the cardinal veins.[136] The VEGFC/VEGFR3 and angiopoietin/TIE2 signaling pathways have also been reported to be vital in the formation and differentiation of SCs and maintenance of SC integrity.[139,140] SC dysfunction decreases drainage of aqueous humor, which leads to increased intraocular pressure, ultimately resulting in glaucoma. Genetic deletion of angiopoietin 1 and 2 (TIE2 ligands) during late embryogenesis in mice resulted in loss of SC and development of glaucoma in early life. Loss of function mutations in TIE2 and angiopoietins have also been observed in human patients with congenital glaucoma.[140,141] The ascending vasa recta (AVR) of the kidney provides another example of a hybrid vascular bed. The AVR is a vascular network that drains large volumes of interstitial fluid from the renal medulla.[142] AVR endothelial cells express blood endothelial cell markers (endomucin, CD34, CD31) and some LEC markers (PROX1 and VEGFR3) but not LYVE1 and podoplanin.[142] High expression of PROX1 and VEGFR3 and abundant fenestration in the AVR may help facilitate its functional roles in fluid re-uptake in the kidney.[142]

Taken together, LEC plasticity and heterogeneity are likely to play in the specialized functions of lymphatic and lymphatic-like vessels in different tissues and organs.

Lymph Node Microscopic Structure and Function

Lymph nodes are soft, lumpy specialized structures that are closely integrated with the lymphatics, serving as filters to prevent reentry of harmful stimuli into circulation and as key immune surveillance centers. These highly organized structures have different cellular compartments that play crucial roles for mounting effective immune responses[1,143] (Fig. 1.4A). The lymph node

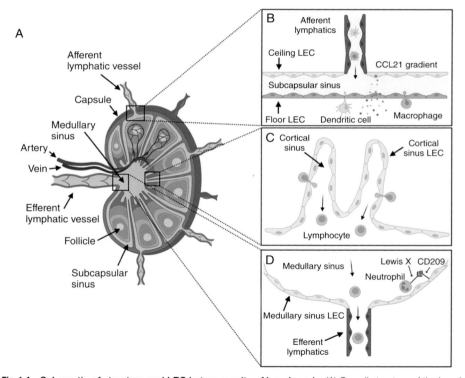

Fig. 1.4 Schematic of structure and LEC heterogeneity of lymph node. (A) Overall structure of the lymph node in cross section. (B) Afferent lymphatic vessels drain into the subcapsular sinus (SCS). The outer layer (ceiling LEC) and inner layer (floor LEC) are molecularly and functionally distinct. A chemokine CCL21 gradient guides transmigration of leukocytes to the parenchyma. (C) Lymphocyte egress from the lymph node takes place via a blind-ended cortical sinus and migration toward medullary sinus. (D) Cortical sinuses emerging at the paracortex of the lymph node drain lymph into medullary sinus, which then exits the lymph node through an efferent lymphatic vessel. Neutrophils adhere to the medullary sinus by interaction between Lewis X (CD15) on neutrophils and CD209 on medullary sinus LECs. (Created with BioRender.com.)

contains multiple lymphoid lobules surrounded by a sinus system filled with lymph enclosed in a collagenous fibrous capsule. The lobules are covered in a dense reticular meshwork that provides a three-dimensional (3D) scaffold with gaps for cellular interactions.[144] The lymph node is composed mainly of leukocytes that account for approximately 95% of cells. Other stromal cell types within the lymph node include BECs, LECs, and fibroblastic reticular cells, which all contribute to adequate organ function.[14,145] The number and structural organization of lymph nodes vary between species. Generally, lymph nodes become more abundant and complex as species size increases. For example, mice have approximately 22 lymph nodes arranged in simple chains, whereas humans have about 450 lymph nodes organized in more complex chains. Larger species also have greater anastomoses of afferent lymphatics compared with smaller species.[144,146]

Lymph nodes receive blood supply through high endothelial venules that facilitate entry of blood antigens, naïve cells, and memory cells. Lymph carrying antigen-presenting cells (APCs), tissue-derived antigens, and immune cells enters the node through the afferent lymphatic vessels (see Fig. 1.4B). By providing an avenue for antigens, APCs, and lymphocytes to converge, the lymph node facilitates effective immune surveillance and activation of adaptive immunity.[1] Upon entering the lymph node, APCs and lymphocytes migrate to distinct subcompartments within the parenchyma. T lymphocytes and dendritic cells traffic to paracortical T-cell areas, whereas B lymphocytes home to the follicles in the cortex (see Fig. 1.4C). This is modulated by stromal cell networks and stromal cell–derived chemokines (CCL21, CCL19, and CXCL13), which play crucial roles in directing immune cells to their respective compartments.[147] Within the reticular meshwork, APCs present antigens to lymphocytes, which become activated and undergo clonal expansion to generate new antigen-specific lymphocytes and plasma cells to initiate an immune response.

After entering the lymph node, afferent lymphatic vessels form branched sinus systems. The basic structure of the lymph node sinus system is conserved across mammalian species.[144,148] Much of our current knowledge about the sinus system was acquired from studies in rodent models. However, human lymph node sinuses differ significantly in structure as a result of the presence of trabeculae and trabecular lymphatic sinuses that are absent in rodents.[149] In general, the afferent lymphatics penetrate the lymph node capsule to open into a subcapsular sinus (SCS) with multiple afferent vessels entering at different positions (see Fig. 1.4A). The SCS is lined by LECs on both sides that cover the entire cortex. LECs facing the capsule are termed *ceiling LECs* and those that border the lymph node parenchyma are known as *floor LECs* (see Fig. 1.4B). Within the sinus lumen, there are both migratory leukocytes of the afferent lymph and tissue-resident leukocytes. SCS macrophages and sinus-resident dendritic cells are associated with floor LECs and have cellular projections that maintain surveillance of the sinus lumen.[14] The SCS macrophages trap large-sized particles, molecules, and microbes in the lymph and present antigens to naïve/memory B and T cells migrating to the follicles and T-cell areas, respectively.[150,151] During infection or inflammation, SCS macrophages can reactivate memory B cells to differentiate into plasma cells in the subcapsular proliferative foci (SPF)—a site of rapid plasma cell differentiation.[151] Small molecules (<70 kDa), however, can penetrate directly through lymph node conduits to reach the B-cell follicles and T-cell areas.[152]

The SCS connects directly to the medullary sinus at the lymph node margin. Although, there is no clear demarcation point between both major sinuses, the ceiling LECs in the medulla have a distinct phenotype.[153] In all mammals, the medullary sinuses converge into a single efferent lymphatic vessel that transports lymph out of the lymph node (see Fig. 1.4D). Medullary sinuses contain slow-flowing lymphocytes emerging from the lymph node and native intralumenal medullary sinus macrophages. Other sinus systems include the transverse and cortical sinuses.

Transverse sinuses are deep radial invaginations of SCS situated in the lymph node fibrous septae. They are present in humans, rats, and other large species but not in mice. Transverse sinuses form shortcut conduits from the SCS to the medullary sinus to enhance subcompartmentalization of the lymph node. Cortical sinuses, on the other hand, are blind-ended sacs that appear at the paracortical zone and drain into the medullary sinuses. They form a compact network of lymphatics through which egressing lymphocytes exit the lymph node parenchyma.[14]

Lymph node organogenesis occurs with a massive LEC remodeling, which starts at embryonic day 12 (E12) in mice as a cup-like projection around the anlage (the future lymph node area).[154-156] Embryonic LECs serve as a primary lymphoid tissue organizer (LTo) and attract hematopoietic lymphoid tissue-inducer (LTi) to the anlage.[156-158] At E15.6–E16.5, LECs from collective lymphatics underneath the lymph node anlage remodel and form a disc-like structure, which is subsequently engulfed by a cup-like LEC sheet at E20.5. Around E16.5, the outer and inner layers of LEC sheets and sinusoidal cords form. At this stage, the outer layer (ceiling LECs) and inner layer (floor LEC) express unique gene expression in adult lymph nodes, suggesting the LEC heterogeneity is already established during embryonic development. Lymph node LECs also secrete growth factors like PDGFβ to recruit SMCs, which is required for capsule formation.[154]

Several studies have suggested the presence of heterogenous populations of LECs in the lymph node.[14,153,159] In mice, LECs lining the SCS express macrophage scavenger receptor 1 (MSR1), whereas cortical sinus LECs express endomucin.[160] Ceiling LECs have also been reported to differentially express atypical chemokine receptor CCRL1, which maintains CCL21 chemokine gradient in the murine SCS.[161] Human LECs, however, lack expression of the general lymphatic marker LYVE1 in the SCS.[149] A single-cell survey characterizing LEC heterogeneity identified six transcriptionally distinct LEC subtypes located in distinct anatomic locations in the human lymph node.[153,159] Floor LECs in the SCS and medullary sinus constitutively express neutrophil chemoattractants. Interestingly, selective expression of C-type lectin CD209 on medullary sinus LECs facilitates neutrophil adhesion via CD209-Lewis X binding, thus mediating neutrophil recruitment into the medullary sinuses.[153] Overall, LEC heterogeneity in the lymph node creates a unique chemokine gradient and provides important niche for immunologic events.

The Lymphatic System and Cancer

Tumor vasculature consists of leaky vessels and the network is formed in nonhierarchical fashion where cancer cells invade into the bloodstream (Fig. 1.5A).[162] In addition to leaky blood vessels, lymphatic vessels are present in the tumor microenvironment, and they play an active role in tumor progression and metastatic spread (see Fig. 1.5A).[1,2,163-166] The dissemination of tumor cells from primary tumors to distant organs via circulation or lymphatics is a key characteristic of malignant cancer progression.[167] Several studies have shown that increased lymphatic vessel invasion increases the risk of lymph node and distant metastasis and is associated with poor patient prognosis.[168-171] Peritumoral lymphatic vessels take up cells and macromolecules from tumors and transport them to sentinel lymph nodes. As a result, tumor-associated lymphatic vessels serve as an important route for metastatic cancer cells to spread from the primary tumor to migrate to regional lymph nodes (see Fig. 1.5B).

Tumor-associated lymphangiogenesis is promoted by lymphangiogenic growth factors produced by tumor cells and other cells in the tumor microenvironment, including stromal cells, tumor-infiltrating macrophages, fibroblasts, and activated platelets.[172-175] VEGFC and VEGFD are believed to be the major growth factors attracting VEGFR3-expressing LECs and accelerating tumor lymphangiogenesis.[176-178] Experimental models suggest that overexpressing VEGFC or VEGFD in tumors stimulates tumor-associated lymphatic vessel growth and increases lymph node metastasis.[177-180] On the other hand, blocking VEGFR3-mediated signaling by using soluble forms of VEGFC and VEGFD decoy peptides that inhibit VEGFR3 signaling[180-182] or neutralizing antibodies targeting VEGFR3[183-187] suppresses tumor lymphangiogenesis and

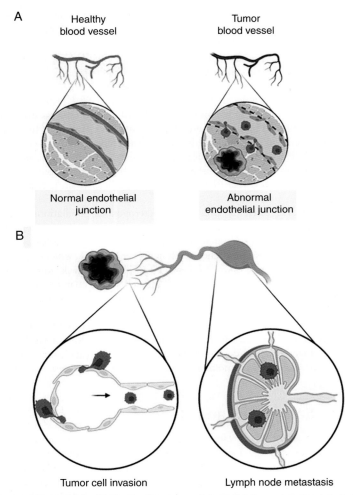

Fig. 1.5 Routes of metastasis. (A) Healthy blood vessels have tightly regulated endothelial junctions that prevent fluid leakage. Endothelial junctions on tumor blood vessels are abnormal and leaky where tumor cells can enter the circulation. (B) Tumor cells use lymphatics to migrate and metastasize to distant lymph nodes. (Created with BioRender.com.)

metastasis. Studies in human tissue and animal models indicate that tumor-secreted VEGFC and VEGFD also regulate enlargement or collapse of tumor lymphatics via misregulation of LEC proliferation and alterations to lymphatic-associated smooth muscle cells.[188-190] VEGFR2 is not involved in new lymphatic vessel sprouting but promotes lymphatic vessel enlargement.[191] Dilated lymphatic vessels enhance lymph flow and facilitate metastatic tumor cell dissemination to the lymph node.[192] Several other growth factor and signaling pathways have also been linked to tumor lymphangiogenesis, including VEGFA, NRP2, angiopoietins, PDGFB, fibroblast growth factor 2 (FGF2), hepatocyte growth factor (HGF), epidermal growth factors (EGF), insulin-like growth factors (IGFs), Ephrin-B2, growth hormone (GH), and adrenomedullin (AM) (for in-depth review, see the literature[163,193,194]).

Tumor-associated lymphatic vessels share molecular profiles similar to those of normal lymphatic vessels but there are significant differences.[120] Comparison of primary LECs isolated from normal tissues and from highly metastatic fibrosarcoma indicated that tumor lymphatics had elevated expression of tight junction regulatory protein endothelial cell-selective adhesion molecule (ESAM), transforming growth factor-beta coreceptor endoglin CD105, angiogenesis-associated leptin receptor, and immunoinhibitory receptor CD200 and reduced expression of subendothelial matrix proteins such as collagens, fibrillin, and biglycan.[120] Such distinct molecular difference suggests that tumor lymphatics can potentially enhance tumor progression and spread.

Lymphatics play important roles in controlling immune trafficking and in chemokine-regulated immune surveillance. CCL21, a chemokine expressed by LECs, has a critical role in attracting CCR7-expressing immune cells through afferent lymphatics to lymph nodes.[112,195,196] Tumor cells take advantage of this mechanism to promote their lymphatic invasion.[197] Tumor cells produce VEGFC to stimulate upregulation of CCL21 in LECs, which in turn serve as a chemoattractant promoting migration of CCR7-expressing tumor cells toward LECs.[198] Cancer cells express receptors that respond to chemokines expressed by lymphatics to increase the rate of metastasis to lymph nodes.[199-203] Particular sets of chemokines and receptors that promote the spread of cancer via lymphatic vessels are being used in cancer immunotherapy to target subsets of tumor cells.[204] Tumor-associated lymphatic vessels take up fluid containing antigens and antigen-presenting cells from the tumor microenvironment and transport them to the lymph nodes. This process recruits immune cells and initiates the adaptive antitumor immune response.[205,206] Enhanced lymphatic function in brain cancers such as glioblastoma can promote cancer clearance. VEGFC-promoted stimulation of lymphatic drainage primes CD8+ T cells in the deep cervical lymph node, allowing migration of CD8± T cells into the tumor in the brain and enhanced glioblastoma clearance.[207] However, it is important to note that although lymphatics are critical for initiating antitumor responses, the immunosuppressive function of LECs in the tumor microenvironment could be compromised and subsequently suppress antitumor immunity and let tumor cells evade immune surveillance.[164] LECs on lymphatic vessels and lymph node express major histocompatibility complex (MHC) class I and class II, which function like antigen-presenting cells to induce some level of self-tolerance.[208,209] Immune tolerance is also promoted by VEGFC in a melanoma model and induces tumor-specific CD8+ T-cell death, protecting tumor cells from antitumor immunity.[210] Moreover, tumor-associated lymphatics increase the expression of the immunosuppressive molecule programmed death-ligand 1 (PD-L1) that targets CD8+ T cells.[211] Taken together, these and other findings highlight the dual roles of lymphatic vessels to both promote and inhibit tumor immunity.[164]

Conclusions

Although lymphatic research has a long history, the development of powerful new tools and methods for visualizing and manipulating the lymphatic system in living animals has led to greatly increased understanding of this previously mysterious system. Many important new aspects of lymphatic vessel development and function in health and disease have been uncovered, and identification of new lymphatic markers, transcription factors, growth factors and receptors, and miRNAs have greatly advanced our knowledge of how lymphatics develop and function. Many new questions are now emerging in this rapidly developing field because of increased awareness of the important role of lymphatics in many diseases, including a key role in cancer biology. Most of our current knowledge regarding the function of lymphatics in cancers is limited to a few cancer types such as melanoma, breast cancer, and glioblastomas, so there is much still to be explored. Better understanding the communication between lymphatics and tumors and their unique organ-specific crosstalk will improve traditional cancer management and lead to the development of new tools for diagnosis and treatment.

Key References

1. Oliver G, et al. The Lymphatic vasculature in the 21(st) century: novel functional roles in homeostasis and disease. *Cell*. 2020;182(2):270-296.
2. Petrova TV, Koh GY. Biological functions of lymphatic vessels. *Science*. 2020;369(6500):eaax4063.
7. Sabin FR. On the origin of the lymphatic system from the veins and the development of the lymph hearts and thoracic duct in the pig. *Am J Anat*. 1902;1(3):367-389.
14. Jalkanen S, Salmi M. Lymphatic endothelial cells of the lymph node. *Nat Rev Immunol*. 2020;20(9): 566-578.
18. Alitalo K, Tammela T, Petrova TV. Lymphangiogenesis in development and human disease. *Nature*. 2005;438(7070):946-953.
19. Baluk P, et al. Functionally specialized junctions between endothelial cells of lymphatic vessels. *J Exp Med*. 2007;204(10):2349-2362.
30. Yaniv K, et al. Live imaging of lymphatic development in the zebrafish. *Nat Med*. 2006;12(6):711-716.
44. Yang Y, Oliver G. Development of the mammalian lymphatic vasculature. *J Clin Invest*. 2014;124(3): 888-897.
48. Wigle JT, Oliver G. Prox1 function is required for the development of the murine lymphatic system. *Cell*. 1999;98(6):769-778.
53. Karkkainen MJ, et al. Vascular endothelial growth factor C is required for sprouting of the first lymphatic vessels from embryonic veins. *Nat Immunol*. 2004;5(1):74-80.
55. Jeltsch M, et al. Hyperplasia of lymphatic vessels in VEGF-C transgenic mice. *Science*. 1997; 276(5317):1423-1425.
104. Weber M, et al. Interstitial dendritic cell guidance by haptotactic chemokine gradients. *Science*. 2013;339(6117):328-332.
142. Qi H, Kastenmuller W, Germain RN. Spatiotemporal basis of innate and adaptive immunity in secondary lymphoid tissue. *Annu Rev Cell Dev Biol*. 2014;30:141-167.
146. Girard JP, Moussion C, Forster R. HEVs, lymphatics and homeostatic immune cell trafficking in lymph nodes. *Nat Rev Immunol*. 2012;12(11):762-773.
157. van de Pavert SA, Mebius RE. New insights into the development of lymphoid tissues. *Nat Rev Immunol*. 2010;10(9):664-674.
161. Folkman J. Tumor angiogenesis: therapeutic implications. *N Engl J Med*. 1971;285(21):1182-1186.
172. Olumi AF, et al. Carcinoma-associated fibroblasts direct tumor progression of initiated human prostatic epithelium. *Cancer Res*. 1999;59(19):5002-5011.
176. Stacker SA, et al. VEGF-D promotes the metastatic spread of tumor cells via the lymphatics. *Nat Med*. 2001;7(2):186-191.
178. Skobe M, et al. Induction of tumor lymphangiogenesis by VEGF-C promotes breast cancer metastasis. *Nat Med*. 2001;7(2):192-198.
203. Nagarsheth N, Wicha MS, Zou W. Chemokines in the cancer microenvironment and their relevance in cancer immunotherapy. *Nat Rev Immunol*. 2017;17(9):559-572.

Visit Elsevier eBooks + (eBooks.Health.Elsevier.com) for complete set of references.

CHAPTER 2

The Chemistry, Structure, and Function of Immunoglobulins

Maria J. Gutierrez ■ Stephen Desiderio

SUMMARY OF KEY FACTS

- Immunoglobulins (Igs) are the soluble mediators of antigen recognition. An Ig that is capable of specifically binding an antigen is termed an *antibody*.
- Immunoglobulins range in molecular weight from 150 kD to 900 kD and are built from tetrameric units consisting of two heavy (H) chains and two light (L) chains, each chain containing one variable (V) domain and one or more constant (C) domains.
- There are five major classes of human Igs (IgM, IgD, IgG, IgA, and IgE), distinguished by their H chain constant regions.
- The Ig classes differ with respect to their effector functions. The antigen-binding sites of Ig are located in the V regions of the paired heavy and light chains.
- Antibody–antigen binding exhibits a range of affinities, from $K_A \approx 10^5$ M^{-1} to $K_A \approx 10^{10}$ M^{-1}.
- Ig genes are assembled from arrays of V, D, and J gene segments by V(D)J recombination.
- Constraints on V(D)J recombination enforce allelic exclusion, the process by which a given B cell expresses only one Ig.
- The affinity of Ig for antigen is increased during B-cell maturation by consecutive rounds of somatic hypermutation (SHM) and selection. SHM is initiated by the enzyme activation–induced deaminase (AID).
- A process related to SHM, class switch recombination (CSR), allows a B cell that expresses IgM and IgD of a defined antigenic specificity to express other Ig classes of the same specificity.
- CSR, like SHM, is initiated by AID.
- Defects in V(D)J recombination, SHM, or CSR are associated with primary immunodeficiency disorders.
- The Ig constant regions are subject to glycosylation and the resulting glycan modifications are structurally diverse.
- Glycosylation modulates the half-life, inflammatory activity, and cytotoxic effector function of Ig. Glycosylation also occurs at somatically mutated sites in Ig variable regions and can promote survival of some B-cell lymphomas.
- The effector functions of Ig include neutralization of antigen, opsonization, recruitment of complement, and recruitment of other immune cells.
- Of particular importance to immuno-oncology is antibody-dependent cellular cytotoxicity (ADCC), a process by which effector cells bearing Ig receptors recognize and lyse target cells coated by specific antibodies.
- The main ADCC effectors are natural killer (NK) cells.

Continued on following page

SUMMARY OF KEY FACTS—cont'd

- Monoclonal antibodies (mAbs), in distinction from the polyclonal antibodies characteristic of a natural immune response, possess a unique primary amino acid sequence and are directed against a single antigenic epitope.
- More than 100 mAbs have been approved for therapeutic use in the United States. They are derived by natural immunization and cellular cloning or by more direct methods of genetic engineering.
- Earlier generations of mAbs were generated in mice and deleterious immune responses in humans were mitigated by synthesis of mouse–human chimeras; more recently the generation of humanized mice and direct cloning from human B cells have obviated the immunogenic properties of mAbs derived from nonhuman sources.

The Structure of Immunoglobulins

OVERALL STRUCTURE

Immunoglobulin (Ig) and T-cell receptors (TCRs), produced by B- and T-lymphoid cells, respectively, are the specific antigen recognition units of the adaptive immune system. Whereas TCRs are exclusively associated with the cell surface, Ig is present in both membrane-bound and secreted forms. This chapter will focus on Ig, although it should be noted that Ig and TCRs share a number of similarities, particularly with respect to the structure and genetic encoding of their antigen-binding sites.

The term *antibody* denotes an Ig capable of recognizing a specific antigen. In soluble form, antibodies are the main effectors of B-cell-mediated adaptive immunity. Antibodies are large, multimeric proteins ranging in molecular weight from about 150 kD (IgG) to 900 kD (IgM).[1-3] All classes of antibodies are built from one or more heterotetrameric, Y-shaped units; the basic unit is depicted in Fig. 2.1 for IgG. Each heterotetramer consists of two identical heavy (H) chains and two identical light (L) chains of molecular weight 50–75 kD and 23 kD, respectively. The H chains are joined covalently by disulfide linkages, as is each L chain to its neighboring H chain (see Fig. 2.1).[1,2]

Historically, partial proteolysis was used to dissect the functional regions of Ig molecules. Some of these proteolytic fragments retain significance today as therapeutic agents. Digestion of IgG with papain cleaves each H chain at the amino-terminal side of the inter-H chain disulfide linkages, thereby releasing two antibody fragments, termed Fab, each containing a single antigen-binding site (see Fig. 2.1). Digestion of IgG with the protease pepsin cleaves each H chain at the carboxy-terminal side of the inter-H chain disulfide bonds (see Fig. 2.1).[1,2] This produces a fragment termed F(ab')$_2$, in which the two antigen-binding sites remain linked, and an Fc fragment, consisting of the paired carboxy-terminal C$_H$ domains. The Fc fragment is responsible for diverse effector functions, including antibody-dependent cytotoxicity (ADCC), opsonization, and complement fixation.[2,3]

STRUCTURES OF THE IG LIGHT AND HEAVY CHAINS

The synthesis of functional antibody light and heavy chains underlies the generation of humoral immune responses. The expression of Ig H and L chains is initiated in an ordered fashion during B-cell development, and this ordering is a consequence of the regulated assembly of Ig heavy chain (IgH) and Ig light chain (IgL) genes, as described in detail below.

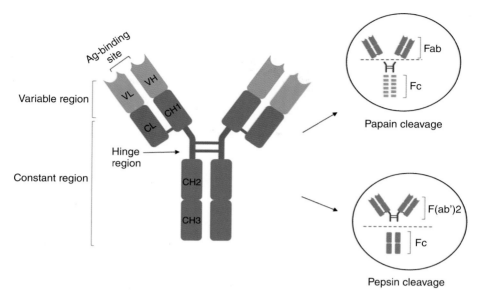

Fig. 2.1 Immunoglobulin and its proteolytic fragments. Left, schematic diagram of IgG. *VL and CL,* light chain variable and constant domains; *VH, CH1, CH2, and CH3,* heavy chain variable and constant domains. Antigen-binding sites and hinge region are indicated. Upper right, cleavage with papain yields two Fab fragments. Lower right, cleavage with pepsin yields an F(ab')2 fragment and an Fc fragment. (Created with BioRender.com)

The Ig chains are built up from globular protein domains, each approximately 110 amino acid residues in length. These domains share a common structure called the *immunoglobulin fold*, consisting of two β sheets linked by a disulfide bond and surrounding a hydrophobic core. Each light chain comprises two immunoglobulin domains, termed V_L and C_L, for variable and constant, because the amino-terminal V_L domain is variable in sequence and the carboxy-terminal C_L domain is constant in sequence for a given class of light chain (see Fig. 2.1).[2,4] The antibody heavy chains contain four or five immunoglobulin domains, depending on the antibody class (see later): V_H and C_H1 through C_H3 or C_H4, where V and C denote variable and constant, as for the light chains. In a folded, heterotetrameric Ig molecule, the V_H and V_L domains are closely associated and form the antigen-binding site; the C_H1 and C_L domains are likewise associated, as are the paired C_H2, C_H3, and, when present, C_H4 domains (Fig. 2.2).[1,2]

Ig molecules are not rigid but contain flexible regions that allow the antibody to conform to the arrangement of binding sites in multivalent ligands. The first of these flexible regions, the elbow, is formed by the relatively unstructured polypeptide sequences that link V_L and C_L and V_H to C_H1 (see Figs. 2.1 and 2.2). All antibody classes except for IgM and IgE contain a second flexible region, the hinge, which permits the Fab arms of the antibody to rotate and bend relative to the Fc.[5] The hinge region also contains the interheavy chain disulfide bonds and differs in length among H chain classes, as will be discussed in the following section.

ANTIBODY–ANTIGEN BINDING

The V regions of Ig H and L chains are highly variable in sequence, but this variability is not evenly distributed along the lengths of the V_H and V_L regions. Rather, in each V region, sequence variability is clustered in three distinct locations called the complementarity-determining regions

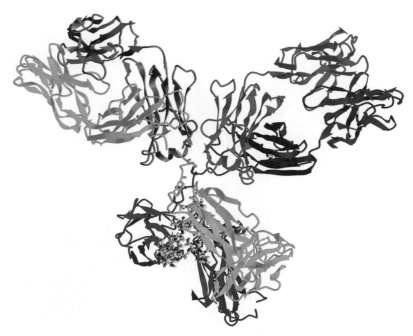

Fig. 2.2 Structure of an IgG1 antibody. Ig heavy and light chains are depicted in ribbon format. Teal and blue, heavy chains; brown and magenta, kappa chains. Carbohydrate is depicted in ball and stick format. (Reproduced from Wang J, Youkharibache P, Zhang D, et al. iCn3D, a web-based 3D viewer for sharing 1D/2D/3D representations of biomolecular structures. Bioinformatics. 2020;36(1):131–135. doi: 10.1093/bioinformatics/btz502.)

1 through 3 (CDR1–CDR3). These hypervariable regions span residues 24 to 34, 50 to 56, and 89 to 97 in the human V_L domains and residues 31 to 35, 50 to 65, and 95 to 102 in the V_H domains.[4,6,7] As a consequence of imprecision in the assembly of Ig genes, as described later, the lengths of the third CDRs are variable. In the folded, assembled tetraheteromeric antibody molecule, the three CDRs of each Ig chain are brought into proximity to form a single surface that constitutes the antigen-binding site (Fig. 2.3). Because the amino acid residues that comprise the CDRs are highly variable in sequence, it follows that the surface that they form is highly variable in shape. Within a given Ig molecule, the two H chains are identical, as are the two L chains; therefore the two antigen-binding sites are identical.

The surfaces formed by the six CDRs are large, with typical areas ranging from 700 to 750 Å.[2] In crystal structures of Fab fragments in complex with protein antigens the interacting antigenic surface, termed an *epitope*, is of a similar area.[8] Binding between these two surfaces is mediated by hydrophobic interactions, van der Waals forces, hydrogen bonds, and electrostatic interactions. The binding of Ig to its cognate antigen is reversible; antibody–antigen affinities are measurable and can be expressed as association constants (K_A). For the binding of an antibody to protein antigens, a wide range of affinities is observed, from $K_A \approx 10^5 \ M^{-1}$ for the lowest affinity interactions to $K_A \approx 10^{10} \ M^{-1}$ for very high-affinity binding. It is important to note that these affinities refer to the binding of an antigen to a single antigen-binding site. Because antibodies are multivalent, the binding of an antibody to a multivalent antigen can involve the simultaneous engagement of two or more antigen-binding sites. The strength of such an interaction is called *avidity* and can greatly exceed the affinity measured for monovalent binding.[9,10]

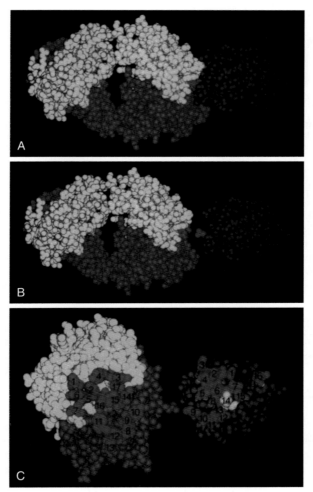

Fig. 2.3 **Binding surface of an antibody with a protein antigen.** (A) Structure of a complex between an antibody Fab fragment and hen egg lysozyme. Blue, H chain; yellow, L chain; green, lysozyme. (B) Separation of the Fab and lysozyme models demonstrating space complementarity. Lysozyme residue Gln121 (red) inserts into a pocket on the Fab surface. (C) Break-apart views of the antibody and antigen interaction surfaces. Contacts are shown in red. Left, 1 through 7, L chain residues that contact antigen; left, 8 through 17, H chain residues that contact antigen. Right, 1 through 16, lysozyme residues that contact antibody. (Reproduced from Amit AG, Mariuzza RA, Phillips SE, Poljak RJ. Three-dimensional structure of an antigen-antibody complex at 2.8 A resolution. Science. 1986;233:747–753.)

Antibody Isotypes

CHARACTERISTICS OF HUMAN ANTIBODY ISOTYPES

In humans, there are five primary immunoglobulin classes: IgM, IgD, IgG, IgA, and IgE; each immunoglobulin class is defined by its heavy chain isotype: mu (μ), delta (δ), gamma (γ), alpha (α), and epsilon (ε), respectively (Fig. 2.4). All immunoglobulin classes employ the same light chain isotypes, which are either kappa (κ) or lambda (λ).[1,2]

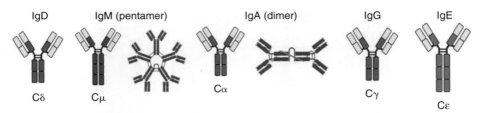

Fig. 2.4   Immunoglobulin classes. Schematic diagrams of IgD, IgM, IgA, IgG, and IgE are shown. IgM and IgA are depicted in their monomeric and multimeric forms, respectively. Teal, green, purple, red, and orange denote regions of each antibody that are encoded by their corresponding H chain constant exons. (Adapted from "Immunoglobulin variations" by BioRender.com (2021). Retrieved from https://app.biorender.com/biorender-templates).

The IgG class contains four subclasses: IgG1, IgG2, IgG3, IgG4. The IgA class comprises two subclasses, IgA1 and IgA2. The IgG and IgA subclasses are differentiated by the structures of their hinge and tail regions, which confer distinct functional characteristics (Table 2.1).[2,11]

In addition to their secreted forms, all Ig classes have corresponding membrane-bound forms in which the heavy chain isotypes differ from those of the secreted forms at the carboxyl terminus: the membrane-bound heavy chains have an extended peptide sequence containing a negatively charged extracellular juxtamembrane domain, a transmembrane domain, and a positively charged anchor sequence. Membrane-bound Ig associates with the Igα/Igβ heterodimer (CD79) to form the B-cell receptor (BCR) complex, which transduces antigenic signals. Mature naïve B-cells and unswitched memory B-cells express two membrane-bound Ig classes, IgD and IgM. Further maturation of B cells is accompanied by class switching, a process by which IgD and IgM are replaced by IgG, IgA, or IgE at the cell surface (see **Class switch recombination and somatic hypermutation**). Ig-bearing memory B cells reside in lymphoid tissues[12] and peripheral blood, where they comprise approximately 21% to 28% of the circulating pool of B cells in adults.[13] Notably, IgA+, IgG+, and IgM+IgD+ B cells are differentially distributed across tissues. For example, human tonsils contain a larger frequency of IgA+ B cells than other organs, IgM+IgD+-expressing naïve B cells are the predominant isotype in peripheral blood, lymph nodes, and the bone marrow, and IgG+ cells seem to be evenly distributed across most tissues.[14] In contrast, IgE+ B cells appear only transiently and in low numbers in germinal centers.[15]

Soluble antibodies are produced by terminally differentiated B cells collectively known as antibody-secreting cells (ASCs), which arise from activated B cells. ASCs include short-lived effector cells that arise early in antibody responses (plasmablasts and short-lived plasma cells) and long-lived plasma cells that are responsible for durable antibody responses. Short-lived ASCs can arise in response to T cell–independent antigens or during the early responses to T cell–dependent antigens. Conversely, the generation of long-lived ASCs requires cell-to-cell interactions with T cells in specialized microenvironments known as *germinal centers* (GCs).[16] GCs are located in the follicles of lymphoid organs and promote the development of high-affinity memory B cells and long-lasting plasma cells, responsible for long-term antibody production. Long-lived ASCs reside in gut-associated lymphoid tissues (GALT) and in the bone marrow, where microenvironmental signals are required for their longevity.[16,17] Long-lived ASCs predominantly produce IgA and IgG. In contrast, IgE+ ASCs are rarely found, perhaps because most IgE+ B cells differentiate into short-lived ASCs.[15]

BIOLOGIC FUNCTIONS OF IG ISOTYPES

IgM. IgM is the first immunoglobulin produced during B cell development and its membrane-bound form is initially found on the surface of naïve B cells. In response to T cell–independent

TABLE 2.1 ■ Characteristics of Soluble Antibody Isotypes and Subclasses

Immunoglobulin	% in Serum (Adults)	Molecular Weight (kD)	Structure	Half-Life (Days)	Amino Acid Residues in Hinge Region	Placental Transfer	Opsonization	Complement Activation
IgG	75						+++	
IgG1	67	146	H2L2	23	15	++++		++
IgG2	22	146	H2L2	23	12	++		+
IgG3	7	165	H2L2	7–21	62	++/+++++		+++
IgG4	4	146	H2L2	23	12	+++		–
IgA	15						–	
IgA1			(H2L2)2	5.5	22	–		–
IgA2			(H2L2)2	5.5	9	–		–
IgM	10	970	(H2L2)5	5–10	–	–	+	+++
IgE	<0.01	188	H2L2	2	–	–	–	–
IgD	<0.5	188	H2L2	2.8	58	–	–	–

antigens and early during the response to T cell–dependent antigens, B cells differentiate into plasmablasts and short-lived plasma cells, which secrete soluble IgM. IgM is usually secreted as a pentamer ((H2L2)5), comprising IgM monomers (H2L2) that are covalently linked by disulfide bonds. The IgM pentamer also contains a 137 amino acid–long polypeptide termed *J-chain* that facilitates IgM multimerization and secretion at mucosal surfaces.[3,18] The pentameric structure of soluble IgM confers high avidity for polyvalent antigens because each IgM molecule contains up to 10 functional antigen-binding sites. The relatively high avidity of such polyvalent interactions can compensate for the relatively low affinity of IgM, which is generated during primary antibody responses before the onset of affinity maturation. Importantly, IgM efficiently supports complement fixation and opsonization of antigen, which are its two main effector functions. Additionally, natural antibodies with innate-like properties are of the IgM class. Specifically, natural IgM is present from birth without external antibody exposure and acts as the first line of defense against invading pathogens. Natural IgM also has an important role in the recognition and clearance of apoptotic cells and regulation of inflammation and self-tolerance, contributing to tissue homeostasis.[19]

IgD. In its membrane form, IgD is expressed on the surface of late transitional and mature naïve B cells, where it is often co-expressed with IgM (IgD+IgM+ B cells). Co-expression of IgD and IgM is regulated through alternative splicing, and the usage of Cμ and Cδ varies widely across B cells.[20] In contrast to IgM, the expression of IgD is transient, and IgD disappears from the cell surface upon B cell activation. Because IgD and IgM co-expression occurs only during a narrow developmental window in B cells, membrane-bound IgD is thought to play an important regulatory role in the fate of naïve B cells.[21] Furthermore, observations that IgD BCRs sense endogenous antigens less efficiently than IgM BCRs suggest that the balance of IgM and IgD co-expression on subsets of mature B cells (e.g., naïve follicular B cells) may contribute to the development of self-tolerance.[21,22]

In humans, a subset of B cells expressing IgD only (IgM−IgD+) is found in the respiratory mucosa and its associated lymphoid organs (e.g., tonsils, cervical lymph nodes) and glands (e.g., salivary and lacrimal).[14,23] IgM−IgD+ B cells originate through a noncanonical form of class switch recombination and, characteristically, use only λ light chains.[12] In addition, the mucosal microbiota regulate IgM-to-IgD CSRs in response to airborne and oral antigens, suggesting an important role of IgM−IgD+ B-lymphoid cells in shaping the antigenic composition of the respiratory tract and their response to pathogens.[12,23]

In its soluble form, IgD is mainly released by IgM−IgD+ plasma cells and is found in most extravascular body fluids (lacrimal, mammary, pancreatic, cerebrospinal, nasal, and bronchial fluids) except for the intestinal mucosa, where only traces of IgD are detected.[23] Although lacking a specific Fc receptor, IgD binds mucosal basophils, mast cells, and to a lesser extent phagocytes, triggering the release of antimicrobial peptides. Secreted IgD may also suppress IgE-mediated degranulation of basophils and mast cells in response to allergens. IgD is also found in very low concentrations in serum, where it accounts for less than 0.25% of all immunoglobulin (see Table 2.1).[12,23]

IgA. IgA, the most abundant Ig isotype in humans, is predominantly secreted at mucosal surfaces. IgA is also present in serum, comprising about 15% of circulating Ig. Serum IgA is monomeric (H2L2), whereas secretory IgA (sIgA) at mucosal membranes and in bodily fluids is usually dimeric ((H2L2)2) where the two IgA monomers are associated with J-chain by means of disulfide bonds. There are two subclasses of IgA that are largely differentiated by their hinge regions. IgA1 has a hinge region of 22 amino acid residues with linked glycans at serine and threonine. The long hinge region of IgA1 is susceptible to degradation by bacterial proteases. In contrast, IgA2 has a hinge region of nine amino acid residues that, although lacking linked glycans, is more stable. Hence IgA2 is the predominant subclass in mucosal surfaces that are rich in bacterial proteases, such as the colonic mucosa.[13,23]

Human B cells may undergo class switching to IgA in the course of T cell–dependent or T cell–independent responses, giving rise to IgA antibodies of high or low affinity, respectively. T cell–dependent class switching is dependent on transforming growth factor beta (TGF-β) and binding of CD40 on the B cell to CD40L on the surface of the T cell. Conversely, T cell–independent class switching involves innate signals from Toll-like receptors and the dendritic cell (DC)-derived factors BAFF and APRIL, which promote B-cell activation and survival. Intestinal epithelial cells produce APRIL upon sensing bacteria through TLRs. APRIL triggers sequential class switching from IgA1 to IgA2 in B cells of Peyer patches, thereby enriching the production of IgA2 in the distal intestinal tract.[24]

Secretory IgA (sIgA) is the main Ig class transferred to infants through breast milk. Indeed, the concentration of IgA reaches 12 mg/mL in antibody-enriched colostrum (up to 50% of the protein conferred to newborns) and averages about 1 mg/mL in mature milk.[25] IgA in breast milk is produced by IgA plasma cells primed in maternal mucosal-associated lymphoid tissues that migrate to the lactating breast.[26] Antibodies are transferred to breast milk through the epithelium of lactiferous ducts and alveoli. This epithelium expresses the polymeric Ig receptor (pIgR), which binds to the J-chain of polymeric IgA to form complexes that undergo endocytosis. Next, IgA is transported in vesicles to the apical epithelial side where the intramembranous domain of pIgR is cleaved, releasing IgA bound to an external fragment of the pIgR called the secretory component. The secretory component protects secreted antibodies from degradation by proteases at mucosal surfaces.[23] In most mammalian species, antibodies from breast milk are absorbed in the distal gut and transported into the neonatal circulation by Fc-mediated transcytosis in entero-cytes. In contrast, in human infants, breast milk antibodies do not enter the circulation and are primarily produced for host defense at mucosal surfaces. Because of its origin in plasma cells primed in maternal mucosa, the IgA transferred in human breast milk is directed primarily against commensal, gut, and respiratory antigens, providing neonates with protection against mucosal antigens found in the mother. Breast milk antibodies also play a critical role in establishing the infant's commensal flora and immune responses during early life.[27,28]

IgG. In humans, IgG is the most abundant Ig in serum and nonmucosal tissues, and it has the longest serum half-life of all immunoglobulin isotypes. IgG antibodies comprise four subclasses: IgG1, IgG2, IgG3, and IgG4. The four subclasses are similar, differing mainly in surface-exposed residues on the constant domains and the structure of their hinge regions. These differences confer specific properties on each subclass, including antigen-binding, half-life, complement activation, and placental transfer (see Table 2.1).

Consequently, IgG subclasses exhibit functional differences. Effector mechanisms include direct neutralization of pathogens and toxins, activation of complement-dependent cytotoxicity (CDC), antigen-dependent cellular phagocytosis (ADCP), and antibody-dependent cell-mediated cytotox-icity (ADCC).[18] IgG-mediated complement activation is initiated by the binding of complement component C1q to the Fc region (CH2 domain), leading to pathogen opsonization by C3b and the formation of the membrane attack complex (C5–C9). IgG Fc domains can also activate complement by interacting with mannose-binding lectin. IgG1 and IgG3 are potent complement activators, whereas IgG2 and IgG4 are less effective.[11] The characteristics of the Fc region also determine the affinity of each subclass for specific Fc receptors (FcγRs), thereby contributing to the regulation of downstream IgG effector mechanisms. There are six types of human FcγRs: I, IIa, IIb, IIc, IIIa, and IIIb. As a class, FcγRs belong to the Ig receptor superfamily and are localized on antigen-presenting and innate immune cells. IgG1 and IgG3 bind to all FcγR subclasses; IgG4 binds most strongly to FcγRI but also binds IIa, IIb, IIc, and IIIa with lower affinity, and IgG2 binds predominantly to FcγRIIa.[3,11]

A distinct IgG Fc receptor, the neonatal Fc receptor (FcRn), is structurally similar to class I major histocompatibility complex (MHC). It is found on hematopoietic cells (namely, myeloid-derived innate immune cells, professional antigen-presenting cells, and vascular endothelia).

FcRn also resides in hepatocytes and some epithelial cells, including podocytes, choroid plexus, and intestinal and respiratory epithelial cells.[29] FcRn binds to IgG with high affinity under acidic conditions (pH < 6.5) but not at physiologic pH. This property plays a key role in IgG transport by defining locations in which IgG is bound or released. Prenatally, FcRn transcytoses IgG from the mother to the fetus across the placental syncytiotrophoblast. Throughout life, FcRn transports IgG at epithelial barriers via Fc-mediated transcytosis. Importantly, in APCs, FcRn governs the intracellular trafficking of IgG and IgG immune complexes into compartments where they are processed for antigen presentation. FcRn also protects IgG from degradation and recycles antibodies in endothelial, hematopoietic, and epithelial tissues, prolonging IgG half-life.[23,29,30]

IgE. IgE mediates immediate hypersensitivity reactions. IgE also participates in protective immune responses against helminths as well as viruses and toxins. IgE is extremely potent and therefore is the most tightly regulated of all Ig isotypes. Class switching to IgE is primarily T cell dependent, requiring interactions with T-follicular helper cells through CD40 and CD40L in addition to soluble signals such as interleukin (IL)-4 and IL-13. Alternatively, IgE can be produced independently by T cells in response to glucocorticoids, the B-cell survival factors BAFF and APRIL, complement C4b-binding protein, or IL-4 in the context of infection by Epstein-Barr virus (EBV). Conversely, class switching to IgE is inhibited by some cytokines (e.g., IL-10, IL-21, TGF-β) and cell surface receptors (e.g., BCR, CD45, CTLA4, FcεRII).[31,32]

IgE+ B cells and IgE-secreting cells are short-lived and are rarely found in the peripheral blood or tissues of healthy individuals but increase under pathologic conditions associated with IgE overproduction, such as allergies, and are positively correlated with plasma IgE levels.[15,33] Soluble IgE, which has the shortest half-life of the circulating immunoglobulins (see Table 2.1), is typically present in serum at concentrations lower than 0.01% of serum Ig. IgE upregulates the expression of its receptors on target cells, which is one of the reasons for its potency. IgE binds with high affinity to FcεRI on the surfaces of mast cells, basophils, Langerhans cells, and eosinophils, stimulating degranulation and the release of inflammatory mediators. A low-affinity receptor for IgE, FcεRII or CD23, is constitutively expressed on B cells, where it promotes cell growth and negatively regulates IgE synthesis. An inducible form of CD23 is expressed on various hematopoietic cells and on epithelial cells, where it transports antigens from the cell surface to the basolateral membrane.[2]

The Genetic Basis of Immunoglobulin Diversity

ORGANIZATION AND ASSEMBLY OF IMMUNOGLOBULIN LOCI

In humans, there are three Ig loci: the heavy chain locus (IGH) on chromosome 14q32, the kappa locus (IGK) on chromosome 2p11, and the lambda locus (IGL) on chromosome 22q11. At each locus, the corresponding Ig variable domain is encoded by an array of gene segments that are brought together during B cell development by a process termed V(D)J recombination. The IGH locus spans approximately 1.3 Mb. The heavy chain variable domains are encoded by three banks of gene segments, termed variable (VH), diversity (D), and joining (JH). At the 5′ end of the IGH locus, as defined by transcriptional orientation, there are about 50 functional VH segments, followed by 27 D segments and 6 JH segments (Fig. 2.5). At the pro-B stage of B cell development, a D segment is joined to a JH segment; subsequently, a VH segment is joined to the DJH unit, thereby forming an intact variable coding sequence. To the 3′ side of the JH cluster are arrayed the exons encoding each of the heavy chain isotypes: μ, δ, γ3, γ1, α1, γ2, γ4, ε, and α2.

Whereas the heavy chain variable regions are encoded in three discrete DNA segments, VH, D, and JH, the variable regions of the kappa and lambda light chains are encoded in two DNA segments, VL and JL. The IGK locus, which spans about 1.7 Mb, contains an array of 44 functional Vκ segments, followed by a cluster of 5 Jκ segments and a single Cκ exon encoding

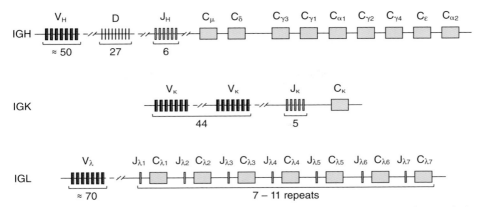

Fig. 2.5 **Organization of the Ig heavy and light chain loci.** IGH, IGK, and IGL, H, κ, and κloci, respectively. Variable (V), diversity (D) and joining (J) segments are indicated. Constant exons are depicted in light blue. The numbers of functional gene segments at each locus are given below each diagram.

the constant domain (see Fig. 2.5). The organization of the human IGL locus, which spans about 1.1 Mb, is more complex than that of IGK, consisting of about 70 Vλ segments and a cluster of from 7 to 11 Cλ exons, each flanked at the 5′ end by a Jλ segment (see Fig. 2.5). Despite the difference in organizational complexity, kappa and lambda light chain genes are assembled by a single recombination event that joins one VL segment to one JL segment.

During B cell development, activation of rearrangement at the light chain loci follows productive rearrangement at the heavy chain locus, which occurs at the pre–B cell stage. Rearrangement of the kappa locus generally precedes that of lambda.

MECHANISM OF V(D)J RECOMBINATION

V(D)J recombination is mechanistically related to bacterial DNA transposition and retroviral integration. Recombination is initiated by a specialized transposase, termed RAG (for recombination activating gene protein), consisting of two RAG-1 subunits and two RAG-2 subunits. Each V, D, or J gene segment is tagged with a recombination signal sequence (RSS) consisting of conserved heptamer and nonamer elements, separated by a less highly conserved spacer of 12 or 23 bp. These RSSs are the functional analogs of transposase binding sites in bacterial transposition and long terminal repeats in retroviral integration. The RAG tetramer brings together a pair of participating gene segments by binding to their RSSs; this process is constrained by the geometry of RAG so that synapsis can only occur between RSSs of differing spacer lengths. Thus the RSSs not only represent binding sites for the RAG complex but also play an essential role in determining which segments can join to each other. Upon synapsis, RAG nicks each gene segment at the junction between a recombination signal sequence and the coding portion of the gene segment. Nicking is followed by a transesterification reaction that produces a coding end, terminating in a hairpin, and a 5′-phosphorylated, blunt signal end (Fig. 2.6).

The two coding ends produced by DNA cleavage are subsequently joined to each other to produce a coding joint; the signal ends are likewise joined to form a signal joint (see Fig. 2.6). Joining is carried out by nonhomologous end joining (NHEJ), one of several pathways for double-strand DNA break repair active in mammalian cells. The DNA ends produced by RAG are bound by a complex of Ku70, Ku80, and the DNA-dependent protein kinase catalytic subunit (DNA-PK$_{CS}$); upon activation, DNA-PK$_{CS}$ phosphorylates Artemis, an adenosine

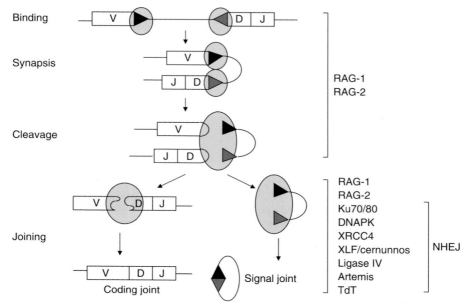

Fig. 2.6 **V(D)J recombination.** Joining of a V segment to a DJ unit is shown. Black and gray triangles, recombination signal sequences (RSSs). The location of RAG is shown in blue. Participants in each phase of the reaction are listed at right. Recombination begins with the binding of RAG to two participating RSSs, followed by synapsis and cleavage of DNA at the junction of each RSS with its accompanying coding segment. Subsequent repair by NHEJ results in formation of coding and signal joints. For details see text.

triphosphate (ATP)-dependent nuclease that opens the hairpins at the coding ends. In the course of joining, variable numbers of base pairs may be removed from either coding end, and untemplated nucleotides may be introduced at random by terminal deoxynucleotidyl transferase (TdT). The DNA ends are made blunt by the action of translesion DNA polymerases Pol μ and Pol λ and then joined through the action of XLF/Cernunnos, XRCC4, and DNA Ligase IV (see Fig. 2.6).

V(D)J recombination introduces antibody diversity by two general means: combinatorial diversity and junctional diversity. Combinatorial diversity arises from the presence of multiple V, D, and J segments and from the property that one member of each class is selected for joining. From the numbers of known gene segments, one can estimate that 8100 combinations of VH, D, and JH segments are possible at the IGH locus; 220 combinations of Vκ and Jκ segments are possible at the IGK locus; and 490 combinations of Vλ and Jλ segments are possible at the IGL locus. If any heavy chain is capable of pairing with any light chain, then the number of combinations that can be generated by V(D)J recombination is 8100 $\times$ (220 + 490) or about 5.8 $\times$ 10^6. Junctional diversity occurs at the VH-D-JH, Vκ-Jκ, and Vλ-Jλ coding joints and is restricted to DNA sequences that encode the third CDRs of Ig H and L chains. Junctional diversity has three sources: the loss of nucleotides from coding joints through the action of nucleases associated with NHEJ, the addition of templated nucleotides at sites of hairpin opening, and the addition of nontemplated nucleotides through the action of TdT. Junctional diversity makes a large contribution to overall antibody diversity. Because coding joints are imprecise with respect to the reading frame, two-thirds of all VH-D-JH and VL-JL junctions are nonproductive; as we will see in the following, selection for in-frame rearrangements is exerted during development.[34-37]

ALLELIC EXCLUSION, ISOTYPIC EXCLUSION, AND RECEPTOR EDITING

Each newly formed B cell is monospecific with respect to Ig expression: it expresses one and only one antibody specificity, thereby ensuring an unambiguous mapping of antigen to immunologic response. Monospecificity is a consequence of two related mechanisms: allelic exclusion and isotypic exclusion. Allelic exclusion is the phenomenon by which expression of Ig heavy and light chain genes is restricted to a single allele. This restriction is enforced largely at the level of V(D)J recombination: each newly formed B cell carries a single productive rearrangement at the heavy chain locus and at one of the two light chain loci. The mechanisms by which this restriction occurs at the IGH, IGK, and IGL loci differ but have two features in common; asynchronous rearrangement and a feedback mechanism by which productive rearrangement is detected. Isotypic exclusion describes the fact that each B cell expresses a single heavy chain and light chain isotype, with the exception that Ig μ and Ig δ are co-expressed on nascent B cells. Light chain isotypic exclusion is enforced at the level of V(D)J recombination and is mechanistically related to allelic exclusion. Heavy chain isotypic exclusion is largely a consequence of class switch recombination, a process that will be described in the section **Class switch recombination and somatic hypermutation**.

In pro-B cells, D-to-JH joining occurs at the IGH locus on both alleles. This is followed by asynchronous VH-to-DJH joining; if the rearrangement is productive—that is, in frame with respect to the V region coding sequence—Ig μ chain is expressed at the cell surface in association with the surrogate light chain proteins VpreB and λ5. The acquisition of Ig heavy chain expression prior to light chain gene rearrangement defines the pre–B cell stage of B cell development. The assembly of μ chain, VpreB, and λ5 is accompanied at the cell surface by the signal transducer proteins Ig α and Ig β; together, this complex is termed the pre–B cell receptor or pre-BCR. Signals emanating from the pre-BCR suppress further VH-to-DJH joining at the IGH locus, suppress apoptosis, drive proliferative expansion of the pre–B cells, and promote differentiation to the stage at which rearrangement begins at the IGK locus. If the initial VH-to-DJH rearrangement is not productive, the pre-BCR is not expressed and rearrangement is permitted at the second allele. Only B-cell progenitors that have productively rearranged one or the other of their IGH alleles survive because a functional pre-BCR is required for further development.

Rearrangement of the IGK alleles developmentally follows that of the IGH alleles and also occurs asynchronously; productive rearrangement results in expression of a κ light chain that pairs with the μ heavy chain to form surface-bound Ig (sIg); the complex of sIg with Ig α and Ig β is termed the B-cell receptor (BCR). Signals emanating from the BCR inhibit further recombination at the IGK locus. If neither IGK allele gives rise to a productive rearrangement, V(D)J recombination is activated at the IGL locus; just as for IGK, rearrangement at the IGL alleles is asynchronous and productive rearrangement initiates a feedback signal that blocks further recombination at the locus.

Most of the antibodies that are produced in the initial wave of B cell development in humans are self-reactive and are removed by several mechanisms, including a process involving V(D)J recombination called receptor editing. Receptor editing is the result of continuing V(D)J recombination in a nascent B cell that already expresses a functional BCR. The recognition of self-antigen by an autoreactive BCR on an immature B cell results in receptor internalization and the extinction of signals that suppress V(D)J recombination. Thus in newly generated, autoreactive B cells, RAG remains active; additional rounds of V(D)J recombination at the light chain loci result in replacement of the self-reactive light chain with a light chain of different specificity.[34-38]

CLINICAL SIGNIFICANCE OF DEFECTS IN V(D)J RECOMBINATION

Defects in V(D)J recombination and DNA repair mechanisms underlie several types of human inborn errors of immunity (IEI). Loss-of-function mutations in *RAG1* and *RAG2* or in genes encoding components of NHEJ (Artemis, DNA-PKcs, Cernunnos, or DNA ligase IV) are associated with severe combined immunodeficiency (SCID).[39] The absence of T and B cells in these patients results from the inability to generate functional B- or T-cell receptors and a concomitant early arrest of lymphocyte development. Characteristically, individuals with defective NHEJ also exhibit radiosensitivity. In contrast to adaptive lymphoid cells, natural killer (NK) cells are unaffected in this group of disorders. One should note that not all debilitating mutations in *RAG1* or *RAG2* result in SCID. Hypomorphic mutations in *RAG*, which permit residual protein function, are associated with atypical SCID and immune dysregulation phenotypes such as Omenn syndrome and combined immunodeficiency with granulomas and/or autoimmunity (CID-G/AI).[40]

CLASS SWITCH RECOMBINATION AND SOMATIC HYPERMUTATION

Naive B cells express IgM and IgD. In such cells, the dual expression of μ and δ heavy chains occurs by alternative splicing of a primary transcript originating upstream of the assembled Cμ gene. Other isotypes are expressed in the course of an immune response, dependent on the nature of the antigen and the mode of immunization. The replacement of IgM and IgD by other Ig isotypes, which occurs principally in germinal centers, is termed class switching, and this process has its basis in a form of DNA rearrangement called class switch recombination (CSR).[41-43]

The human IGH locus contains an array of CH exon clusters, occurring in the following order: Cμ, Cδ, Cγ, Cε, and Cα. CSR is the translocation of the variable domain coding sequences from their initial position upstream of the Cμ and Cδ exon clusters to a position upstream of one of the downstream CH exon clusters, with deletion of the intervening DNA. The resulting recombined heavy chain gene retains the same variable domain coding sequence as the original μ and δ chains but includes CH exons encoding γ, ε, or α heavy chains (Fig. 2.7).

CSR occurs between pairs of sites called switch (S) regions, which lie upstream of the exons encoding Cμ and Cδ and each of the remaining CH exon clusters. Each switch region is preceded by an IGH intervening region (I_H) that contains an RNA polymerase II promoter. Any given CSR event involves two S regions; for example, class switching from μ to γ4 involves recombination between the Sμ region that precedes the Cμ exons and the Sγ4 region that lies before the Cγ4 exons. CSR requires transcription from the I_H promoters through the corresponding S regions and the downstream CH exons. The requirement for transcription provides a way by which external signals can direct switching a particular Ig class; for example, IL-4

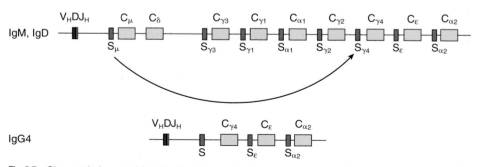

Fig. 2.7   Class switch recombination. Switching of Ig isotype from IgM and IgD to IgG4 is accomplished by recombination between the Sμ and Sγ4 regions. This results in the translocation of a V_HDJ_H exon from a position upstream of the Cμ exons to a position upstream of the Cγ4 exons.

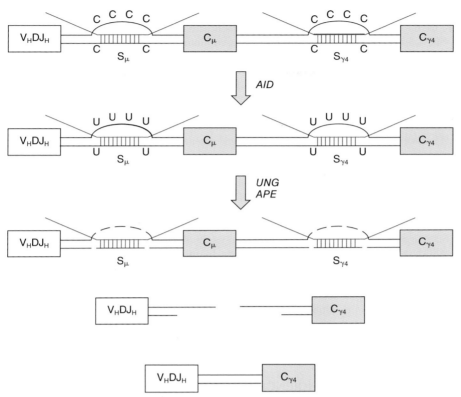

Fig. 2.8 **Mechanism of targeted DNA cleavage at S regions during class switch recombination.** DNA cleavage at Sμ and Sγ4 is shown, corresponding to the recombination event depicted in Fig. 2.7. Noncoding transcripts traversing the Sμ and Sγ4 regions anneal to the template DNA strands, forming R-loops. AID deaminates C residues in the displaced single strands and on the template strand at the single- to double-strand transition. UNG removes the uracil residues resulting from deamination and APE introduces nicks at the abasic sites. The density of nicking is sufficient to produce staggered, double-strand breaks.

directs switching from IgM to IgG4 and IgE. The resulting RNA transcripts hybridize to the template DNA strand of the participating S regions, displacing a loop of single-stranded DNA (Fig. 2.8). CSR is initiated at these structures, termed R-loops, by the enzyme activation-induced cytidine deaminase (AID), which deaminates cytosine (C) on the displaced DNA strand and at the single- to double-strand transition to produce uracil (U). Uracil is removed by uracil N-glycosidase (UNG), a component of the base excision repair (BER) machinery and the resulting abasic sites are cleaved by apurinic/apyrimidinic endonucleases (APEs) to produce staggered double-strand breaks in the participating S regions (see Fig. 2.8). The breaks are then repaired by the NHEJ machinery in such a way that the variable region exons are moved from upstream of the Cμ exons to a position upstream of a Cγ, Cε or Cα exon cluster.[41]

In the course of a typical T cell–dependent antibody response, the average affinity of immunoglobulin for antigen increases by as much as a thousand-fold or more. This increase, termed *affinity maturation*, results from mutation of the antigen-binding site, followed by selection of B cells that express Ig of increased affinity for antigen. In activated germinal center B cells, Ig genes are subject to mutation at a rate of about 10^{-3} mutations per base pair per cell division, a million times higher than the background rate of 10^{-9}. The term *somatic hypermutation* (SHM) is used to describe the process by which mutations are introduced into Ig genes at elevated frequency.

SHM, like CSR, is initiated by AID in transcriptionally active Ig genes, where it associates with RNA polymerase II and the transcription elongation factor SPT5. AID preferentially deaminates C residues in single-stranded DNA, which forms transiently during transcription, and exhibits a bias for WRC sequence motifs, where W is A or T and R is A or G. Thus deamination of C by AID occurs preferentially at specific hotspots within transcribed Ig genes.[44] The action of AID is not entirely restricted to Ig loci, however, and off-target activity of AID can promote the development of B lymphoid malignancies.

The deamination of C to U by AID has several potential consequences whose overall effect is the introduction of transition (pyrimidine to pyrimidine or purine to purine) and transversion (pyrimidine to purine or purine to pyrimidine) mutations.[45,46] If the U residue resulting from deamination of C is not removed by BER, replication across U ultimately results in a C/G > T/A transition mutation. If the U residue is removed by UNG in the absence of DNA cleavage by APE, replication across the resulting abasic site is accomplished by an error-prone, translesion DNA polymerase, resulting in C/G > T/A, C/G > A/T, or C/G > G/C. Additionally, DNA mismatch repair activity near the site of C deamination can result in mutagenesis of A/T base pairs.

SHM increases the affinity of Ig for antigen by producing structural changes that reside largely but not exclusively in the antigen-binding site. Some of these changes increase the number of hydrogen bonds or van der Walls contacts between antibody and antigen; it takes only a few additional hydrogen bonds to increase affinity by three orders of magnitude. Other structural alterations are evident in antibody–protein complexes, including increases in the buried hydrophobic surface and closer shape complementarity at the antigen-antibody interface. In some cases, increased affinity is the result of greater structural rigidity at the interface with antigen to optimize the shape of the antigen.[43,47]

PRIMARY IMMUNODEFICIENCIES ARISING FROM DEFECTS IN CSR AND SHM

Defects in CSR and SHM are associated with a number of primary immunodeficiency syndromes in humans.[39] Specifically, defects in proteins that mediate T cell–B cell interactions required for CSR (e.g., CD40 and CD40 ligand), in *AICDA*, the gene that encodes AID, or in components of the base excision repair machinery (e.g., UNG) are associated with hyper IgM syndromes. These syndromes are a clinically heterogeneous group of primary immunodeficiencies characterized by elevated levels of IgM, severe reductions in serum IgG and IgA (although residual IgG production may be seen in UNG deficiency), and normal numbers of total B cells in the absence of switched memory (IgD− CD27+) B cells. Typically, loss-of-function mutations in *AICDA* and *UNG* present predominantly as antibody deficiencies accompanied by recurrent bacterial sinopulmonary infections, lymphoid hyperplasia, and autoimmunity. A similar phenotype has been associated with autosomal recessive defects in INO80, the catalytic ATPase subunit of a chromatin remodeling complex required for S-region synapsis and DNA repair during CSR. In contrast, defects in CD40 and CD40 ligand (CD40L) are associated with combined immunodeficiencies that exhibit diminished antigen-specific T-cell responses in addition to defective CSR and present clinically with severe and opportunistic infections. Characteristically, patients with CD40 and CD40L defects lack germinal centers in peripheral lymphoid tissues. Often, patients with CD40L deficiency also exhibit neutropenia and increased risk of malignancies, particularly lymphomas and tumors of the gastrointestinal tract, the hepatobiliary tree, and the pancreas.[48] Likewise, inborn errors of immunity with defects in SHM occur. For example, autosomal recessive MSH6 deficiency is known to cause partial impairment of CSR and abnormalities in SHM.[49] Clinically, patients with MSH6 deficiency may have elevated serum IgM levels but only mildly decreased IgG. Notably, severe infections are not present, although patients with MSH6 defects exhibit radiosensitivity with defective DNA repair and elevated risk of malignancies.[39]

Glycosylation of Ig Heavy Chains

Ig is modified posttranslationally by the addition of glycans to each of the heavy chains. Glycans are complex oligosaccharides containing up to 15 monosaccharide residues. The types of glycosylation that occur on Ig are depicted in Fig. 2.5. Glycans are structural components of each Fc region and exert effects on antibody conformation, solubility, half-life, interactions with receptors, and antigenicity. Notably, antibody glycosylation is highly conserved and the heritability of certain patterns (e.g., sialylation) suggests that some glycans are under strict genetic regulation.[18,50] Conversely, although glycosylation of Ig is under genetic control, it is subject to change during development and aging. For example, IgG exhibits higher glycosylation and lower bisection levels in infants and toddlers than in older children. In addition, decreased galactosylation of IgG is seen upon aging. Antibody glycosylation may also be influenced by sex, biologic processes such as pregnancy, nonheritable factors like diet and environment, and diseases.[51,52]

IGG GLYCOSYLATION CONFERS COMBINATORIAL DIVERSITY ON THE IG FC REGION

In IgG molecules, glycans are assembled and attached to the amide group of Asn297 in the γ chains. This posttranslational modification occurs in the endoplasmic reticulum and the Golgi during IgG synthesis. Glycosylation proceeds through a glycan precursor attached to Asn297, composed of two sequential N-acetylglucosamine (GlcNAc) moieties and a mannose residue, followed by branching mannose antennae, each capped with an additional GlcNAc residue (see Fig. 2.5).[18]

Additional fucose, galactose, sialic acid, and a bisecting GlcNAc (b-GlcNAc) can be added to this core structure and, as the nascent antibody transits through the Golgi apparatus, antibody glycans are modified by glycosyltransferases, glycosidases, and other enzymes (Fig. 2.9). This

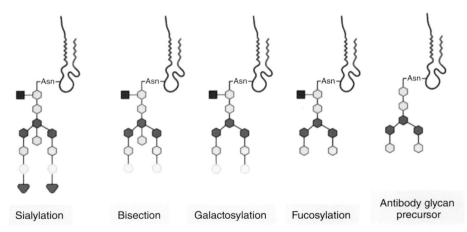

Fig. 2.9 Types of IgG glycosylation. In the Golgi apparatus an antibody glycan precursor (right) can be modified by four distinct glycosyltransferases that add sialic acid (ST6GAL1), a bisecting N-acetylglucosamine (MGAT3), galactose (B4GALT1), or fucose (FUT8). (Adapted from "Protein Glycosylation in the ER" by Biorender.com (2021) Retrieved from. https://app.biorender.com/biorender-templates).

process generates a known repertoire of 36 unique glycans that may be added to secreted IgG. Considering the diversity added by glycosylation and the fact that humans possess four IgG subclasses, at least 144 distinct Fc regions are associated with IgG. Moreover, because the two heavy chains may be glycosylated asymmetrically, the combinatorial diversity of the IgG Fc region can be even greater. In a single antibody molecule, the glycan on one heavy chain may match the glycan on the opposing side (homologous pairing) or differ (heterologous pairing). In humans, approximately 70% of IgG molecules are asymmetrically glycosylated, allowing many glycan combinations with diverse effects on antibody conformation and Fc binding.[18]

Monogenic defects in antibody glycosylation associated with inborn errors of immunity have helped to uncover the roles of individual glycosylation pathway components. For example, the gene *MOGS* encodes mannosyl-oligosaccharide glucosidase, which catalyzes the initial step in glycan trimming during IgG processing in the endoplasmic reticulum. Patients deficient in *MOGS* present with a complex primary immunodeficiency syndrome characterized by neurologic complications (e.g., global developmental delay, seizures) and severe hypogammaglobulinemia due to reduced IgG half-life.[53]

Non-monogenic glycosylation abnormalities are also associated with human disease. Glycosylation modulates the inflammatory activity of IgG, and defects in glycosylation have been linked to several types of chronic immunologic disorders. Notably, aberrant IgG galactosylation can result in an abundance of IgG antibodies that lack terminal galactose and sialic acid residues and instead carry a fucose residue, the so-called IgG-G0F isoform. This isoform is associated with autoantibody-dependent diseases such as rheumatoid arthritis (RA), systemic lupus erythematosus (SLE), and systemic vasculitis.[54] Decreased levels of galactosylated IgG glycoforms are also reported in various cancers, including solid tumors (e.g., gastric, lung, prostate, and ovarian cancers) and hematologic malignancies (e.g., multiple myeloma), and an abundance of agalactosylated IgG glycoforms is positively correlated with disease progression and metastatic disease.[51] Conversely, IgG sialylation is associated with antiinflammatory properties. In autoimmune diseases, for example, a high level of IgG galactosylation and sialylation, as well as elevated fucosylation, is associated with a diminution in the proinflammatory effects of disease-associated autoantibodies, explaining at least in part why serum levels of known pathogenic autoantibodies alone do not necessarily correlate with disease severity.[54] In some malignancies, higher sialylation IgG levels are also associated with better survival rates. Under physiologic conditions, highly sialylated IgG has antiinflammatory effects and may protect against autoimmune and inflammatory diseases.[51]

About 85% of IgG is fucosylated and the fucose residue, which is attached to the core glycan, interferes with the interaction of IgG with FcγRIIIa, thereby suppressing modulating antibody-dependent cell-mediated cytotoxicity (ADCC; see section **Antibody Dependent Cellular Cytotoxicity**). This property has been exploited therapeutically, and afucosylated IgG glycoforms, which display increased binding affinity to the FcγRIIIa and enhanced ADCC activity, are now engineered for clinical use in the treatment of cancer.[55,56]

In addition to glycosylation of the Fc region, about 20% of human IgG has additional glycosylation sites within the variable regions, introduced by SHM.[18,57] Glycosylation of the variable domains may affect Ig stability, half-life, and binding properties. Moreover, variable domain glycans can also modulate the antiinflammatory activity of intravenous immunoglobulins and may be modified in physiologic and pathologic conditions.[57]

Importantly, some diffuse large B-cell lymphomas exhibit glycosylation of the surface Ig variable regions. These cells acquire N-glycosylation sites through somatic mutations affecting the complementarity-determining regions (CDRs). Typically, those sites are occupied by oligomannose structures that interact with the C-type lectin DC-SIGN (dendritic cell-specific intercellular adhesion molecule-3 grabbing non-integrin) on macrophages and dendritic cells in the tumor microenvironment. This interaction activates BCR signaling on the lymphoma cells, contributing to their survival; clinically, the presence of acquired BCR N-glycosylation sites is associated with more rapid disease progression. A similar feature has been described for follicular lymphoma, suggesting a close relationship between these two lymphoma subgroups. Because BCR activation contributes to the survival of these lymphomas, disruption of the interaction between DC-SIGN and N-glycosylated BCR may have merit as a therapeutic strategy.[58]

GLYCOSYLATION OF IGM, IGA, IGD, AND IGE

In contrast with IgG, other Ig classes (IgM, IgA, IgD, and IgE) have more than one glycosylation site on each heavy chain and are more heavily glycosylated. In the case of IgM, each μ chain has five potential glycosylation sites. In an IgM pentamer, there are 51 potential glycosylation sites: 50 sites contributed by the 10 μ chains and an additional site on the associated J chain. An IgM hexamer, which lacks a J-chain, has 60 potential glycosylation sites. Notably, the glycosylation of human IgM is site specific, with a distinct glycosylation pattern at each of the five μ chain glycosylation sites. Sites 1 through 3 are predominantly fucosylated and sialylated, whereas sites 4 and 5 are oligomannosidic.[59] These properties may affect the binding of IgM to antigen and complement. IgA is also heavily glycosylated with patterns that have low interindividual variability but differ depending on the IgA subclass and site of secretion.[60] The α1 and α2 chains of IgA1 and IgA2 contain two and four N-glycosylation sites, respectively. Interestingly, IgA2 has less sialic acid than IgA1, which may contribute to the greater propensity of IgA2 to promote inflammation. In contrast to all other Igs, IgA1 has several O-linked glycosylation sites in its hinge region, predominantly galactosylated or sialylated. The O-glycans seem to serve as bacterial interaction sites under physiologic conditions and may be aberrantly recognized by autoantibodies in diseases such as IgA nephropathy.[60] O-linked glycosylation sites are also seen in the IgD hinge region (up to seven O-linked glycans in humans), in addition to three N-linked glycosylation sites found at positions Asn^{354}, Asn^{445}, and Asn^{496} in the IgD Fc region.[61] Human IgE molecules are also heavily glycosylated as seven potential N-linked glycosylation sites are distributed across each ε chain. A single N-linked oligomannose glycan at N394 contributes to the folding of IgE folding and its binding to FcεRI. In addition, there are five sites occupied by complex antennary glycans and the remaining site, N383, is usually unoccupied. Although relatively poorly characterized, IgE glycosylation patterns seem to modulate allergic responses. For instance, increased IgE sialylation was observed in peanut-allergic individuals relative to healthy controls; conversely, removal of sialic acid from IgE was associated with attenuation of effector-cell degranulation and anaphylaxis in several models of allergy.[62] In summary, the glycosylation patterns of human IgM, IgA, IgD, and IgE, like those of IgG, are important determinants of antibody function.

Antibody-Dependent Cellular Cytotoxicity

Antibody-dependent cellular cytotoxicity (ADCC) is an adaptive immune defensive mechanism in which immune effector cells bearing Fc receptors recognize and lyse target cells coated by antibodies bound to antigens expressed on their surfaces. ADCC plays an important role in antitumoral and antiviral immunity and represents a mechanism of action for therapeutic antibodies used in cancer treatment.

THE ROLE OF FC RECEPTORS IN ADCC

The most important triggers of ADCC are IgG antibodies acting through Fcγ receptors (FcγR). FcγR involved in ADCC responses are categorized as stimulatory (FcγRI, FcγRIIa, FcγRIIc, FcγRIIIa) or inhibitory (FcγRIIb), depending on whether their intracellular domains carry the immunoreceptor tyrosine-based activating motif (ITAM) or the immunoreceptor tyrosine-based inhibitory motif (ITIM).[5,6] The main ADCC effectors are natural killer (NK) cells, which induce target cell apoptosis in various ways. First, NK cells express high levels of FcγRIIIa (CD16), which recognizes IgG on target cells.[3] Next, the cross-linking of FcγRIIIa on NK cells triggers ITAMs phosphorylation and downstream signaling, inducing cytoskeletal reorganization, cellular polarization, and release of cytotoxic granules. Direct killing of target cells occurs through the uptake of NK-derived perforin- and granzyme-containing granules when this pathway is activated. Notably, although CD16-mediated ADCC is mostly executed by NK cells, FcγRIIIa and perforin are also expressed by small subpopulations of antigen-experienced cells; for example, αβ effector memory T cells.[63] NK cells may also trigger apoptosis of target cells via tumor necrosis receptor superfamily death receptors such as Fas and TRAIL. The surface expression of death receptors on target cells is induced by NK cell–derived factors such as interferon (IFN)-γ, enhancing antigen presentation and adaptive immune responses by nearby immune cells.[64] Subpopulations of CD16-expressing monocytes and macrophages also have ADCC capabilities and may kill cancer and virus-infected cells via tumor necrosis factor (TNF)-α-mediated cell death.[65]

Other FcγR-bearing innate immune cells include granulocytes and dendritic cells (Table 2.2).[3,44,45] On neutrophils and other granulocytes, FcγRIIa (CD32a) activates direct killing of IgG-coated target cells through the release of inflammatory mediators (e.g., prostaglandins, reactive oxygen species, lysosomal species) and cytokines (e.g., IFN-γ, TNF-α, IL-1, and IL-6). In contrast, FcγRIIb (CD32b) plays a negative regulatory role by counteracting stimulatory FcγR.

In addition to IgG, IgA and IgE may mediate ADCC. Indeed, the binding of cells opsonized with monomeric IgA to FcαRI (CD89) on neutrophils elicits vigorous antitumor ADCC responses.[46] Activation of the high-affinity IgE receptor (FcεRI) on effector cells, particularly eosinophils, triggers cell activation in antiparasitic responses.

EFFECTS OF GLYCOSYLATION ON ADCC

Alterations in glycosylation can cause conformational changes in the Ig Fc domains that alter their affinity for Fc receptors and exert changes in Ig effector function, including ADCC. For example,

TABLE 2.2 ■ **Expression of FcγR on ADCC Effector Innate Immune Cells**

FcR	Neutrophils	Eosinophils	Basophils	Monocytes	Macrophages	DC	NK
FcγRI	I	I	I	+	+/−	I	−
FcγRIIa	+	+	+	+	+	+	−
FcγRIIb	+	+	+	+	+	+	−
FcγRIIc	+/−	−	−	−	−	−	−
FcγRIIIa	−	−	−	+/−	+/−	−/I	+/−
FcγRIIIb	+	I	+/−	−	−	−	−
FcαRI	+	+	−	+	+	+/−	−
FcεRI	−	+	+			+	−

Abbreviations: +, ε constitutive expression; −, no expression; I, inducible expression.
Adapted from Bournazos S, Gupta A, Ravetch JV. The role of IgG Fc receptors in antibody-dependent enhancement. Nat Rev Immunol. 2020;20(10):633–643. doi:10.1038/s41577-020-00410-0; Bakema JE, van Egmond M. The human immunoglobulin A Fc receptor FcaRI: a multifaceted regulator of mucosal immunity. Mucosal Immunol. 2011;4(6):612–624. doi:10.1038/mi.2011.36; Prussin C, Metcalfe D. 5. IgE, mast cells, basophils, and eosinophils. J Allergy Clin Immunol. 2006;117(2):S450–S456. doi:10.1016/j.jaci.2005.11.016.

on IgG antibodies, hypergalactosylation and afucosylation enhance FcγRIIIa binding. Notably, b-GlcNAc also enhances ADCC through an indirect effect on fucosylation. Specifically, because bisection and fucosylation are mutually exclusive, b-GlcNAc seems to strengthen the binding of antibody to FcγRIIIa by promoting afucosylation. Conversely, fucosylation destabilizes the interaction between antibody and a glycan on FcγRIIIa, thereby impairing Ig binding.[18] Furthermore, sialylation decreases antibody affinity for classical Fc receptors but enhances affinity for DC-SIGN, a noncanonical Fc receptor. The binding of Ig to DC-SIGN culminates in the upregulation of the inhibitory FcγRIIb on macrophages, which exerts an antiinflammatory effect.[49,66]

The effect of glycosylation on ADCC and other Ig effector functions has been exploited in the engineering of therapeutic monoclonal antibodies (mAbs). Specifically, Ig glycosylation patterns have been manipulated to enhance mAb efficacy. As one example, several therapeutic IgG mAbs are designed to be afucosylated to increase binding to FcγRIIIa. Glycosylation may also be used to alter the pharmacokinetic properties of mAb. For example, IgG-bearing terminal sialic acid residues have a longer half-life than nonsialylated antibodies, and antibodies with a higher content of terminal mannose are cleared more quickly from the blood. In addition, Ig glycosylation may contribute to the safety profile of mAb. For example, antibodies produced in nonhuman cells may have immunogenic glycoforms in humans, resulting in the formation of antidrug antibodies and allergic reactions.

Therapeutic Monoclonal Antibodies

PRODUCTION OF MONOCLONAL ANTIBODIES

Antibodies produced during a natural immune response are typically polyclonal. As products of multiple B-cell clones, they bear a variety of CDR structures, recognize multiple antigenic epitopes, exhibit different affinities for the immunogen, and are not restricted to a single class or subclass. In contrast, monoclonal antibodies are so named because historically they were isolated from a single antibody-producing B cell clone; they comprise heavy and light chains each of a single defined protein sequence; their antigen-binding sites are therefore identical and they recognize the same epitopes.

The production of monoclonal antibodies usually begins with an antigenic exposure that elicits a polyclonal response in the recipient host—whether that is an unmodified animal, an animal bearing modified Ig loci, or a human subject (Fig. 2.10). In all of these cases, immunization is followed by isolation of a clone of cells expressing a single Ig or identification of DNA sequences encoding a single Ig of interest. In some instances, DNA sequences encoding the desired antigen-binding domains are isolated from combinatorial libraries, bypassing immunization altogether.

Monoclonal antibodies can be generated by immunizing a mouse with the target antigen. After examination of serum for the presence of a polyclonal response, splenocytes are harvested and immortalized by fusion to a myeloma cell line that has lost the ability to synthesize its own antibody; the resulting hybrid cells are termed *hybridomas*.[67] The myeloma line is typically marked genetically to permit selection for products of fusion with splenic B cells. Most commonly, the myeloma fusion partner is defective for the enzyme hypoxanthine-guanine phosphoribosyltransferase (HGPRT), which renders it unable to grow in the presence of aminopterin, an inhibitor of de novo nucleotide synthesis. Hybridoma cells, in contrast, are able to grow in the appropriate medium because HGPRT is supplied by the B-cell fusion partner.[67] More recently, it has become feasible to bypass the need to generate hybridomas: B cells expressing BCRs of the desired specificity can be enriched by fluorescence-activated cell sorting (FACS) using fluorophore-tagged antigens and DNA encoding the corresponding Ig chains can be constructed by recombinant methods such as the polymerase chain reaction.

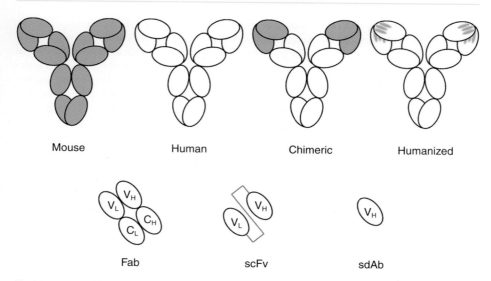

Fig. 2.10 Monoclonal antibodies and some of their derivatives. Intact mouse and human mAbs are shown at top left in blue and white, respectively. Chimeric antibodies are produced by domain swapping between mouse (blue) and human (white) precursors. Humanized antibodies were historically made by engrafting smaller portions of mouse mAbs—for example, CDRs—onto a human backbone. An Fab fragment, a single-chain variable fragment (scFv), and a single-domain antibody (sdAb) are diagrammed below.

The utility of mouse monoclonal antibodies as therapeutic agents in humans is greatly limited because, as foreign proteins, they elicit pathogenic immune responses in the recipient. These responses are mitigated by the use of chimeric or humanized monoclonal antibodies (see section **Major monoclonal antibody variants)** More recently, the ability to generate wholly human monoclonal antibodies has largely bypassed the issue of foreignness. One route to human monoclonal antibodies involves the isolation and enrichment of reactive B cells from immunized or convalescent patients; B cells whose surface Ig is directed against an antigen or epitope of interest are isolated by FACS, and sequences encoding the desired Ig domains are isolated. Another route to human monoclonal antibodies has been made possible by the generation of transgenic or knock-in mice in which portions of the murine Ig loci are replaced by the corresponding human genomic sequences. In one iteration of this approach, the mouse IGH and IGK V clusters are replaced by genomic DNA encoding the corresponding human V segments. Immunization of these humanized mice elicits antigen-specific B cells whose V regions are specified by human DNA; by cell sorting and subsequent genetic engineering, it is possible to obtain DNA encoding human monoclonal antibodies of the desired specificity. An additional means of obtaining human antigen-binding domains avoids immunization altogether. A library of human single-chain variable fragments (scFvs; see section **Major monoclonal antibody variants)** or Fab is constructed in a filamentous bacteriophage in which the antigen-binding regions are expressed as fusions to a viral coat protein; phage-bearing DNA sequences encoding the desired variable regions are isolated through sequential rounds of enrichment for antigen binding.

The monoclonal antibodies obtained by the routes described above can be subsequently produced in a variety of ways. Immortalization of an antibody-secreting cell by generation of hybridomas or by infection with Epstein-Barr virus provides one way of obtaining functional monoclonal antibodies. Alternatively, monoclonal antibodies can be expressed from genetically engineered, Ig-encoding DNA sequences by transfection or transduction into recipient hosts such as the Chinese hamster ovary (CHO) mammalian cell line.[68]

MAJOR MONOCLONAL ANTIBODY VARIANTS

Thirty-five years after approval of the first monoclonal antibody for clinical use, over 100 therapeutic mAbs have become available in the United States. These fall into several main types. The first mAbs were generated in mice and produced from hybridomas. The first licensed therapeutic mAb was Orthoclone OKT3 (muromomab-CD3), a mouse anti-CD3 antibody approved in 1986 to suppress renal transplant rejection.[69] The utility of mouse mAbs in humans is limited, however, by their immunogenicity of nonhuman proteins. Chimeric and humanized mAbs were developed to overcome these limitations (see Fig. 2.10). Their production employs recombinant DNA technologies to combine human amino acid sequences with mAbs derived from rodents and other nonhuman species. The first chimeric mAbs were engineered by fusing mouse variable domains to human Ig constant regions. Examples of chimeric mAbs include abciximab,[70] an anti-GPIIb/IIIa antibody approved for the inhibition of platelet aggregation, and rituximab, an anti-CD20 mAb, originally approved for the treatment of non-Hodgkin lymphoma and now used to treat several oncologic and inflammatory diseases. The generation of humanized mAbs involves complementary-determining region (CDR) grafting, by which nonhuman CDR sequences are inserted into an otherwise human antibody. The first humanized mAb was daclizumab, an anti-IL-2 receptor antibody approved in 1997 to prevent transplant rejection.[71] The availability of humanized mAbs has allowed the treatment of chronic diseases requiring long-term therapy. More recently, as described in the previous section, the development of fully human antibodies was made possible by the use of phage display technologies or genetically modified mice. The first fully human therapeutic antibody, adalimumab, is directed against tumor necrosis factor α (TNF-α) and was approved in 2002 for the treatment of rheumatoid arthritis.[72] Currently, over 30 human antibodies have been approved in the United States, including mAbs used to treat infections (e.g., gram-negative sepsis, anthrax, *Clostridium difficile*, Ebola, and severe acute respiratory syndrome coronavirus 2 [SARS-CoV-2]), autoimmune and autoinflammatory disorders (e.g., inflammatory arthritides, systemic lupus erythematosus, psoriasis, NLRP3-associated autoinflammatory disorders, primary hemophagocytic lymphohistiocytosis), metabolic diseases (e.g., familial hypercholesterolemia, X-linked hypophosphatemia), Alzheimer disease, atopic dermatitis, asthma, and a number of hematologic and solid malignancies.[73]

Therapeutic antibodies can be modified to produce bifunctional antibodies, antibody–drug conjugates, Fc-fusion proteins, and antibodies with engineered Fc regions to enhance specific Fc functions. Bifunctional antibodies, also called bispecific, are mAbs in which two paired immunoglobulin chains of different antigen specificity are incorporated into a single antibody molecule, allowing it to bind two distinct antigens and thereby providing additional functionality. Examples of bifunctional mAbs include blinatumomab, an anti-CD3 and anti-CD19 mAb that assists cytotoxic T cells in killing CD19-positive acute lymphocytic leukemia (ALL) cells. Antibody–drug conjugates carry drugs or toxins and are used for targeted delivery to specific cells or sites. Fc-fusion antibodies are composed of Ig Fc domains directly attached to another protein with beneficial immunologic function, conferring the ability to bind native Fc receptors to the fusion partner. The antibody Fc region can also be modified to alter function. For example, Fc receptor binding regions can be modified to increase antibody half-life (by promoting binding to the FcRn) and to enhance or prevent ADCC and complement activation (e.g., by using interchanging IgG1, IgG2, IgG3, and IgG4 backbones, which differ in their ability to activate FcR). Because most therapeutic antibodies are of the IgG class, the glycosylation of the Fc region can also be manipulated to produce antibodies with enhanced or silenced Fc effector functions.[74]

Antibody engineering methods additionally allow the manufacture of antibody fragments of reduced size and altered pharmacologic properties compared with full-length antibodies. The most common types of antibody fragments in therapeutic use include Fab (fragment antigen binding) fragments, comprising a variable domain and the first constant domain of the heavy and light chains, and single-chain variable fragments (scFvs), consisting of the variable domains of a light and a heavy chain connected by a linker[74] (see Fig. 2.10). As a general feature, antibody fragments permit better tissue penetration in comparison to full-sized antibodies. Small scFvs may also be directed against cell organelles and, although with some limitations (e.g., reduced stability because of decreased disulfide bond formation in the cytoplasm), can be used to target intracellular proteins. In addition, because of their reduced size, antibody fragments may be easier to manufacture because prokaryotic systems may be employed in their production, and, in the absence of the Fc portion, glycosylation is not required. Nonetheless, antibody fragments lacking an Fc domain are rapidly degraded, resulting in a short circulating life and, importantly, are unable to induce Fc-mediated functions.[74]

Another group of small antibodies, termed *single-domain antibodies* (sdAbs), comprise a single variable domain derived from an antibody heavy or light chain. The first sdAbs were engineered from the heavy chain–only antibodies found in camelids (e.g., llamas, alpacas, vicuñas, and camels) and also identified in cartilaginous fish. This novel class of small antibodies is about 1/10th the size of intact human antibodies and is easily modifiable. sdAbs also have several advantageous biophysical characteristics. For example, many require no disulfide bond formation or glycosylation to retain antigen-binding properties, and they are highly soluble and remarkably stable to temperature or chemical denaturation. Together, these properties make sdAbs attractive for a number of biotechnological, diagnostic, and therapeutic applications, including their use as crystallization chaperones, for manipulation of intracellular signaling, for antibody delivery to immune-privileged sites (e.g., the blood-brain-barrier), for in vivo imaging, and for the engineering of chimeric antigen receptor (CAR) T cells.[74]

NOMENCLATURE

Therapeutic monoclonal antibodies are identified following the World Health Organization (WHO) International Nonproprietary Names (INN) nomenclature.[75] In this system, mAbs end with the stem *-mab,* and word substems are used to designate the mAb target (tumors, organ systems, bacteria, viruses), and conjugated mAbs are assigned a two-word name to indicate that a second substance is attached (e.g., alacizumab pegol). Until 2017, substems were also used to identify the mAb source (e.g., animal, chimeric, humanized, human; Table 2.3). In a revised nomenclature system published in November 2021, the suffix *-mab* is replaced by stems that divide mAbs into four groups: group 1 uses the stem *-tug* for full-length unmodified immunoglobulins, group 2 uses *-bart* for full-length artificial antibodies, group 3 has the stem *-mig* for multiimmunoglobulins of any length (e.g., bispecific antibodies), and group 4 assigns the stem *-ment* for monospecific antibody fragments.[75]

MODES OF ACTION

The therapeutic effects of mAbs are exerted in two general ways: first, by the direct targeting of an antigen, determined by the affinity of the CDR regions for the relevant epitope, and second, by the antibody's ability to recruit other immune cells (e.g., NK cells, phagocytes) or activate

TABLE 2.3 ■ **World Health Organization (WHO) International Nonproprietary Names (INN) Nomenclature for Monoclonal Antibodies**

Source Substem[a]		Target Substem		Stem	
-a	Rat	-ami	Serum amyloid protein	-mab	All mAbs (until 2021)
-e	Hamster	-ba	Bacterial	-tug	Unmodified Ig
-i	Primate	-ci	Cardiovascular	-bart	Artificial antibody
-o	Mouse	-de	Metabolic or endocrine pathway	-mig	Multiimmunoglobulin
-u	Human	-eni	Enzyme inhibition	-ment	Ig fragment
-xi	Chimeric	-fung	Fungal		
-zu	Humanized	-gro	Skeletal muscle mass relates growth factors and receptors		
		-ki	Cytokine and cytokine receptor		
		-ler	Allergen		
		-pru	Immunosuppressive		
		-sto	Immunostimulatory		
		-ne	Neural		
		-os	Bone		
		-ta	Tumor		
		-toxa	Toxin		
		-vi	Viral		
		-vet	Veterinary use		

[a]In use until 2017.

immune factors (e.g., complement) to kill target cells. Accordingly, in the treatment of infectious diseases, mAbs may interrupt viral multiplication by targeting specific viral antigens. Examples include anti-SARS-CoV-2 mAbs, directed against the virus's spike protein, or palivizumab, directed against the respiratory syncytial virus (RSV) fusion (F) glycoprotein. In addition, some mAbs can target key proteins and toxins (e.g., the protective antigen of *Bacillus anthracis*) on bacterial surfaces, impairing the pathogen's survival or mitigating its pathogenicity. In the treatment of noninfectious diseases, therapeutic mAbs may interfere with receptor–ligand interactions by means of cell surface receptor blockade or by ligand sequestration, hindering cell-to-cell interactions or cell signaling. Other mechanisms of action involve effector functions of mAbs and promote killing of targets; these mechanisms include antibody-dependent cytotoxicity (ADCC), complement-dependent cytotoxicity (CDC), and antibody-dependent phagocytosis (also known as *opsonization*). These effects are mediated by the Fc portion of the antibody (heavy chain second and third constant regions in IgG) and, notably, are absent from mAb fragments engineered without the Fc region.

Key References

1. Cohen S, Milstein C. Structure of antibody molecules. *Nature.* 1967;214(5087):449-452. doi:10. 1038/214449a0.

3. Bournazos S, Gupta A, Ravetch JV. The role of IgG Fc receptors in antibody-dependent enhancement. *Nat Rev Immunol.* 2020;20(10):633-643. doi:10.1038/s41577-020-00410-0.

10. Wedemayer GJ, Patten PA, Wang LH, Schultz PG, Stevens RC. Structural insights into the evolution of an antibody combining site. *Science.* 1997;276(5319):1665-1669. doi:10.1126/science.276.5319.1665.

14. Glass DR, Tsai AG, Oliveria JP, et al. An integrated multi-omic single-cell atlas of human B cell identity. *Immunity.* 2020;53(1):217-232.e5. doi:10.1016/j.immuni.2020.06.013.

16. Halliley JL, Tipton CM, Liesveld J, et al. Long-lived plasma cells are contained within the CD19− CD38hiCD138+ subset in human bone marrow. *Immunity.* 2015;43(1):132-145. doi:10.1016/ j.immuni.2015.06.016.

17. Landsverk OJB, Snir O, Casado RB, et al. Antibody-secreting plasma cells persist for decades in human intestine. *J Exp Med.* 2017;214(2):309-317. doi:10.1084/jem.20161590.

18. Jennewein MF, Alter G. The immunoregulatory roles of antibody glycosylation. *Trends Immunol.* 2017;38(5):358-372. doi:10.1016/j.it.2017.02.004.

23. Chen K, Magri G, Grasset EK, Cerutti A. Rethinking mucosal antibody responses: IgM, IgG and IgD join IgA. *Nat Rev Immunol.* 2020;20(7):427-441. doi:10.1038/s41577-019-0261-1.

29. Borghi S, Bournazos S, Thulin NK, et al. FcRn, but not FcγRs, drives maternal-fetal transplacental transport of human IgG antibodies. *Proc Natl Acad Sci USA.* 2020;117(23):12943-12951. doi:10.1073/ pnas.2004325117.

34. Schatz DG, Swanson PC. V(D)J recombination: mechanisms of initiation. *Annu Rev Genet.* 2011;45: 167-202. doi:10.1146/annurev-genet-110410-132552.

35. Gellert M. V(D)J recombination: RAG proteins, repair factors, and regulation. *Annu Rev Biochem.* 2002;71:101-132. doi:10.1146/annurev.biochem.71.090501.150203.

36. Zhang L, Reynolds TL, Shan X, Desiderio S. Coupling of V(D)J recombination to the cell cycle suppresses genomic instability and lymphoid tumorigenesis. *Immunity.* 2011;34(2):163-174. doi:10.1016/ j.immuni.2011.02.003.

38. Yan CT, Boboila C, Souza EK, et al. IgH class switching and translocations use a robust non-classical end-joining pathway. *Nature.* 2007;449(7161):478-482. doi:10.1038/nature06020.

42. Alt FW, Yancopoulos GD, Blackwell TK, et al. Ordered rearrangement of immunoglobulin heavy chain variable region segments. *EMBO J.* 1984;3(6):1209-1219.

43. Muramatsu M, Kinoshita K, Fagarasan S, et al. Class switch recombination and hypermutation require Activation-Induced Cytidine Deaminase (AID), a potential RNA editing enzyme. *Cell.* 2000;102(5): 553-563. doi:10.1016/S0092-8674(00)00078-7.

58. Chiodin G, Allen JD, Bryant DJ, et al. Insertion of atypical glycans into the tumor antigen-binding site identifies DLBCLs with distinct origin and behavior. *Blood.* 2021;138(17):1570-1582. doi:10.1182/ blood.2021012052.

67. Taggart RT, Samloff IM. Stable antibody-producing murine hybridomas. *Science.* 1983;219(4589):1228- 1230. doi:10.1126/science.6402815.

69. Ortho Multicenter Transplant Study Group. A randomized clinical trial of OKT3 monoclonal antibody for acute rejection of cadaveric renal transplants. *N Engl J Med.* 1985;313(6):337-342. doi:10.1056/ NEJM198508083130601.

74. Ingram JR, Schmidt FI, Ploegh HL. Exploiting nanobodies' singular traits. *Annu Rev Immunol.* 2018;36(1):695-715. doi:10.1146/annurev-immunol-042617-053327.

75. Balocco R, De Sousa Guimaraes Koch S, Thorpe R, Weisser K, Malan S. New INN nomenclature for monoclonal antibodies. *Lancet.* 2022;399(10319):24. doi:10.1016/S0140-6736(21)02732-X.

Visit Elsevier eBooks+ (eBooks.Health.Elsevier.com) for complete set of references.

CHAPTER 3

The Role of the Complement System in Cancer Etiology and Management

Stefan E. Sonderegger ■ Silvia Manzanero ■ Trent M. Woodruff
■ Jad Farouqa ■ Jamileh Nabizadeh ■ Nadya Panagides
■ Barbara E. Rolfe

SUMMARY OF KEY FACTS

- The complement system is a key component of the innate immune system, responsible for facilitating immune defense mechanisms, regulating inflammation, and maintaining tissue homeostasis.
- The complement system is a proteolytic cascade, comprising more than 50 highly regulated soluble proteins and membrane-bound receptors. The cascade is initiated by recognition of pathogen-associated patterns (PAMPs), damage-associated molecular patterns (DAMPs), and binding to immune complexes and proceeds via three distinct pathways: the classical, the lectin, and the alternative pathways.
- Complement activation results in production of important immune mediators, including C3a, C3b, C5a, and C5b-9, which mediate innate immune responses against foreign invaders, attraction of immune effector cells, phagocytosis, and formation of the membrane attack complex (MAC) resulting in cell lysis. This process is tightly controlled by a range of soluble and membrane-bound regulatory proteins.
- Though essential to immune function, dysregulated complement activation contributes to a diverse range of disease pathologies, including atypical hemolytic uremic syndrome, C3 glomerulopathies, age-related macular degeneration, rheumatoid arthritis, sepsis, atherosclerosis, ischemia-reperfusion injury, and cancer.
- Complement-targeting drugs have been FDA-approved for mostly orphan conditions such as paroxysmal nocturnal hemoglobinuria, yet several more are in clinical trials or under development.
- Complement is activated in response to cancer cells, and complement activation products are deposited within tumor tissue. Bioinformatics analysis indicates a negative correlation between complement signaling pathways and prognosis in many cancer types.
- Complement mediators including C3a, C5b, and sublytic C5b-9 have been implicated for roles in promoting tumor growth and metastasis.
- Research in preclinical models suggests the therapeutic potential of complement-targeting drugs, either alone or in combination with current cancer therapeutics.

Introduction

The complement system is critical to proper immune function, but inappropriate or excessive complement activation contributes to many pathologic inflammatory conditions including cancer. Traditionally regarded as contributing to the antitumor response through complement-dependent cytotoxicity (CDC), there is growing evidence that complement activation products including C3a, C5a, and C5b-9 can also promote tumor growth. Indeed, complement proteins have been shown to regulate primary tumor growth and metastasis, *indirectly* via the antitumor immune response, angiogenesis, and formation of the premetastatic niche and *directly* by promoting tumor cell proliferation and migration. The availability of complement-targeting drugs, with more in the developmental pipeline, suggests the potential for novel immunotherapeutic strategies to target both innate and adaptive immunity and boost the antitumor response.

Complement Activation Pathways

A key component of innate immunity, the complement system forms the first line of defense, aiding in the elimination of pathogens and damaged cells. The complement system is a proteolytic cascade, comprising more than 50 highly regulated soluble proteins and membrane-bound receptors.[1] Complement activation elicits a range of proinflammatory effects, including increased vascular permeability, modulation of cytokine release, recruitment of innate immune cells such as neutrophils and macrophages to damaged tissues, enhanced phagocytosis, and lysis of pathogens and damaged cells.[1,2] Although it has been traditionally regarded as a mediator of innate immune activities, the complement system also contributes to efficient adaptive immune responses.[3-5]

The complement cascade is activated in response to danger signals (damage- or pathogen-associated molecular patterns; DAMPs and PAMPs) via three pathways (Fig. 3.1), depending on the stimuli.[6] The classical pathway is activated via interaction of antigen–antibody complexes with the multimeric collectin C1q[7] leading to conformational changes in the C1q molecule and complex formation with serine proteases C1r and C1s. The lectin pathway is initiated by the binding of mannan-binding lectin (MBL), ficolins, and other pattern recognition molecules that recognize aberrant carbohydrates on the surfaces of pathogens[8] and damaged or necrotic cells,[9] allowing for the recruitment of MBL-associated serine proteases (MASPs)-1 and -2. The alternative pathway is triggered by interaction with foreign antigens on pathogen surfaces.[6] The activation of classical and lectin pathways, leading to formation of the C1qrs complex and activation of MASP-2, respectively, results in proteolytic cleavage of C4 into C4a and C4b and then C2 into C2a and C2b. C4b then binds to C2b, generating the classical/lectin C3 convertase (C4b2b complex).[8,10] The alternative pathway, however, is in a constant state of low-level activation (tickover), in which spontaneous hydrolysis of a labile thioester bond converts C3 to a bioactive form $C3(H_2O)$ in the fluid phase.[9] This pathway proceeds directly through C3 cleavage to generate an alternative pathway C3 convertase (C3bBb), thus allowing an immediate response to microbial challenge.

Once generated, C3 convertases cleave C3 to produce the important effector molecules anaphylatoxin C3a and opsonin C3b. Formation of C3b also enables binding of the protease factor B (FB). The resulting proconvertase (C3bB) is quickly transformed by factor D (CFD) into an active C3 convertase (C3bBb) that by itself can cleave more C3 into C3b, thereby creating an amplification loop for C3b deposition.[11] C3 convertases from the classical or alternative pathways also bind to C3b to generate C5 convertases (C4b2b3b and C3bBb3b, respectively). These in turn cleave the downstream component C5 to generate anaphylatoxin C5a and C5b, which initiates formation of the membrane attack complex. These products of complement pathway activation (i.e., C3a, C3b,

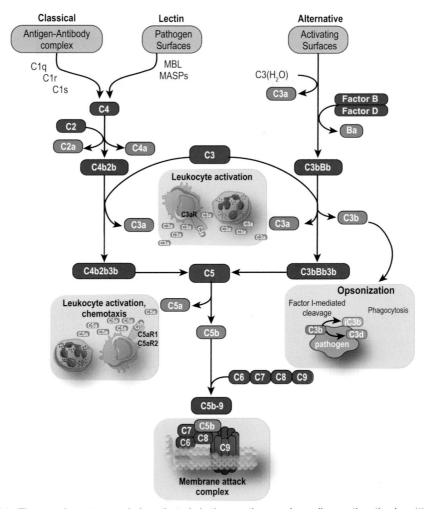

Fig. 3.1 **The complement cascade is activated via three pathways, depending on the stimulus.** (1) The classical pathway activated by immune complexes; (2) the lectin pathway, activated by carbohydrate structures on pathogens and damaged and dead cells; and (3) the alternative pathway, activated by foreign surfaces. All pathways converge at the central protein C3, which is cleaved to produce active fragments; opsonin **C3b**, which aids recognition and clearance of foreign material by macrophages (opsonization); and anaphylatoxin **C3a**. Downstream component C5 is cleaved by C5 convertases to generate anaphylatoxin **C5a** and **C5b**; C5b combines with C6, C7, C8 and multiple units of C9 to form the membrane attack complex formation (MAC; **C5b-9**), which destroys invading pathogens. A fourth pathway, the extrinsic pathway, is triggered by serine proteases of the coagulation cascade, which cleave C3 and C5 to generate C3a and C5a, respectively.

C5a, C5b) are responsible for mediating many of the effects of the complement system (described in **Complement effector molecules**).

Finally, although its role in human physiology and pathology has yet to be clearly demonstrated, complement activation can be triggered directly by proteolytic enzymes that cleave C3 and C5 to form C3a and C5a, respectively.[12] This fourth extrinsic pathway can be initiated by

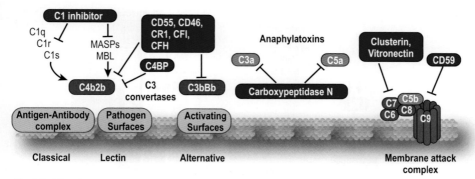

Fig. 3.2   Regulators of the complement pathway. Complement activation is tightly controlled by membrane-bound and -soluble complement regulatory molecules (green boxes). C1 inhibitor prevents excessive activation of both classical and lectin pathways by inhibiting the classical pathway C1 complex and inactivating lectin pathway MASP-1 and -2. The C3 convertases, C4b2b and C3bBb, are regulated by complement receptor 1 (CR1), C4 binding protein (C4BP), CD55 (decay-accelerating factor; DAF), CD46 (membrane cofactor protein; MCP), and factor I (CFI); C3bBb is also regulated by factor H (CFH). The anaphylatoxins C3a and C5a are degraded by carboxypeptidase N. Formation of the C5b-8 complex is inhibited by vitronectin and clusterin, and CD59 (protectin) inhibits C9 insertion into the membrane attack complex (MAC).

enzymes of the coagulation cascade such as factors IX, X, XI/XIa, plasmin, and thrombin, as well as other enzymes, including cathepsin D, granzyme B, and β-tryptase, which are secreted by damaged cells or leukocytes.[13,14] Notably, there is also evidence for intracellular generation and function of complement activation fragments.[15]

To maintain the balance between efficient destruction of pathogens and prevention of unwanted damage to host tissue, complement activation is tightly controlled by soluble and membrane-bound regulatory proteins.[16] These include soluble factors such as carboxypeptidases; complement factors (CF)H, CFB, CFD, and CFI; C4b-binding protein (C4BP) and C1 inhibitor (C1inh); and membrane complement regulatory proteins (mCRPs) such as CD35 (complement receptor type-1; CR1), CD46 (membrane cofactor protein; MCP), and CD55 (decay-accelerating factor; DAF; Fig. 3.2). These CRPs protect both normal and neoplastic cells from damage by accelerating decay of convertases or cleaving activation fragments to inactive forms. Another membrane-bound protein, CD59 (protectin), binds to C8 and C9 to prevent assembly of the membrane attack complex (MAC).[9,17]

Complement Effector Molecules

Activation of the complement cascade leads to generation of potent effector molecules, including C3a, C3b, C5a, and C5b.[10]

OPSONIN C3B

C3b not only amplifies the complement response via convertase formation (see **Complement activation pathways**) but also acts as a mediator of innate and adaptive immunity. Cleavage of C3 induces a conformational change in the C3b fragment, allowing it to bind to proteins or carbohydrates present on cell membranes and foreign structures in a process called *opsonization*. C3b binding to CR1 on immune cells enables opsonized cells to be shuttled to the spleen and liver[18] where C3b binds to the complement receptor of the immunoglobulin family (CRIg) expressed on tissue-resident macrophages such as Kupffer cells and induces phagocytosis.[19]

In addition to its role as an opsonin, C3b mediates adaptive immune functions, improving the contact between effector and target cells and potentiating antibody-dependent cell-mediated cytotoxicity (ADCC)[20] and CDC.[21] Additionally, C3b deposited on antigen-presenting cells interacts with CR1/CR2 expressed on antigen-specific T cells to promote their proliferation.[22]

ANAPHYLATOXINS C3A AND C5A

C3a and C5a are powerful immune mediators through which the complement system exerts many of its effects. Small polypeptides comprising 77 and 74 amino acids, respectively,[23] the anaphylatoxins have ~36% overall homology but higher homology in the C-terminal "active" regions of the molecules.[24] C5a binds two specific receptors, C5a receptor (R)1 (CD88) and C5aR2 (C5a-like receptor 2; C5L2),[8] and C3a binds to a single receptor, C3aR.[25,26] All three receptors (C5aR1, C5aR2, and C3aR) belong to the superfamily of seven transmembrane spanning G protein–coupled receptors and are expressed primarily by myeloid cells, including monocytes, macrophages, eosinophils, basophils, and neutrophils.[27-30] Expression by nonmyeloid cells has also been reported, especially in lung and liver.[31-33] C5a binds both C5aR1 and C5aR2 with high affinity, but is thought to exert most of its biologic activity via the former.[34]

C5a binding to C5aR1 downregulates cyclic adenosine monophosphate (cAMP)/protein kinase A (PKA) signaling and activates signaling pathways such as phosphatidylinositol-3-kinase (PI3K)/Akt and mitogen-activated protein kinase (MAPK)[35] to induce a range of proinflammatory responses. These include chemoattraction of macrophages, neutrophils, basophils, and mast cells[8,36]; enhanced phagocytosis[23]; and modulation of cytokine release.[35] C5a triggers histamine release from basophils and mast cells,[37] which in turn stimulates vasodilation and increased vascular permeability.[38] It also stimulates neutrophil degranulation and release of toxic mediators such as reactive oxygen species (ROS)[39] and neutrophil extracellular trap (NET) formation after priming with interferon (IFN)-γ.[40] Additionally, C5a has been reported to stimulate angiogenesis by promoting the migration of microvascular endothelial cells.[41] It also links to the adaptive immune system, influencing the trafficking and migration of B-cell populations[42,43] and modulating T-cell responses; it provides survival signals for naïve CD4[+] cells,[44] inhibits induction and function of regulatory T cells (Tregs),[45] and promotes T-cell activation during interaction with antigen-presenting cells (APCs) in vitro and in vivo.[46] The alternate receptor C5aR2 lacks G protein coupling and thus was originally thought to be a "decoy" or scavenger receptor, binding excess C5a without exerting direct physiologic effects.[34] However, there is emerging evidence to suggest that C5aR2 can independently induce and moderate biologic functions of C5a through β-arrestin and p90RSK activation.[47-50]

C3a has been reported to exert effects in mast cells, macrophages/monocytes, T cells, and APCs. It induces calcium mobilization from intracellular stores,[51,52] activation of extracellular signal-regulated kinases (ERK)1/2, and release of extracellular adenosine triphosphate (ATP) in monocytes and macrophages.[53] Despite the lack of evidence for C3aR expression by T cells,[28] C3a/C3aR has been reported to activate phosphoinositide-3-kinase (PI3K)-γ and induce phosphorylation of Akt, upregulating the antiapoptotic protein Bcl-2 and downregulating the proapoptotic molecule Fas, to decrease T cell apoptosis and enhance proliferation.[54] However, the activity of C3a is short-lived, because it is rapidly cleaved at the C-terminal arginine to form C3a des-Arg, which can no longer bind to C3aR.[55]

Compared with C5a, C3a is a much weaker chemoattractant[56] but has been reported to exert a range of immunomodulatory functions including degranulation of eosinophils, basophils, and mast cells.[23,57] C3aR is thought to negatively regulate the mobilization of hematopoietic stem and progenitor cells from the bone marrow[58,59] and has also been shown to prevent neutrophil egress into the circulation, thus reducing acute tissue injury after ischemia[60] or neurotrauma.[61] Like C5a,

C3a signaling may contribute to the regulation of adaptive immunity,[62] inhibiting natural (n)Treg function[54] and enhancing the survival and function of effector Th1 and Th17 cells.[44] Conversely, the absence of C3aR signaling in CD4$^+$ T cells is reported to be associated with enhanced interleukin (IL)-10, transforming growth factor (TGF)-β expression, and Foxp3$^+$-induced (i)Treg-mediated immunosuppression.[45]

Both C3aR and C5aR have been shown to regulate Toll-like receptor (TLR)-induced cytokine production, with C5aR1 synergizing with TLR-2 and TLR-4 to elicit stronger inflammatory responses and C3aR regulating TLR9 signaling.[63,64] Moreover, TLR-induced inflammatory cytokines such as interleukin (IL)-6 can upregulate the expression of C3aR and C5aR.[65]

Despite their critical roles in the development of effective immune responses, excess production of C5a and C3a can contribute to pathogenic proinflammatory responses, resulting in tissue damage and, eventually, multiorgan failure.[34] Indeed, the anaphylatoxins are implicated in a range of inflammatory diseases including arthritis,[66] ischemia-reperfusion injury,[67] sepsis,[68] neurodegenerative diseases,[69] and cancer.[70]

THE MEMBRANE ATTACK COMPLEX (MAC; C5B-9)

The membrane attack complex (MAC) is typically formed on the surface of pathogen membranes. Insertion of the MAC into the membrane of gram-negative bacteria, enveloped viruses, and parasites induces calcium ion influx and activation of lytic signals, which ultimately lead to cell death.[71] Although insertion of the MAC into nucleated host cells can lead to membrane disruption and death by apoptosis[72] or cell lysis,[73] mammalian cells are typically resistant.[74] This is because of either the shedding of MAC complexes deposited on the cell surface[75] or the expression of regulatory factors, such as CD46, CD55, and CD59, which inhibit early complement activation and amplification and thus prevent MAC pore assembly.[76]

In the absence of lysis, so-called sublytic MAC has been reported to signal through multiple pathways, including PI3K, Akt, and ERK, to exert different effects in different cell types. This includes effects on cell cycle and proliferation, apoptosis, protein synthesis, and membrane lipid composition (for in-depth review, see Morgan[77]). Sublytic MAC has also been reported to induce inflammatory cytokine production, trigger degranulation of neutrophils and macrophages,[78] and induce platelet activation.[79]

Complement Therapeutics

Complement-targeting drugs have provided researchers with important tools to dissect the roles of the complement system in health and disease and also led to the development of powerful new therapeutic strategies (for in-depth review, see Mastellos et al.,[80] Ricklin et al.,[81] and Zelek et al.[82]). To date a number of complement therapeutics have been approved for clinical applications, mostly for rare (orphan) diseases such as paroxysmal nocturnal hemoglobinuria (PNH). These include drugs targeting serine proteases C1r, C1s, and MASPs (Cinryze, Cetor, Berinert, Ruconest), C3 (compstatin analogs such as pegcetacoplan), C5 (e.g., eculizumab), and C5aR1 (avacopan; Table 3.1).

Compstatin is a 13-residue cyclic peptide that selectively binds to human and primate forms of C3 and C3b,[83] preventing propagation and amplification of complement activation and effector generation via all three pathways.[84] Although the efficacy of the original drug was hampered by its limited in vivo half-life and the high plasma concentration of C3 (0.75–1.35 mg/mL),[85] more potent and stable analogs have been developed, including AMY-101 (Amyndas Pharmaceuticals) and APL2 (Apellis Pharmaceuticals), which are in clinical trials for diseases such as periodontal, renal, neurologic, and ophthalmic diseases.[86,87] Indeed, APL2 (Pegcetacoplan or Empaveli; Apellis) was recently approved by the U.S. Food and Drug Administration (FDA) for the rare hematologic disorder PNH.[88]

TABLE 3.1 ■ **Selected Therapeutic Agents That Target the Complement Pathway, Approved or on the Discovery Pathway**

Target	Class	Agent(s)	Translational Status—Cancer	Translational Status—Other Conditions
C1r, C1s, MASPs	Serine protease inhibitor	C1-INH (Cinryze)	Not yet trialed	U.S. FDA and EU EMA approved for hereditary angioedema
C5	Monoclonal antibodies	Eculizumab (Soliris), ravulizumab (Ultomiris)	Not yet trialed	U.S. FDA and EU EMA approved for PNH, aHUS, myasthenia gravis, neuromyelitis optica spectrum disorder
C5	Oligonucleotide	Aptamer – ARC1905	Not trialed	Trials discontinued
C5aR1	Small-molecule antagonists	PMX53 (3D53, JPE1375), PMX205	Preclinical	Phases Ia and Ib/IIa successful
C5aR1	Small-molecule antagonists	CCX168 (avacopan)	Not yet trialed	U.S. FDA and EU EMA approved for antineutrophil cytoplasmic autoantibody (ANCA)-associated vasculitis
C5aR1	Monoclonal antibodies	IPH5401 (avdoralimab)	STELLAR-001, Phase I study of IPH5401, in combination with durvalumabin for advanced solid tumors	Phase II trial for severe COVID-19-related pneumonia unsuccessful
C5a	Monoclonal antibodies	IFX-1 (vilobelimab)	Not yet trialed	Sepsis, hidradenitis suppurativa, and COVID-19 Phase II trials completed
C5a and c5a desArg	Monoclonal antibodies	MEDI7814	Not yet trialed	Preclinical
C3 and C3b	Compstatin analogs	Pegcetacoplan, AMY-101, APL2	Not yet trialed	U.S. FDA and EU EMA approved for PNH
C3a	Competitive agonist	SB290157	Preclinical	Preclinical

FDA, Food and Drug Administration; *EMA,* European Medicines Agency.

Eculizumab (Soliris)[89] and ravulizumab (Ultomiris)[90] are humanized monoclonal antibodies (mAbs) that target C5, blocking C5 cleavage to C5a and C5b and thereby preventing formation of the downstream MAC complex. The first complement therapeutic to be FDA-approved, eculizumab was approved for treatment of PNH in 2007, atypical hemolytic uremic syndrome (AHUS) in 2011,[81] and more recently for generalized myasthenia gravis[91] and neuromyelitis optica spectrum disorder.[92]

Because they inhibit many of the main functions of the complement system (see Fig. 3.1), C3 and C5 inhibitory drugs are associated with an increased risk of infections.[93] For example, approximately 50% of patients treated with eculizumab experience serious adverse events, including an increased risk of meningococcal disease.[94] Additionally, because eculizumab is unable to block C5 cleavage mediated by the extrinsic protease pathway or in tissues that reside behind a restrictive barrier, a C5a-targeted approach may be preferable for specific conditions.[95] The PMX family drugs are potent and highly selective C5aR1 antagonists developed at The University of Queensland, Australia.[36,96] These cyclic hexapeptides have properties favorable for clinical development, including small molecular weight (<1000 Da), nanomolar potency, plasma stability, oral bioavailability, and high receptor selectivity.[97] The original drug, PMX53 (initially referred to as 3D53), was shown to effectively reduce C5a-mediated inflammatory responses in numerous animal models of disease, including ischemia-reperfusion injury,[98] stroke,[99] inflammatory bowel disease,[100] atherosclerosis,[101] arthritis,[36] and epilepsy.[102] Although Phase Ia and Ib/IIa safety/efficacy trials showed PMX53 to be safe, with no signs of toxicity,[103] its poor oral bioavailability and short circulation half-life (around 20 minutes in humans) limited its clinical development. Medicinal chemistry improvements led to development of a lipophilic analog, PMX205, with enhanced efficacy and in vivo stability compared with its parent molecule.[104,105] A linear analog of PMX53 (JPE1375) has in vitro potencies comparable to those of PMX53, with improved receptor specificity, microsomal stability, and antagonistic potency in mouse but not human cells[106]; however, it also has a reduced in vivo half-life and pharmacodynamics.[107] Other C5aR1 antagonists reported in the literature[35] include CCX168 (avacopan), which is orally bioavailable, has a good safety profile, and was recently FDA-approved for the treatment of antineutrophil cytoplasmic antibody–associated vasculitis.[108]

In addition to small-molecule drugs, monoclonal antibodies targeting C5aR1 have been shown to reverse inflammatory arthritis in a mouse model,[109] and one of these antibodies, IPH5401 (avdoralimab), is being developed by Innate Pharma for the treatment of inflammatory diseases, including cancer. However, a Phase II clinical trial for treatment of severe coronavirus disease 2019 (COVID-19)-related pneumonia was suspended when it failed to meet primary endpoints.[110] Antibodies targeting C5a are also in development, including IFX-1 (vilobelimab), which recently completed Phase II trials for treatment of sepsis,[111] hidradenitis suppurativa (clinicaltrials.gov identifier NCT03001622), and COVID-19.[112] Another antibody, MEDI7814, inhibits the binding of C5a and its less active desarginated metabolite (C5a des-Arg^{25}) to both C5aR1 and C5aR2 receptors.[95] Originally proposed as a potential therapeutic for acute inflammatory conditions, the antibody did not progress past Phase I clinical trial. However, it may be a useful tool to understand the interaction between C5a and the C5aR2 receptor. Finally, Mehta and co-workers used a mouse arthritis model to show that targeting C5 and C5aR1 simultaneously may be more effective than targeting either component separately.[113]

Although a number of C3a agonists have been reported,[114] the development of effective C3a inhibitors has proven more elusive. SB290157 is a nonpeptide arginine analog that acts as a competitive antagonist with high affinity for the C3a receptor.[115] Antiinflammatory activity has also been demonstrated in animal models through a reduction in neutrophil numbers.[116] However, like PMX53, SB290157 has a short circulation half-life.[117] It has also been reported to have agonist properties and other off-target effects in a number of cellular systems,[118] possibly depending on the level of receptor expression. New approaches to molecule development are underway and will potentially lead to efficacious and safe therapeutic agents. Of note, Lohman et al. reported a method (heterocyclic "hinge") to convert small-molecule C3a agonists to antagonists by inducing conformational changes in the core structure.[119] However, until the in vivo specificity, stability, and safety of these drugs can be confirmed, their therapeutic potential remains unknown.[120]

Complement Response to Cancer

Bioinformatics analysis has identified the complement cascade as one of the key pathways associated with initiation and progression of cancers such as lung cancer,[121] glioma,[122] and hepatocellular[123] and clear cell renal carcinoma.[124] These findings are of great clinical interest, not only for identification of therapeutic targets but also for identification of potential biomarkers that could be used for screening, diagnosis, prognosis, and monitoring responses to therapy. The clinical potential of complement components as cancer biomarkers was highlighted by Lawal et al whose analysis of clinical data from 33 human cancer types showed that C3, C5, C3AR1, and C5AR1 expression is associated with tumor immune evasion via dysfunction or loss of T-cell phenotypes[125]; high C3 expression is also associated with shorter progression-free survival in several cancer types.[126]

Evidence of complement activation in response to tumors comes from the detection of activation products including C3a, C4d, C5a, and C5b-9[127] in tumor tissue and plasma from human breast,[128,129] thyroid,[130] lung,[131,132] oropharyngeal,[133] esophageal,[134] gastric,[135] colorectal,[136] and hepatic[137] tumors. Complement proteins have also been detected in the ascitic fluid of ovarian carcinoma patients and C1q and C3 cleavage products deposited on the surface of tumor cells isolated from this fluid.[138]

Tumor cells have been reported to activate all three pathways of the complement system, depending on the tumor type and the nature of the antigens expressed.[139] Natural IgM leads to activation of the classical pathway through the recognition of tumor-specific antigens resulting from posttranslational modifications. For example, the expression of gangliosides GD3 and GD2 on the surface of melanoma and neuroblastoma cells leads to complement mediated cell lysis in vitro through this pathway.[140] Local complement activation through the classical pathway has also been demonstrated in a murine lung cancer model.[141] High mannose expression in glioma cell lines has been reported to activate the lectin pathway,[142] and aberrant glycosylation patterns in murine sarcoma models activate classical or lectin pathways.[143] Conversely, the alternative pathway may be activated by aberrantly expressed viral carbohydrates on the surface of virally transformed tumors such as Burkitt lymphoma[144] or human immunodeficiency virus (HIV)-infected cells.[145] The research thus far supports the core, but complex, role of complement in cancer progression and highlights the numerous therapeutic approaches available to modify tumor growth.

Complement Dependent Cytotoxicity and Cancer

The complement system has traditionally been assumed to play a beneficial role in immune surveillance against tumors, contributing to antitumor defense mechanisms via CDC[146] and ADCC.[147] ADCC is mediated through the engagement of Fc receptors on natural killer (NK) cells and antibody mediated phagocytosis.[148] CDC is initiated by binding of the Fc region of cell-bound antibodies to C1q, triggering classical pathway activation, MAC assembly, and direct cell lysis; at the same time, opsonic fragments (e.g., C3b, iC3b, and C3dg) deposited on tumor cells are recognized by complement receptors (CR1, CR3, CR4, or CRIg) on phagocytic cells,[149] inducing phagocytosis and modulating the function of antigen-presenting cells.[10] The release of inflammatory mediators such as C5a also contributes to the antitumor response by promoting recruitment of phagocytic cells to the tumor[8] and upregulating the expression of Fc receptors on leukocytes to enhance antibody-dependent cellular cytotoxicity.[150]

Unfortunately, naturally occurring antibodies to tumor-associated antigens are relatively weak and incapable of inducing efficient complement-mediated cytotoxicity.[151] Moreover, vaccination attempts to induce production of high-affinity antibodies against tumor antigens have met with limited success in patients with cancer.[152] However, the introduction of recombinant antibodies for cancer treatment has led to renewed interest in complement to promote antitumor defense

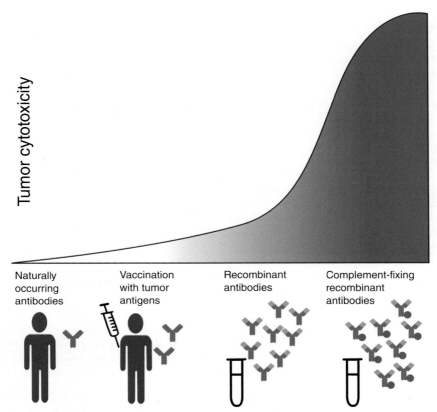

Fig. 3.3 Schematic representation of cytotoxic potential for different strategies for antibody response to tumor-associated antigens.

(Fig. 3.3). C5a agonists have been used as molecular adjuvants to induce antigen-specific antibody[153] and cytotoxic T-lymphocyte (CTL)[154] responses to weak antigens. For example, the C5a agonist (YSFKDMP(MeL)aR) was used in the murine B16 melanoma model to target C5aRs present on dendritic cells (DCs). This improved presentation of poorly immunogenic tumor-related antigens to T cells for subsequent cytotoxic T cell–mediated killing and reduced tumor growth.[155] Another study[156] demonstrated that the tumoricidal effect of a monoclonal antibody against human epidermal growth factor receptor 2 (HER2/neu) was augmented by fusion with C5a through enhanced recruitment of human granulocytes, the primary immune effector cells responsible for facilitating ADCC.

A successful strategy to optimize the therapeutic efficacy of mAb-based immunotherapies is the use of structural modifications to enhance complement activation and production of the MAC as an effector to kill tumor cells.[151,157] For example, the ability of anti-CD20 mAbs including rituximab to eliminate cancerous B cells in patients with chronic lymphocytic leukemia (CLL) through CDC is now well established.[148,158] Despite this, only a small number of the more than 35 mAbs approved by the FDA for anticancer treatment[159] are complement-fixing, highlighting a possible window of opportunity to increase the efficiency of current immunotherapies (see Fig. 3.3). However, the efficacy of CDC for tumor targeting mAbs may be limited because of production of CRPs by cancer cells.[151]

Complement Regulatory Proteins and Cancer

Tumor cells are thought to escape immune attack by upregulating CRPs (for in-depth review, see Fishelson and Kirschfink[160]). These proteins act variously by inhibiting complement activation, blocking MAC assembly or insertion into the cell membrane, or facilitating removal of the MAC from the cell surface to protect against complement mediated lysis of tumor cells.[161-163] High expression of membrane regulatory proteins such as CD46,[164-166] CD55,[164,167] and CD59[164,165,168] on tumor cells is associated with increased metastatic potential and poor prognosis in many cancers (for in-depth review, see Geller and Yan[139]). Elevated expression of soluble regulators, CFH, and factor H-like protein (FHL)-1 in biologic fluids is also associated with poor outcomes in cancers such as ovarian,[169] bladder,[170] lung,[171] and hepatic[137] cancers. Other soluble regulators such as clusterin,[172] factor I,[173] and C4b-binding protein (C4BP)[174] are secreted by tumor cells (Table 3.2).

CRPs may also limit the efficacy of therapeutic mAbs.[17] For example, Golay and co-workers showed in freshly isolated patient's cells that the efficacy of cell killing by the anti-CD20 mAb rituximab was dependent on the balance between levels of CD20 and CRPs such as CD55 and CD59.[175] Accordingly, therapeutic strategies to block or silence CRP expression using monoclonal antibodies, RNA interference, or small peptides have been evaluated as a means of improving the therapeutic efficacy of antibodies such as rituximab.[176] To this end, neutralization of CD55 and CD59 has been shown to enhance the antitumor efficacy of rituximab against leukemia[177] and non-Hodgkin lymphoma cells.[178] Neutralization of these same CRPs has also been reported to increase Herceptin-mediated complement cytotoxicity against lung cancer cells[179] and eradicate micrometastases and small solid tumors from breast carcinoma and ovarian teratocarcinoma cell lines by complement-mediated mechanisms.[180] Though this approach is limited by the ubiquitous expression of CRPs by normal cells as well as tumor cells, Macor and co-workers showed that bispecific Abs to CD20 and CD55 or CD59 specifically neutralized membrane CRPs on Burkitt lymphoma cells, enhancing their susceptibility to complement-mediated lysis in vitro and preventing tumor growth in a mouse model.[181]

TABLE 3.2 ■ **Soluble and Membrane-Bound Complement Regulatory Proteins Implicated for a Role in Cancer Evasion**

Regulator	Function	Location	References
CD46 (MCP)	Cofactor for CFI–mediated cleavage of C3b and C4b	Membrane-bound	164-166
CD55 (DAF)	Destabilizes C3/C5 convertases of the classical and alternative pathway	Membrane-bound	164,167
CD59 (protectin)	Inhibits the formation of MAC by binding C8 and C9	Membrane-bound	164,165,168
CFH	Decay accelerating activity and CFI cofactor in the alternative pathway	Plasma	137,169-171
Clusterin	Binds to C5b-7 and inhibits generation of C5b-9	Plasma	173
CFI	Cofactor dependent degradation of C3b and C4b.	Plasma	174
C4BP	C3 convertase inhibitor in the classical and lectin pathway	Plasma	172

C4BP, C4 binding protein; CFH, complement factor H; CFI, complement factor I, DAF, decay accelerating factor; MCP, membrane cofactor protein

Complement Activation in the Tumor Microenvironment Enhances Tumor Growth

Although the complement system was originally thought to play an important role in cancer immunosurveillance, research over the past 15 years has revealed that complement activation within the tumor microenvironment suppresses effective antitumor immune responses and promotes tumor growth. Indirect evidence that complement activation products may contribute to tumor growth was provided in 2006 by Nozaki and co-workers, who showed that both C3aR- and C5aR1-deficient mice had reduced levels of neovascularization, vascular endothelial growth factor (VEGF) production, and blood vessel formation, all critical factors for tumor perfusion and invasion.[182] However, the first direct evidence that complement proteins promote tumor growth came from a seminal study by Markiewski and co-workers in 2008[183].

ROLE FOR C5A IN REGULATING TUMOR GROWTH

Markiewski et al. used a mouse cervical cancer model to show that C5a enhanced tumor growth via recruitment of myeloid-derived suppressor cells (MDSCs), leading to increased production of ROS and reactive nitrogen species (RNS) and suppression of $CD8^+$ T cell–mediated responses.[183] Since then, the tumor-promoting effects of C5a–C5aR signaling has been corroborated in numerous other murine cancer models, including lung,[131] breast,[184] ovarian cancer,[185] lymphoma,[186] and melanoma.[187] The majority of studies suggest that C5a acts by promoting immunosuppressive myeloid cells, although the detailed mechanisms may differ between tumor types. For example, Corrales et al. demonstrated that C5aR1 antagonism with PMX53 inhibited lung cancer growth by reducing MDSCs and immunosuppressive molecules, including ARG1, CTLA4, IL-6, IL-10, LAG3, and PDL1 (genes for arginase 1, cytotoxic T-lymphocyte associated protein 4, interleukin-6, interleukin-10, lymphocyte-activation protein 3 and programmed death-ligand 1), within the tumor microenvironment. Although they showed that C5a induced endothelial cell chemotaxis and blood vessel formation in vitro, they found no differences in tumor vascular density in PMX53-treated mice.[131] In contrast, Nunez-Cruz and co-workers found that C5a stimulates angiogenic activity by endothelial cells and that the absence of complement signaling impaired ovarian cancer growth, primarily by reducing tumor vascularization.[185] Similar to previous reports, our laboratory showed that inhibition of C5aR1 signaling slowed the growth of B16 melanoma tumors by reducing tumor-infiltrating immunosuppressive leukocyte populations (MDSC, macrophages and Tregs) and increasing $CD4^+$ T lymphocytes.[187] We also provided evidence of a minor protective role for the alternate receptor, C5aR2, in modulating the effects of C5a on tumor growth, a result corroborated by Ding and co-workers, who showed that colorectal tumorigenesis was reduced in C5aR1-deficient mice but exacerbated in the absence of C5aR2.[188]

C3A AS A REGULATOR OF TUMOR GROWTH

The first direct evidence that C3a contributes to tumor growth was provided by our laboratory,[189] with the demonstration that growth of primary B16 melanoma was significantly reduced in C3aR-deficient mice. Daily treatment of established melanomas with the C3aR antagonist SB290157 also slowed tumor growth, suggesting the potential of C3aR as a therapeutic target. Investigations into the cells responsible for the antitumor responses showed that neutrophils and $CD4^+$ T lymphocyte subpopulations were increased in the absence of C3aR signaling, whereas macrophages were reduced. The central role of neutrophils in the antitumor response was confirmed by antibody depletion experiments that reversed the tumor inhibitory effects observed in C3aR-deficient mice; tumor-infiltrating $CD4^+$ T cells were returned to control levels, suggesting that neutrophils mobilized in response to C3aR inhibition may promote T-cell infiltration of the tumor.[189]

Similar protective effects of C3aR deficiency/inhibition have been observed in other murine cancer models, including breast, colon,[189,190] lung,[141] and sarcoma,[143] although the cellular mechanisms may differ. An association between neutrophils and C3aR signaling in tumorigenesis was confirmed by Guglietta et al.,[191] who showed in a mouse model of spontaneous intestinal tumorigenesis that circulating lipopolysaccharide (LPS) induced complement activation and increased coagulation, neutrophil polarization, and neutrophil extracellular trap (NET[192]) formation. This group also demonstrated a correlation between neutrophilia and hypercoagulation in patients with cancer of the small intestine, suggesting the clinical potential of this research.[191] The contribution of macrophages to the tumor-promoting effects of C3aR signaling has also been corroborated in mouse models of sarcoma and colon cancer, with C3aR deficiency shown to confer resistance to sarcoma and colon cancer growth via reduced macrophage accumulation, functional skewing toward M1-like phenotypes, upregulation of IFN-γ-associated genes, and enhanced T-cell responses.[143,193]

As reported for C5aR, cellular responses to C3aR inhibition may vary, depending on the tumor type. For example, in orthotopic murine lung cancer models, C3aR inhibition was found to have no effect on myeloid cells, but increased IFN-γ$^+$/tumor necrosis factor (TNF)-α$^+$/IL-10$^+$ CD4$^+$ and CD8$^+$ T cells.[141] In contrast, the regression of murine mammary and colon tumors was attributed to increased cytotoxic NK cells.[190] To gain further insight into the roles of cell populations within the tumor microenvironment, Davidson and co-workers used single-cell RNA sequencing to demonstrate that stromal cells play a key supporting role, producing C3 and promoting the recruitment and induction of immunosuppressive macrophages via C3aR signaling.[126] Although they found no direct effects of C3a signaling on T cells, the authors suggested that disruption of signaling between stromal cells and infiltrating myeloid populations has the potential to affect subsequent interactions between the innate and adaptive compartments and thus improve the antitumor immune response.

Although the majority of studies have demonstrated protumor effects of C3a/C5a signaling, antitumor effects have been reported in some tumor types, most notably breast cancer models. For example, Kim and co-workers demonstrated that overexpression of C5a protected against the growth of EMT6 mammary tumors in mice.[194] Tumor inhibitory effects of complement proteins were confirmed in an another (HER2/neu-driven) breast cancer model, in which C3 deficiency accelerated carcinogenesis.[195] Further evidence that complement proteins protect against mammary tumor growth was provided by our laboratory; whereas C3aR/C5aR1 agonism slowed the growth of EMT6 and 4T1 mammary tumors, C5aR1 inhibition promoted their growth.[196,197] These results suggest that complement proteins can have different effects, depending on the cancer type, the site of the tumor, and the immune phenotype of the host. Compared with other common tumor models, 4T1 and EMT6 tumors have a low mutational load and are relatively immunogenic, with high levels of immune filtration.[198,199] The site of tumor cell injection may also influence the response because of differences in the nature of the tumor microenvironment and the ability of immune cells to infiltrate the site. Whereas 4T1 and EMT6 cells are injected orthotopically into the mouse mammary fat pad, many other commonly used tumor models are injected subcutaneously. The background immunophenotype of the host is also likely to be an important determinant of the response to immunotherapy.[200] Whereas many tumor models are on a proinflammatory T helper lymphocyte (Th)1/M1 macrophage-oriented C57Bl/6 background, the HER2/neu transgenic model used by Bandini's group,[195] along with 4T1 and EMT6 mammary tumor models, is on an anti-inflammatory Th2/M2-oriented BALB/c background.[201] Although C57Bl/6 and BALB/c mice have normal complement function,[202] differences in complement activation levels within the tumor microenvironment are possible. As demonstrated by Gunn and co-workers in a mouse lymphoma model, low C5a levels promoted Th1 cell differentiation and reduced tumor burden, whereas high C5a levels promoted Treg differentiation and accelerated tumor progression.[186] The complex role of complement proteins in cancer has been highlighted by Roumenina et al., who performed bioinformatics analysis of complement gene expression in 30 different cancers. This analysis showed that cancers could be classified into four groups, based on prognostic effect: (1) protective complement (favorable prognosis associated with high expression of complement genes), (2) protective C3 (favorable prognosis associated with high expression of C3 but not other genes), (3) aggressive complement (poor prognosis associated with high expression of complement genes), and (4) uncertain significance of complement (no obvious association with complement genes).[203] Thus, understanding how different tumors and their microenvironments affect the response to complement-targeting (and other) immunotherapeutic strategies may provide critical insights relevant to future clinical application. This would include the identification of biomarkers to develop diagnostic tests that enable the stratification of patients for complement targeting therapies suited to their individual needs.

SUBLYTIC MAC IN CANCER

The MAC (C5b-9) was originally thought to play an antitumor role through CDC.[148] However, as described in **Complement regulatory proteins and cancer**, tumor cells have multiple strategies by which to protect themselves from MAC-mediated lysis. This includes the expression of high levels of CRPs CD46, CD55, and CD59, which act to limit complement activation and prevent assembly of the MAC. MAC can also be removed from nucleated cells by either budding off (ectocytosis) or engulfment (endocytosis).[78,204] These protective mechanisms may lead to low (sublytic) levels of MAC deposition that is insufficient to kill the target tumor cells but can affect cells in many ways. The assembly of sublytic levels of C5b-9 in the cell membrane increases cytosolic calcium and activates signal transduction pathways such as protein kinase C (PKC),[205] PI3K-Akt, and ERK,[127] increasing cell survival and proliferation[206] and inhibiting apoptosis.[207] It has also been reported to induce the release of inflammatory mediators such as ROS and RNS, leukotrienes, prostaglandins,[208] inflammatory cytokines,[78] adhesion molecules, growth factors, and matrix metalloproteinases (MMPs)[209] and stimulate inflammasome activation[210] by cells in vitro.

In the context of cancer, sublytic MAC has been shown to protect prostate cancer cell lines from TNF-mediated killing[211] and induce the production of angiogenic growth factors by osteosarcoma cell lines.[212] Vlaicu and co-workers have identified a downstream gene product, the response gene to complement-32 (RGC-32), as a potential regulator of tumor growth. RGC-32 contributes to cell cycle regulation by activating Akt and CDC2 kinases and is upregulated in many cancers, including colon and pancreatic cancers.[127,213] It has been shown to induce epithelial–mesenchymal transition (EMT) and to promote cancer cell migration and invasion in lung adenocarcinoma cells via reduction of matrix metalloproteinase activity. The limited in vivo studies suggest that RGC-32 is tumor suppressive in immunocompetent mice,[214] but this effect may be reversed in tumors carrying TP53 mutations.[215] Additional evidence that sublytic MAC contributes to tumor cell activation has been provided by Towner and co-workers,[209] who used a bioinformatics approach to analyze the effects of sublytic MAC on the patterns of gene expression in MC38 colon cancer and B16 melanoma cells. The results revealed a downstream gene expression response likely to alter tumor behavior through induction of proliferative, migratory, and survival pathways, including a central role for EGFR signaling.

ROLES FOR OTHER COMPLEMENT COMPONENTS IN CANCER

Other complement proteins may also contribute to tumor growth. For example, deposition of C1q within the tumor microenvironment has been shown to accelerate tumor growth by promoting angiogenesis and regulating tumor cell motility and proliferation.[216] In another study, C3 was shown to promote tumorigenesis independent of C3aR, C5aR1, C5aR2, C5, or terminal MAC, possibly through pathways mediated by iC3b/C3b on tumor-infiltrating myeloid cells.[217] Indeed, iC3b has been shown to induce the expression of IL-10 and TGF-β2[218] and promote the generation of MDSCs from mouse bone marrow–derived dendritic cell cultures.[219]

As described in **Complement regulatory proteins and cancer**, complement regulatory proteins can promote tumor growth by inhibiting complement activation and complement-mediated tumor cell killing. However, there is also evidence that negative complement regulators can protect against tumor development. For example, the negative complement regulator CFH has been shown to play a critical role in controlling spontaneous complement activation in the liver, with the absence of CFH leading to chronic inflammation and increased risk of hepatic carcinogenesis in mice; increased CFH expression is also associated with improved survival in patients with hepatocellular carcinoma.[137] These results are in accord with a previous study investigating the role of pentraxin-related protein 3 (PTX3), a pattern recognition molecule that activates and regulates the complement cascade by interacting with C1q and CFH. PTX3 deficiency in mice was shown to increase susceptibility to mesenchymal (3-methylcholanthrene; MCA) and epithelial (7, 12-dimethylbenzanthracene; DMBA)/12-O-tetradecanoylphorbol-13-acetate; TPA) carcinogenesis via excessive complement activation, enhance C-C motif chemokine ligand 2/monocyte chemoattractant protein-1 (CCL2/MCP-1) production, and recruitment of tumor-promoting macrophages, leading Bonavita and co-workers to propose that PTX3 acts as an extrinsic oncosuppressor to limit tumor-promoting inflammation.[220]

AUTOCRINE EFFECTS OF COMPLEMENT PROTEINS

The majority of studies suggest that complement proteins influence tumor growth indirectly by modulating the immune response. However, tumor intrinsic effects are also possible. Evidence for a role for C5a–C5aR signaling in cancer cell invasion was provided by Nitta and co-workers, who demonstrated C5aR expression in human tumor tissue and human cancer cell lines, and that C5aR signaling enhanced cancer cell invasion in vitro by stimulating MMP release.[221] A subsequent study by Cho et al.[222] demonstrated expression of both C3aR and C5aR by ovarian cancer cells and that these receptors were capable of autocrine signaling via the PI3K/Akt pathway, leading to increased cell proliferation, migration, and invasion. This group also identified a role for Twist Family BHLH Transcription Factor (TWIST)1 in regulating C3 expression and suggested that C3a–C3aR signaling mediates EMT.[223] Further support for a role for C5a in EMT came from Hu and co-workers,[224] who showed that C5aR1 signaling downregulates epithelial markers E-cadherin and claudin-1 expression in hepatocellular carcinoma cells and upregulates the transcription factor Snail, a key inducer of EMT. C3a and C5a receptors have also been detected on human malignant hematopoietic cell lines and patient blasts; C3a and C5a stimulation of these cells enhances cell motility via activation of p38 MAPK and downregulation of heme oxygenase 1 (HO-1).[225]

Autocrine signaling through the C3a receptor has also been implicated in the growth of some lung cancers[141] and cutaneous squamous cell carcinomas, possibly via activation of the Wnt β-catenin pathway.[226] Another study has suggested that reciprocal C3a-mediated paracrine signaling between cancer cells, cancer-associated fibroblasts (CAFs), and (possibly) myeloid cells promotes tumor progression and potentiates chemotherapy resistance.[227] Though the majority of studies have focused on C3, C5, and their activation products, other complement proteins may also exert autocrine effects. For example, endogenous expression of C1r by cutaneous squamous cell carcinoma cells has been shown to promote tumor cell invasion through induction of MMP-13.[228]

The Role of Complement Activation in Cancer Progression

Tumor metastases are the primary cause of cancer deaths.[229] In addition to effects on primary tumor growth, complement activation may contribute to metastasis at several stages: (a) modifying behavior of primary tumor cells via induction of EMT, leading to loss of cell–cell adhesion and increased motility[223,224]; (b) enabling tumor cell invasion into blood or lymphatic vessels so

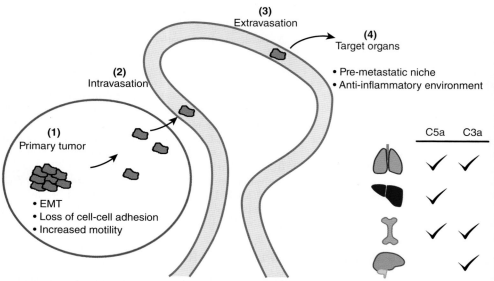

Fig. 3.4   Complement activation facilitates tumor metastasis. (1) At the primary tumor by inducing EMT, loss of cell–cell adhesion, and increased motility; (2) enabling tumor cell to enter the circulation and travel to distant sites; (3) increasing vascular permeability to facilitate tumor cell extravasation into target organs; and (4) at target organs, by contributing to the "premetastatic niche" and facilitating seeding by the arriving tumor cells. These effects have been described for both C5a and C3a in diverse organs such as lung, liver, bone, and brain.

they can enter the circulation and travel to distant sites; (c) increasing vascular permeability to facilitate tumor cell extravasation into organs such as lung, liver, and brain; and (d) contributing to the "premetastatic niche" in target organs by activating and recruiting immunosuppressive cells to facilitate seeding by the arriving tumor cells[230,231] (Fig. 3.4).

The first direct evidence that C5a promotes tumor metastasis was provided by Vadrevu and co-workers.[184] Although C5aR1 blockade did not influence the growth of primary murine breast cancers, it reduced lung metastasis by downregulating MDSCs, Treg cells, and immunosuppressive cytokines such as TGF-β and IL-10 but increasing CD4[+] and CD8[+] T cells in the lung premetastatic niche. This group subsequently used the same model to show that the accumulation of resident alveolar macrophages in the premetastatic niche is due to C5aR1-mediated proliferation; they showed that along with recruited MDSC, alveolar macrophages suppress antitumor T-cell immunity in the lungs and facilitate lung metastasis.[232] Subsequent studies have shown that C5a–C5aR1 signaling endows a prometastatic phenotype in other cancer models. For example, Piao and co-workers showed that C5a contributed to hepatic metastasis of colon cancer by increasing expression of chemokines and antiinflammatory cytokines and promoting infiltration of macrophages, neutrophils, and dendritic cells.[233] Similarly, in lung cancer models, C5aR1 activation increased tumor cell invasion, migration, and osteolysis, via induction of osteoclastogenic and angiogenic factors such as IL-8, CCL2, VEGF, and C-X-C motif chemokine ligand (CXCL)16 to promote bone metastasis.[234]

Like C5a, C3a has also been reported to contribute to metastasis of sarcomas[143] and breast and lung[141] cancers; for example, by modulating the expression of prometastatic cytokines such as TGF-β by CAFs.[235] Another interesting study in a leptomeningeal metastasis model showed that the interaction of cancer cell–derived C3/C3a with C3aR in the choroid plexus disrupted the blood–cerebrospinal fluid barrier, allowing access to nutrients that adapt the cerebrospinal fluid (CSF) for growth of metastatic cancer cells.[236] The clinical significance of these results was revealed in patients with primary tumors, where high C3 levels in CSF were shown to be associated with leptomeningeal metastasis. This work opens the door to C3 targeting as a therapeutic strategy to suppress leptomeningeal metastases that are refractory to current therapeutic approaches.

Another complement regulatory protein implicated for a role in promoting tumor metastasis is PTX3. In contradiction to the work (described in **Complement regulatory proteins and cancer**) of Bonavita and co-workers, who proposed that PTX3 acts as an oncosuppressor,[220] Rathore et al. showed that PTX3 is upregulated in human metastatic and chemotherapy-resistant melanoma. They further showed that autocrine production of PTX3 by melanoma cells promotes migration, invasion, and expression of the EMT factor TWIST1 via inflammation-related pathways.[237]

Potential Application of Anticomplement Cancer Therapies (C3aR/C5aR/IL-10 Pathway)

The development of the checkpoint inhibitors, anti-CTLA-4, and anti-programmed death-1 (PD-1)/PD-L1 has revolutionized the treatment of cancers such as lymphoma, melanoma, lung, and renal cancers.[238] Although rates vary widely between cancers, it is estimated that only around 12% of patients respond to checkpoint inhibitors.[239] The lack of response in the remaining patients is thought to be at least partly due to a large suppressive myeloid cell population within tumor tissue[240] and the absence of T-cell populations capable of responding to checkpoint inhibition.[241] Hence, there is a search for strategies to convert so-called cold (T cell–poor) tumors into hot (T cell–rich) tumors[242] and thus improve immunotherapy response rates.

As described in previous sections, preclinical studies suggest the potential of complement-targeting drugs for cancer treatment. Given their ability to reduce immunosuppressive cell populations (MDSCs, macrophages, and Tregs) and increase effector (CD4$^+$ or CD8$^+$) T-cell numbers within the tumor microenvironment, these drugs may also improve the efficacy of existing immunotherapeutic approaches. Indeed, inhibition of C5aR1 signaling has been reported to reduce expression of the checkpoint inhibitors, including CTLA-4, PD-L1, and PD-1, by cells within the tumor microenvironment.[131,243]

The potential of combination therapeutic approaches has been demonstrated in melanoma, colon, and lung cancer models, with combination PD-1/C5aR1 blockade markedly reducing tumor growth and metastasis by reducing MDSCs, increasing CD8$^+$ T cells, and reducing expression of exhaustion markers.[244,245] Inhibition of tumor cell–derived C3 also enhanced the efficacy of anti-PD-L1, resulting in upregulated expression of IFN-γ-associated genes and long-term tumor-specific immunity.[193] Because C3aR and C5aR1 appear to promote tumor growth by different mechanisms, combined blockade of C3aR/C5aR1 signaling may be even more effective. Indeed, combination C3aR/C5aR inhibition has been reported to enhance the clinical efficacy of anti-PD-1 mAb therapy via the upregulation of IL-10 production by CD8 T cells.[246] Following on from these preclinical studies, a Phase I trial to investigate the efficacy of an anti-C5aR monoclonal antibody (IPH5401), in combination with the anti-PD-L1 antibody durvalumab, in patients with advanced solid tumors *(STELLAR-001)* was commenced in September 2018. Preliminary results suggested a manageable toxicity profile,[247] but the trial was terminated in 2021 due to minimal anti-tumor activity.[248]

Complement targeting therapies may also influence the tumor response to conventional therapies such as chemotherapy and radiotherapy. Inhibition of C3a signaling was shown to restore tumor sensitivity to docetaxel in a murine prostate cancer model.[227] Another study used a transgenic model of squamous carcinogenesis to show that C5aR1 inhibition improved the efficacy of paclitaxel by reprogramming macrophages to recruit cytotoxic CD8$^+$ T cells.[249] Conversely, local production of C3a and C5a has been demonstrated to be critical to radiotherapy-induced tumor-specific immunity and therapeutic efficacy in a murine melanoma model.[250] Interestingly, dexamethasone, which is often administrated in combination with radiotherapy, was shown to limit complement activation and reduce antitumor efficacy.

Conclusions

The complement system is an essential part of the innate immune system, regulating inflammation, facilitating immune defense mechanisms, and maintaining tissue homeostasis. Commensurate with the cancer-promoting role of inflammation, complement proteins have emerged as key contributors to cancer growth and metastasis (Fig. 3.5). Complement is activated within tumor tissue, and bioinformatics analysis has identified a relationship between complement signaling

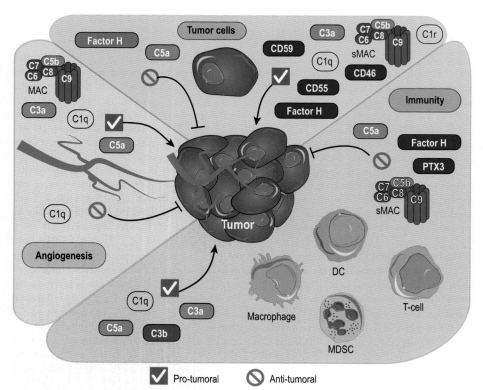

Fig. 3.5   Roles of complement proteins in tumor growth. Antitumor: C3 plays a critical role in immunosurveillance[195]; **C5a** promotes direct tumor cell killing and antitumor immune response[194,196]; the **MAC (C5b-9)** mediates tumor cell lysis via CDC[151]; **PTX3** regulates complement activation and limits tumor promoting inflammation.[220] **Protumor: CRPs** expressed on tumor cells (e.g., **CD46, CD55, CD59**) or in biologic fluids (e.g., **CFH**) limits MAC-mediated tumor cell lysis[160]; **C1q** promotes angiogenesis, tumor cell motility, and proliferation[216]; **C3b/iC3b** induces IL-10 and TGF-β2 and promotes MDSC generation[217]; **C3a** promotes M2/N2 polarization of macrophages and neutrophils, leading to suppression of effector T-cell and NK cell responses[141,143,187,190]; **C5a** recruits immunosuppressive myeloid cells (MDSCs, macrophages, and Tregs), suppresses cytotoxic T-cell responses,[131,183] stimulates angiogenesis,[185] and supports formation of the premetastatic niche[184]; **sublytic (s)-MAC** induces proliferative, migratory, and survival pathways, through release of inflammatory mediators and production of angiogenic growth factors[127]; autocrine production of **C1r, C3a, C5a,** and **PTX3** by tumor cells promotes EMT, proliferation, migration, and invasion.[223,228,237]

and prognosis in a range of cancers. Though most evidence points to the contribution of complement regulatory proteins and the anaphylatoxins C5a and C3a, other components such as sublytic MAC and C3b may also play a role in regulating tumor growth.

Although the majority of studies suggest that the effects of complement proteins on tumor growth are indirect, via immune modulation and promotion of angiogenesis, tumor intrinsic effects are also possible. Moreover, the experience in animal models suggests that responses may differ, depending on tumor type, tumor site, host immune phenotype, and baseline levels of complement activation. Consideration of the tumor type and stage of disease, along with an understanding of the complement effectors at play, may allow for the careful coordination of complement targeting approaches within the overall clinical management of the patient. Clearly, further research is required to fully understand the mechanisms by which complement proteins influence tumor growth, the consequences of targeting these proteins, and how complement targeting drugs interact with other cancer therapies. Nevertheless, preclinical studies highlight the potential of complement proteins as therapeutic targets for cancer, either as monotherapy or in combination with current cancer therapeutics. The availability of complement-targeting drugs, with more in the developmental pipeline, will facilitate progression of this research to clinical trials. To quote Demaria and colleagues,[250] "Given the crucial role of innate immune responses in (antitumor) immunity, harnessing these responses opens up new possibilities for long-lasting, multilayered tumor control."

Key References

64. Zhang X, Kimura Y, Fang C, et al. Regulation of Toll-like receptor-mediated inflammatory response by complement in vivo. *Blood*. 2007;110(1):228-236.
125. Lawal B, Tseng SH, Olugbodi JO, et al. Pan-cancer analysis of immune complement signature C3/C5/ C3AR1/C5AR1 in association with tumor immune evasion and therapy resistance. *Cancers (Basel)*. 2021;13(16):4124.
126. Davidson S, Efremova M, Riedel A, et al. Single-Cell RNA sequencing reveals a dynamic stromal niche that supports tumor growth. *Cell Rep*. 2020;31(7):107628.
131. Corrales L, Ajona D, Rafail S, et al. Anaphylatoxin C5a creates a favorable microenvironment for lung cancer progression. *J Immunol*. 2012;189(9):4674-4683.
139. Geller A, Yan J. The role of membrane bound complement regulatory proteins in tumor development and cancer immunotherapy. *Front Immunol*. 2019;10:1074.
143. Magrini E, Di Marco S, Mapelli SN, et al. Complement activation promoted by the lectin pathway mediates C3aR-dependent sarcoma progression and immunosuppression. *Nat Cancer*. 2021;2(2): 218-232.
160. Fishelson Z, Kirschfink M. Complement C5b-9 and cancer: mechanisms of cell damage, cancer counteractions, and approaches for intervention. *Front Immunol*. 2019;10:752.
183. Markiewski MM, DeAngelis RA, Benencia F, et al. Modulation of the antitumor immune response by complement. *Nat Immunol*. 2008;9(11):1225-1235.
184. Vadrevu SK, Chintala NK, Sharma SK, et al. Complement C5a receptor facilitates cancer metastasis by altering T-cell responses in the metastatic niche. *Cancer Res*. 2014;74(13):3454-3465.
187. Nabizadeh JA, Manthey HD, Panagides N, et al. C5a receptors C5aR1 and C5aR2 mediate opposing pathologies in a mouse model of melanoma. *FASEB J*. 2019;33(10):11060-11071.
189. Nabizadeh JA, Manthey HD, Steyn FJ, et al. The complement C3a receptor contributes to melanoma tumorigenesis by inhibiting neutrophil and CD4+ T cell responses. *J Immunol*. 2016;196(11): 4783-4792.
193. Zha H, Wang X, Zhu Y, et al. Intracellular activation of complement C3 leads to PD-L1 antibody treatment resistance by modulating tumor-associated macrophages. *Cancer Immunol Res*. 2019;7(2): 193-207.

203. Roumenina LT, Daugan MV, Petitprez F, Sautes-Fridman C, Fridman WH. Context-dependent roles of complement in cancer. *Nat Rev Cancer*. 2019;19(12):698-715.

220. Bonavita E, Gentile S, Rubino M, et al. PTX3 is an extrinsic oncosuppressor regulating complement-dependent inflammation in cancer. *Cell*. 2015;160(4):700-714.

223. Cho MS, Rupaimoole R, Choi HJ, et al. Complement component 3 is regulated by TWIST1 and mediates epithelial-mesenchymal transition. *J Immunol*. 2016;196(3):1412-1418.

236. Boire A, Zou Y, Shieh J, Macalinao DG, Pentsova E, Massague J. Complement component 3 adapts the cerebrospinal fluid for leptomeningeal metastasis. *Cell*. 2017;168(6):1101-1113.e13.

244. Ajona D, Ortiz-Espinosa S, Moreno H, et al. A combined PD-1/C5a blockade synergistically protects against lung cancer growth and metastasis. *Cancer Discov*. 2017;7(7):694-703.

245. Zha H, Han X, Zhu Y, et al. Blocking C5aR signaling promotes the anti-tumor efficacy of PD-1/PD-L1 blockade. *Oncoimmunology*. 2017;6(10):e1349587.

246. Wang Y, Sun SN, Liu Q, et al. Autocrine complement inhibits IL10-dependent T-cell-mediated antitumor immunity to promote tumor progression. *Cancer Discov*. 2016;6(9):1022-1035.

250. Surace L, Lysenko V, Fontana AO, et al. Complement is a central mediator of radiotherapy-induced tumor-specific immunity and clinical response. *Immunity*. 2015;42(4):767-777.

Visit Elsevier eBooks+ (eBooks.Health.Elsevier.com) for complete set of references.

CHAPTER 4

Cancer and the Science of Innate Immunity

Melanie Rutkowski

SUMMARY OF KEY FACTS

- The innate immune system is the host's first line of immune defense against challenges of the environment.
- The innate immune system response is a nonrestricted, rapid response.
- Innate immunity is required for the establishment of adaptive immunity, or immune memory.
- Cellular components comprising the innate system include monocytes, macrophages, dendritic cells, and granulocytic cell types such as neutrophils, mast cells, eosinophils, and basophils.
- Myeloid cells are phenotypically plastic, modulated by multiple systemic signals associated with inflammation.
- In a cancer setting, myeloid cells can either promote tumor growth or have antitumor functions.
- Chronic inflammation associated with cancer results in emergency myelopoiesis and emergence of myeloid precursors from the bone marrow and other extramedullary sites.
- Tumors, tumor-produced cytokines and chemokines, tumor-associated leukocytes, restricted nutrient supply, and oxidation of lipids alter the phenotype and function of myeloid cells entering the tumor microenvironment.
- Therapies aimed at genetically or epigenetically reprogramming myeloid cells in vivo or in vitro have shown promise as novel immune therapies.

Introduction

Innate immune cells are extraordinarily sensitive to the environment of the tissues in which they reside, phenotypically and functionally adjusting according to the chemokine and cytokine milieu, changes in tissue metabolism, and changes in the tissue architecture. Because of their functional adaptability, innate immune cells are central for the protection and maintenance of tissue homeostasis in response to inflammation, infectious disease, and cancer. This chapter will highlight critical developmental, transcriptional, and functional aspects of the innate immune system and how each of these pathways can be coopted by or contribute to cancer initiation, tumor growth and metastasis, antitumor immunity, and therapy response. Finally, this chapter will highlight therapeutic targets within the innate immune system that have shown promise as cancer therapies.

The Cellular Components of the Innate Immune Response

The immune system is divided into two branches, the innate immune system (nonrestricted rapid response) and the adaptive immune system (acquired cellular and humoral response). Innate immune cells comprise macrophages, monocytes, dendritic cells, and other myeloid- and lymphocyte-derived subsets that initiate and/or regulate host immune responses so that the adaptive arm of the immune system can eventually be triggered. Innate immune cells are not restricted by antigen and are functionally attenuated through signaling via immune receptors located on the surface or cytoplasm of the cells. These receptors recognize chemokine and cytokine signals, lipids and other signaling molecules, pathogen-associated molecular patterns (PAMPs), and dead and dying cells (damage-associated molecular patterns or DAMPs). To understand how the innate immune system functions in response to cancer, we will first define elements of innate immunity that are relevant to cancer, with an emphasis on myeloid subsets, given their significant contribution to tumor initiation, growth, immune evasion, and metastasis. Understanding the origins and functional potential of myeloid cells in the context of homeostatic or acute inflammatory settings will provide insight into the role of myeloid cells during cancer.

MONOCYTES

Monocytes are mononuclear-derived cell subsets that reside within the bone marrow, patrolling the blood and tissues for pathogens or abnormal cells. Monocytes were originally considered a short-lived precursor to tissue macrophages[1]; however, with the advent of more robust single-cell analysis technologies, fate mapping, and novel investigational model systems to study myeloid ontogeny and function, the origins and contribution of monocytes to tissue inflammation and homeostasis have become more nuanced. Indeed, monocytes do give rise to macrophages during specific inflammatory contexts. However, unlike macrophages, monocytes do not have the capacity for self-renewal, nor are they long-lived, like tissue macrophages derived from embryonic precursors that are maintained into adulthood. Studies have indicated that monocytes can give rise to dendritic cells[2,3] and demonstrated that monocytes are able to function as an individual and transient effector populations. For example, monocytes recruited to the liver by the proangiogenic factor vascular endothelial growth factor (VEGF) were educated to remodel the tissue vasculature without differentiating into macrophages.[4] Monocytes recruited into skin and lungs did not terminally differentiate into macrophages or dendritic cells but instead participated in steady-state tissue surveillance and transport of antigen to draining lymph nodes via the lymphatics.[5] Another study highlighted a critical role for monocytes in the expansion of brown adipose tissue.[6] These studies have challenged the dogma that monocytes solely function to repopulate macrophage and dendritic cell pools but instead demonstrate that in multiple inflammatory contexts monocytes contribute to angiogenesis, tissue remodeling, and antigen trafficking to lymph nodes, all of which are pathways involved in cancer initiation and progression. The relevance and contribution of monocytes to cancer progression will be highlighted in the next section.

Monocyte Ontogeny

In mice, monocytes consist of at least two functionally and phenotypically distinct subsets. Classic monocytes, or inflammatory monocytes, are Ly6C^{high} (GR-1$^+$) with proinflammatory properties, migrating to injured[7,8] or infected[9] tissues from the blood or bone marrow via signaling through chemokine receptor CCR2.[10] Nonclassical Ly6C^{neg} (GR-1^{neg}), or patrolling, monocytes reside in the vasculature and crawl along the luminal vessel surfaces of endothelial cells to surveil tissues during the resolution of inflammation.[8] Ly6C^{neg} monocytes enter into tissues during the latter phase of infection, via CX3CR1 signaling,[11] exerting a tissue repair immune regulatory program.

Ly6C[hi] monocytes have a short-lived half-life of 20 hours[12] but constitute the steady-state precursors to the blood-residing Ly6C[neg] migratory pool[12] such that the abundance of Ly6C[hi] monocytes dictates the pool of Ly6C[neg] progeny.[12] Monocytes are thought to be derived from the common monocyte progenitor (cMoP), a myeloid precursor population found in the bone marrow in mice,[13] and phenotypically defined as CLEC12A[hi]CD64[hi] subsets in humans. Progenitor populations were originally thought to derive in a hierarchical progression from common myeloid progenitor (CMP)- granulocyte-monocyte progenitor (GMP)- monocyte-macrophage dendritic cell progenitor (MDP)-cMoP-monocyte. However, it has been demonstrated that under specific inflammatory contexts a bifurcation in the pathway occurred whereby CMP arose independently from MDP into GMP-derived neutrophil-like monocytes whereas MDP differentiated into monocyte-derived DCs.[14] Thus, distinct ontogenies likely underlie observed functional heterogeneity in monocyte populations. Besides originating from the bone marrow, large pools of monocytes reside in the spleen[15] and lungs,[16] where they are maintained and are recruited en masse in response to inflammation, injury, or other systemic insults.

Most studies investigating monocyte origins and deployment throughout the body have used murine models. Human counterparts exist and have both similar and distinct functional attributes compared with their murine counterparts, which are outlined in Table 4.1. In humans, monocytes represent 10% of the nucleated cells in the blood, whereas in mice monocytes represent 4% of nucleated blood cells.[16] In humans, monocytes are defined based on CD14 and CD16 expression.[17] CD14[++] CD16[−] monocytes are more similar in function and phenotype to Ly6C[hi] monocytes in mice, including having high expression of CCR2 and CD115 while also having lower CD16 expression levels. On the other hand, CD14[+] CD16[+] monocytes also appear to have similar attributes to Ly6C[neg] monocytes, including having elevated CX3CR1 expression.[18] Despite these similarities, important differences between murine and human monocytes have been identified. For example, comprehensive transcriptional and flow cytometric profiling of murine monocytes and their human equivalents revealed that murine monocytes had high PPARγ expression signatures, whereas human monocytes had opposed patterns of surface receptors responsible for recognition and uptake of apoptotic cells and phagocytosis.[19]

Monocyte Function: Differentiation During Homeostasis and Inflammation

Monocytes are recruited in waves, where short-lived Ly6C[hi] monocytes contribute to early inflammation and Ly6C[neg] monocytes specialize in tissue repair and immune regulation. Ly6C[neg] monocytes are longer-lived, with a half-life of up to 2 weeks.[12] Upon entering tissues, and depending on the signals present within a given tissue environment, monocytes will either act as terminally differentiated effectors, as outlined previously, or differentiate into tissue macrophage and dendritic cell populations.

In steady-state conditions, little evidence exists to indicate that classic Ly6C[hi] monocytes contribute significantly to the pool of tissue-resident macrophages.[5,12,20] In the context of pathologic inflammation, Ly6C[hi] monocytes repopulate both tissue-resident macrophage and dendritic cell pools[21] (for in-depth review, see Wynn et al.[21]). One interesting exception to this paradigm is the lamina propria myeloid cells residing in the intestines. Using macrophage depleted conditions, monocyte fate mapping, adoptive transfer of monocytes, and parabiosis experiments, Varol et al. and Bogunovic et al. both demonstrated that circulating inflammatory Ly6C[hi] monocytes replenish the pool of immune-regulatory CX3CR1[+] macrophages but not of CD103[+] lamina propria migratory dendritic cell subsets.[22,23] This process occurs during homeostasis and is thought to differ from other steady-state macrophage pools because of the low-level tonic signaling by the commensal microbiota. Follow-up studies demonstrated that signals from the commensal microbiota were essential for monocyte-driven repopulation of luminal macrophages, because antibiotic treatment significantly depleted monocyte recruitment into the intestines, whereas germ-free mice

TABLE 4.1 ■ Monocyte Subsets in Mice and Humans

Monocyte Subset	Species	Classic Markers	Recruitment	Phenotype	References
Classic monocyte (inflammatory)	Mouse	$CD115^+$ $CD11b^+$ Ly6Chi $CCR2^+$ CX3CR1lo	Recruited early during inflammation Egress from bone marrow to CCL2	Short-lived Proinflammatory Steady-state precursor to nonclassic monocytes	7–10, 12, 17, 18, 19
	Human	$CD14^{++}$ $CD16^-$ $CD115^+$ $CCR2^+$ CX3CR1lo		Proinflammatory	17, 18, 19
Nonclassic (patrolling)	Mouse	$CD11b^+$ Ly6Clo $CCR2^-$ CX3CRhi	Patrol vessels Enter into tissues to CXCR3 ligands	Long-lived Tissue homeostasis/repair Immune regulatory PPAR gamma signature	8, 11, 17, 18, 19
	Human	$CD14^+$ $CD16^+$ $CD115^+$ $CCR2^-$ CX3CR1hi		Immune regulatory Tissue homeostasis/repair	17, 18, 19

exhibited a significant reduction in luminal macrophage levels.[24] Thus, the chronic signals derived by the gut microbiota were central for continued recruitment of Ly6C^{hi} monocytes into the lamina propria. During acute inflammation, such as during colitis, Ly6C^{hi} monocytes respond to bacterial products and give rise to proinflammatory effectors that eventually differentiate into migratory antigen-presenting dendritic cell subsets.[25] On the other hand, noninflammatory patrolling monocytes in both mice[2] and humans[26] directly give rise to migratory dendritic cell subsets in homeostatic settings. This occurs in the absence of acute inflammation, where Ly6C^{hi} monocytes recirculate back to the bone marrow and are converted into Ly6C^{neg} populations that replenish depleted dendritic cell populations in mucosal, but not splenic, tissues.[2]

Monocytes are versatile cell types and, similar to other myeloid-derived counterparts, exhibit sensitivity to the environment in which they reside. Functionally, monocytes exhibit plasticity and have a broad functional repertoire and differentiation potential that is dictated by the signals present in the tissues that they are recruited into. These properties endow monocytes with the potential to elicit robust inflammatory responses or participate in tissue remodeling and repair. Understanding the basis for monocyte fate and function in specific inflammatory contexts will be important for targeting these functionally diverse subsets for the treatment of various diseases, including cancer.

MACROPHAGES

Macrophages, in Greek meaning "the big eater," were originally identified as large phagocytic cells of the myeloid lineage having a critical role in maintaining tissue homeostasis and protection during sterile insults or disease. Macrophages are highly plastic phagocytic cells that have tremendous sensitivity to signals within their microenvironment, endowing them with broad functional diversity in terms of cytokines, chemokines, and other effector molecules. Macrophages occupy all tissues of the body, many of which are seeded into tissues during embryogenesis from the yolk sac and fetal liver. In most circumstances, tissue macrophages are long-lived and self-renew to maintain tissue residency throughout adulthood. Because of these properties, there is a significant effort to define the signaling pathways associated with macrophage recruitment and function within tumor-associated tissues and the tumor itself. To appreciate how macrophages function in the context of tumor initiation, metastasis, antitumor immunity and therapy response, we will first review macrophage ontogeny and function during homeostasis and acute inflammation, summarized in Fig. 4.1.

Macrophage Ontogeny

Macrophages populate tissues throughout the body in distinct waves during embryogenesis, with inputs from the yolk sac, fetal liver hematopoietic stem cells, or bone marrow. The first wave originates from the yolk sac, where erythroid–myeloid precursors either populate tissues directly or establish a niche of embryonic hematopoietic stem cells in the fetal liver. Monocytes originating from the fetal liver constitute the second wave of macrophage seeding into embryonic tissues. With the exception of the intestinal and cardiac macrophages, the latter of which are renewed by adult monocytes during aging,[27] tissue macrophages are able to self-renew into adulthood. Brain microglia are the only population of tissue macrophages seeded exclusively by yolk sac embryonic precursors,[28-31] whereas heart macrophages, liver Kupfer cells, and skin Langerhans cells are seeded by both the yolk sac and fetal liver.[28,29] Alveolar macrophages,[32] kidney macrophages, and red-pulp macrophages are seeded only by fetal liver monocytes.[28,29]

Macrophage Cellular Functions: Tissue-Specific Functions and the Spectrum Model of Activation

Macrophages are considered professional phagocytes, a cell that specializes in phagocytosis,[33] deriving from the Greek words *phago* (to devour) and *cytos* (cell). Phagocytosis is a cellular process in

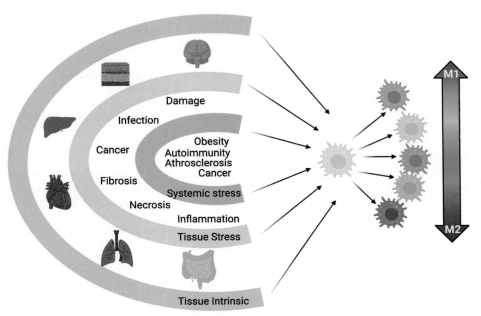

Fig. 4.1 Multispectral model of macrophage activation. The multispectral model of macrophage activation accounts for both tissue ontogeny and signals present within the local tissue environment during homeostatic conditions or during stress. These signals in addition to systemic signals are integrated into the macrophage developmental program to yield phenotypically and functionally distinct macrophage populations. As macrophages receive more complex signals, their functional trajectory becomes less linear and multispectral, with phenotypes more diverse than the bimodal M1 versus M2 distinctions. (Source: Figure generated in Biorender.)

which innate immune cells engulf and ingest large materials (greater than 0.5 μm in size) such as dead and dying cells, pathogens, or other particulate materials. Phagocytosis by macrophages and other professional phagocytes is essential for immune homeostasis and host defense, a process that was first described by Elie Metchnikoff, who received a Nobel Prize for his work in 1908[34] (for in-depth review, see Gordon[34]). Phagocytosis occurs in multiple phases beginning with sensing of the particle to be ingested through receptors on the cell surface,[35,36] internalization of the particle through the plasma membrane and into a distinct cellular compartment termed the *phagosome*,[37] and fusion of the phagosome with lysosomes, an organelle responsible for degradation of phagocytosed macromolecules.[38]

Tissue-resident macrophages exhibit multiple specialized functions for distinct tissue compartments and are identified by specific transcription factors that are induced in response to the tissue microenvironment. Several functionally nonredundant macrophage populations reside in the spleen. Macrophages residing in the red pulp are regulated by the transcription factor PU.1, enabling localization to red pulp for phagocytosis of damaged and dying red blood cells scavenging released iron to maintain iron homeostasis.[39] On the other hand, marginal zone splenic macrophages are dependent on LXRa signaling,[40] where they specialize in the clearance of apoptotic cells while also regulating selective uptake of apoptotic cells by CD8a dendritic cells, a subset in the spleen responsible for regulating autoreactivity to self-antigens.[41] Alveolar macrophages express the transcription factor B lymphoid transcription repressor BTB and CNC homology 2 (Bach2), which enables lipid handling and clearance of surfactant in the alveolar spaces of the lungs.[42] They also facilitate gas exchange and prevent against hypoxia during infection.[43]

Although there are multiple additional examples of tissue specification for macrophages, these studies underscore that macrophage function and phenotype are dictated by the signals present within the tissues that they reside. The advent of single-cell technologies to measure differences in gene expression, protein production, and chromatin regulation have enabled discovery of specific signaling pathways contributing to macrophage heterogeneity during health and disease. This concept is central to the heterogeneity of macrophages observed in disease settings such as cancer. Through transcriptional and epigenetic profiling of tissue-resident macrophages, Lavin et al. identified that aside from lineage-specific transcription factors, tissue-specific microenvironmental signals regulated macrophage identity and function through the induction of core transcription factors and specific chromatin modifications.[44] Tissue signals were so robust that transplanted macrophage precursors or mature macrophages were effectively epigenetically "reprogrammed" when transferred into new tissue environments,[44] exemplifying macrophage functional and transcriptional plasticity. Macrophage plasticity and the ability to be reprogrammed in response to changes in the microenvironment are key considerations when developing anticancer therapies, as will be outlined in the following.

The conceptual framework of macrophage activation has long maintained that macrophages can be polarized into two opposing states: M1, or classically activated inflammatory macrophages, and M2, or alternatively activated immune regulatory macrophages.[45] Studies evaluating macrophage response to acute infection, allergies, obesity, and asthma supported the paradigm that macrophages existed in one of two polarized states. However, this model did not account for the specialized functions of tissue macrophages, macrophages during sterile inflammation and tissue repair, and resolution of inflammation, nor did it encompass macrophage functional changes during chronic and complex disease states such as autoimmunity, chronic infection, and cancer. This paradigm has evolved coincident with the work related to macrophage ontogeny, with elegant studies demonstrating that macrophages have a broad functional repertoire with multiple, distinct, activation programs. Using ex vivo–derived human macrophages, Xue et al. differentiated macrophages in 29 distinct conditions ranging from stimuli associated with M1 and M2 activation axis to stimuli associated with free fatty acids, high-density lipoprotein, or combinations associated with chronic inflammation. Using transcriptomics and network analysis, it was found that in conditions diverging from the classical M1 and M2 paradigm, macrophages had a broad spectrum of activation signatures.[46] These studies support the framework that macrophage activation is multidimensional, where macrophages receive input from tissue environments and external stimuli such as sterile insult, pathogens, or cancer, culminating in a broad range of activation phenotypes. The multispectral model is highlighted in Fig. 4.1.

DENDRITIC CELLS

Dendritic cells were first discovered by Ralph Steinman and Zanvil Cohn in 1973, with Ralph Steinman receiving the Nobel Prize in Physiology or Medicine for this discovery in 2011. Dendritic cells were first identified as a unique cell subset, distinct from macrophages, based upon their extensively branched dendrites, multiple mitochondria, motility, lack of robust phagocytic activity compared with macrophages, and a robust ability to activate T cells.[47,48] After years of skepticism, it is now well accepted that dendritic cells are instrumental for inducing adaptive immune responses to self- and foreign antigens, highlighting their critical role in the initiation of tolerance and protective immunity. Macrophages are professional phagocytes, and dendritic cells are considered professional antigen-presenting cells, a sentinel of immune activation and host memory responses. Given these attributes, much work has gone toward understanding dendritic cells to therapeutically enhance adaptive immune responses against pathogens and tumors and to suppress responses during autoimmunity.

Most subsets of dendritic cells, with the exception of Langerhans cells, are constantly replenished from hematopoietic precursors in the bone marrow. Dendritic cells are subdivided into three subsets based upon lineage precursors, expression of core transcription factors, and functional attributes (summarized in Fig. 4.2). Subsets of dendritic cells are as follows: classic dendritic cells (cDCs), plasmacytoid DC (pDCs), and monocytic DCs (moDC).

cDCs are the most well-characterized subsets, given their ability to activate CD4 and CD8 T cells. cDCs derive from the common dendritic cell progenitor (CDP),[49-51] with precursors

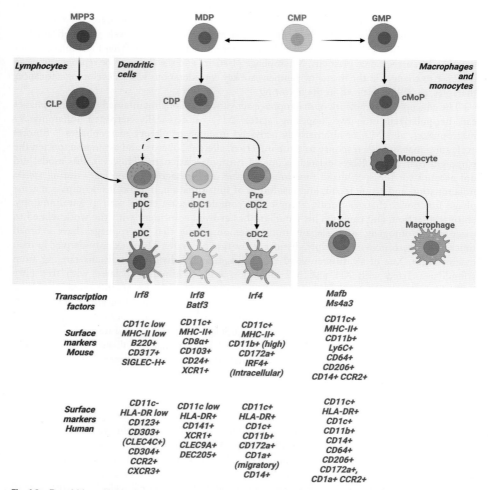

Transcription factors	Irf8	Irf8 Batf3	Irf4	Mafb Ms4a3
Surface markers Mouse	CD11c low MHC-II low B220+ CD317+ SIGLEC-H+	CD11c+ MHC-II+ CD8a+ CD103+ CD24+ XCR1+	CD11c+ MHC-II+ CD11b+ (high) CD172a+ IRF4+ (Intracellular)	CD11c+ MHC-II+ CD11b+ Ly6C+ CD64+ CD206+ CD14+ CCR2+
Surface markers Human	CD11c- HLA-DR low CD123+ CD303+ (CLEC4C+) CD304+ CCR2+ CXCR3+	CD11c low HLA-DR+ CD141+ XCR1+ CLEC9A+ DEC205+	CD11c+ HLA-DR+ CD1c+ CD11b+ CD172a+ CD1a+ (migratory) CD14+	CD11c+ HLA-DR+ CD1c+ CD11b+ CD14+ CD64+ CD206+ CD172a+, CD1a+ CCR2+

Fig. 4.2   Dendritic cell development and classification in human and mice. Hierarchy of differentiation for dendritic cell subsets. Starting from common myeloid progenitors, classic dendritic cells are derived from monocyte dendritic cell precursors (MDPs). Common dendritic cell precursors (CDPs) have the potential to become cDC1 or cDC2. The origin of pDCs is controversial, with studies demonstrating that pDCs arise from common leukocyte progenitors (CLPs), not CDPs, designated by a dotted line. Monocytic dendritic cells (MoDCs) arise from granulocyte-macrophage progenitors (GMPs) and then from common monocyte progenitors (cMoPs). Transcription factors listed are associated with speciation of each dendritic cell subset and can serve as lineage markers to distinguish each population from other myeloid cells, in addition to the surface markers (with the exception of IRF4, which is an intracellular/nuclear stain) listed. (Source: Figure generated in Biorender.)

entering into the lymph nodes to disperse via high endothelial venules where they form an integrated network of DCs.[51] cDCs are subdivided further based upon distinct developmental pathways, expression of core transcription factors, and functional attributes. cDCs are considered a heterogenous population, but the two most well-characterized subsets are cDC1 and cDC2. cDC1 express XCR1 and CLEC9A and can cross-present antigen to CD8 T cells, having an outsized role during antitumor immunity in both mice and humans, as detailed later. cDC2 are more heterogenous and have been identified to represent multiple distinct and heterogenous transcriptional programs[52] (for in-depth review, see Chen et al.[52]). cDC2 typically activate CD4 T cells and, depending on the subset, can be proinflammatory or immune regulatory. A third cDC subset has been identified in humans, termed cDC3, which primes a subset of tissue-homing CD8+ T cells expressing CD103.[53,54]

Plasmacytoid dendritic cells (pDCs) produce large amounts of type I interferon in response to viral infection or inflammation.[55] The origins of pDCs are not as well-defined compared with their classical counterparts. Original studies demonstrated that pDCs can be derived from CDP.[49-51] However, studies tracking progenitor subsets from the lymphoid lineage using the expression of yellow fluorescent protein (YFP) discovered that a majority of pDCs in the thymus and spleen were marked by YFP expression, indicating that the YFP-expressing pDCs derived from lymphoid progenitors.[51] Dress et al. explored this paradigm further by combining single-cell mRNA sequencing with in vivo fate mapping and in vitro single cell–based clonal assays to demonstrate that pDCs arose from a subset of common lymphoid-like progenitors, indicating that pDCs are a distinct lymphoid-derived dendritic cell subset.[56] Monocyte-derived DCs also do not arise from CDP but instead form monocytic precursors in inflamed settings.[14]

OTHER INNATE IMMUNE CELL SUBSETS

Natural Killer Cells

Natural killer (NK) cells are central for host defense against virally infected or transformed cells. NK cells are widely distributed throughout the body, present within secondary lymphoid tissues such as lymph nodes, spleen, and mucosal associated lymphoid tissue in addition to tissues such as the lung, uterus, and liver.[57] In the blood and lymph nodes, NK cells represent approximately 5% to 15% of total lymphocytes,[58] whereas in the liver, lung, and uterus they are represented in higher frequencies.[57] NK cells derive from common lymphocyte progenitors in the bone marrow. However, unlike B- and T-cell lymphocytes, NK cells do not require sensitization to kill target cells because of the lack of expression of antigen-specific receptors. Instead, NK cells express a series of germline-encoded activating and inhibitory receptors that enable distinction between self and nonself, a process referred to as *education* or *licensing*. Although NK cells are generally considered an innate lymphocyte subset, NK cells are also distinct from innate myeloid cells because they do not have the ability to phagocytose cells. Instead, NK cells possess effector capabilities resembling that of T cells, including the secretion of perforin, granzymes, and interferon gamma (IFN-γ). NK cells also express FasL and TRAIL on the cell surface, both of which bind to death receptors on recipient cells, leading to the induction of apoptosis. NK cells also produce a multitude of effector cytokines and chemokines, including tumor necrosis factor alpha (TNF-α), interleukin (IL)-10, GM-CSF, G-CSF, IL-3, CCL2, CCL3, CCL4, CCL5, XCL1, and CXCL8.[59]

NK cells are derived from common lymphoid precursors in the bone marrow prior to populating peripheral lymphoid and nonlymphoid tissues.[60] Commitment to the NK lineage coincides with expression of CD122, a receptor for IL-15, followed by the induction of transcription factors such as STAT5, EOMES, Nfil3, Ets, T-bet, Id2, Tox, and Tcf1. As NK cells mature, they upregulate expression of receptors such as NKp46 and CD49b, a point at which they are considered to be mature because of their potential to exert cytotoxic functions.[61] NK cells continue to progress through a four-stage process of maturation, consisting of transcriptional and functional changes and defined in mice by upregulation of CD11b and gradual loss of CD27, with terminally differentiated CD11b$^+$ CD27$^-$ effectors having potent cytolytic capabilities and reduced potential for expansion.[62] In humans, NK-cell maturation is thought to associate with diminishing levels of surface CD56 expression. Using single-cell RNA sequencing, CD56^{bright} populations were found to have gene expression similar to that of the less differentiated CD11b$^-$ CD27$^+$ subset, whereas CD56^{dim} populations resembled CD11b$^+$ CD27$^-$ populations.[63] However, it remains unknown whether CD56 expression truly identifies human NK subsets from the same lineage, progressing through distinct maturation states, or whether its expression defines subpopulations with unique developmental trajectories.

Central to NK cell function is the expression of a broad array of membrane proteins that calibrate NK cell interactions between other cells, resulting in inhibition or induction of cell cytotoxicity. NK receptors are broadly categorized into activating, inhibitory, and costimulatory receptors.[64] Licensed NK cells express inhibitory receptors that contain immunoreceptor tyrosine-based inhibitory motifs (ITIMs) in their cytoplasmic domains. Upon recognition of self-MHCI, ITIM domains are phosphorylated by SH2 domain–containing protein tyrosine phosphatase 1 (SHP1),[64] effectively inhibiting intracellular signaling pathways controlling NK cell activation. Many NK-activating receptors contain immunoreceptor tyrosine-based activation motif (ITAM)-signaling molecules that, upon receptor crosslinking, lead to activation of the ITAM motif and downstream signaling events associated with NK cytotoxicity and effector function[64] (for in-depth review, see Yokoyama and Plougastel[64]).

Mast Cells

Mast cells are evolutionarily conserved innate immune cells found in connective tissues throughout the body, such as perivascular sites, brain, smooth muscle, peritoneal cavity, gastrointestinal tract, and respiratory tract.[65] Mast cells are known for initiating inflammatory responses during allergic diseases. Although mast cells are often neglected in cancer research because of their low abundance in tissue and tumor microenvironments, it has become clear that in cancer and non-cancer settings, mast cells are pivotal regulators of immune function.

Non-tissue-resident mast cells develop from hematopoietic progenitor populations in the bone marrow[66] where precursor populations are recruited to distal sites via chemokine gradients into the tissue[67] and undergo division,[66,68] followed by maturation and activation by tissue microenvironmental factors. On the other hand, tissue-resident mast cells are derived from yolk sac progenitors.[69-71] Tissue mast cells are long-lived[72-74] and can be replenished from precursors residing in the tissue.[75,76] However, very little is known how progenitor tissue-resident mast cells are matured. For bone marrow–derived mast cells, progenitors differentiate from common myeloid progenitors (CMPs), a process that is tightly controlled by CCAAT/enhancer binding protein α (C/EBPα), GATA-binding factor 2 (GATA-2), GATA-binding factor 3 (GATA-3), Hes-1, and melanocyte-inducing transcription factor (MITF).[66] The downregulation of C/EBPα in GMP along with upregulation of GATA-2, GATA-3, and Hes-1 allows GMP to differentiate into bipotent progenitors, which have the potential to become mast cells and basophils. The subsequent upregulation of MITF and further downregulation of C/EBPα lead to the commitment of progenitors into mast cells.

A tremendous amount of work has been done to identify subtypes of mast cells in animals and humans, where the classification of mast cell subsets is based on the anatomic location and/or the protein contents in the secretory granules. In mice, the most well-characterized subtypes of mast cells are connective tissue mast cells (CTMCs) and mucosal mast cells (MMCs). CTMCs are found in skin, the peritoneal cavity, and the gastrointestinal tract, whereas MMCs usually populate at mucosal sites. CTMCs have granules that contain heparin, histamine, tryptase, and chymase, whereas the granule contents of MMCs mainly comprise chymase and have low levels of histamine and undetectable levels of heparin.[77] In humans, mast cells are classified as MC_T (mast cells containing mainly tryptase) and MC_{TC} (mast cells containing both tryptase and chymase).[77] MC_T reside in the external mucosa of the gastrointestinal and respiratory tracts, whereas MC_{TC} are usually found in the submucosa and perivascular tissues.[78,79] Distinct tissue tropisms give rise to distinct functional attributes, with MC_T critically regulating the immune responses and MC_{TC} being involved in tissue repair.[78,79] Although human and murine mast cells share multiple protein signatures,[80] mast cells from each species also produce a distinct repertoire of proteases[77] and respond differently in the presence of the mast cell stabilizer cromolyn.[81] Host-intrinsic and/or tissue microenvironment–driven variations can also contribute to phenotypical differences in mast cells.[81,82]

Neutrophils

Neutrophils, or polymorphonuclear leukocytes, are the most abundant cell type in the peripheral blood, approximating 50% to 70% of cells in human blood and 10% to 25% of cells in murine blood.[83] Neutrophils are phagocytic and granulocytic cells considered one of the first lines of defense against pathogens. On the other hand, neutrophils also have a central role during immune homeostasis and tissue repair. The neutrophil life cycle is still an intense area of debate, owing to a lack of reliable techniques to accurately trace the path of neutrophil differentiation, circulation, tissue seeding, and eventual death in vivo. Compared with other innate immune cell populations, it is generally accepted that neutrophils are short-lived, surviving only hours to days once in the periphery. Given their critical role for innate immune defense, the numbers of neutrophils circulating in the periphery, and their short half-life, there is a significant requirement for de novo production of progenitors from the bone marrow daily. It is estimated that approximately 60% of all leukocytes produced daily in the bone marrow are granulocytic precursors,[84] with 10^9 neutrophils produced and released from the bone marrow in humans and 10^7 neutrophils produced in mice daily.[85] During inflammation, as many as 10 billion neutrophils can be produced in humans.[86]

Neutrophils are derived from the multipotent progenitors in the bone marrow, undergoing commitment prior to entrance into the blood. Prior to the work by Evrard et al., it was unknown what factors contributed to the phenotypic and functional heterogeneity of peripheral neutrophils. Evrard et al. demonstrated that neutrophils arise from CMPs, transitioning into GMPs and eventually into a previously unrecognized precursor population they termed *preneutrophils*.[87] In homeostatic conditions, commitment of GMP into preneutrophils is driven by expression of the transcription factor C/EBPε and expression of cKit and CXCR4.[87] Preneutrophils are highly proliferative and reside in the bone marrow and spleen. During inflammatory stress, such as sepsis or cancer, preneutrophils rapidly expand to meet the increased demand, giving rise to two distinct neutrophil subsets: nonproliferative immature Ly6G$^{lo/+}$ CXCR2$^-$ CD101$^-$ neutrophils and Ly6G$^+$ CXCR2$^+$ CD101$^+$ mature neutrophils within the blood.[87] Other studies have identified that multipotent progenitors could act as a source of neutrophils in response to hematopoietic demands,[88] whereas Cugurra et al. identified that the skull and vertebral bone marrow can supply the meninges with neutrophils under pathologic conditions such as spinal cord injury and neuroinflammation.[89] Altogether, these studies have begun to establish the underlying mechanisms of neutrophil heterogeneity, underscoring that neutrophil phenotype and function are dependent on systemic inflammatory factors in addition to the tissue of origin.

The production, trafficking, and egress of mature neutrophils from the blood was demonstrated to occur in a diurnal pattern, where the exit of CD62L^{low} CXCR4^{high} "aged" neutrophils from the blood back into the bone marrow and other tissues peaked during resting phases and was followed by emergence of "fresh" neutrophils during awake hours.[90] Casanova-Acebes et al. went on to demonstrate that the circadian clock gene *Artnl1* (BMAL1) was responsible for the diurnal regulation of neutrophil migration.[90] BMAL1 was found to be a cell-intrinsic regulator of CXCL2 production and subsequent signaling through the ligand CXCR2, initiating transcriptional and migratory changes in neutrophils that trigger the aging cascade. On the other hand, the chemo-kine receptor CXCR4 antagonized aging via CXCR2 signaling. Although immature neutrophils express high levels of CXCR4 while being retained in the bone marrow, CXCR4 is paradoxically expressed at high levels in aged neutrophils, a process that is hypothesized to signify a return into the bone marrow and other sterile tissues to bolster to tissue immunity.[91]

Functionally, neutrophils exhibit a broad range of capabilities that are dictated by the tissue environments into which they migrate, by the signals in the tissue or systemic environment they are exposed to, and by a culmination of physiologic factors that differently prime neutrophils in their functional response.[92] For example, neutrophils in an obese setting can metabolize lipids and affect energy expenditure,[93] whereas neutrophils in the spleen provide help to B cells.[94] During inflammation, neutrophil longevity is increased upon activation,[95] which can occur via recognition of tissue insults through expression of multiple innate signaling receptors. Neutrophils are highly phagocytotic cells; they can release potent amounts of reactive oxygen species and proteases from their granule contents and can release neutrophil extracellular traps, or NETs. NETs are an extra-cellular release of neutrophil DNA into a net-like configuration, effectively trapping microorgan-isms. NETs contain a high concentration of antimicrobial molecules and other molecules that are toxic to the captured microbes.[96] As discussed below, the heterogeneity of neutrophil effector function and sensitivity to systemic signals result in significant heterogeneity in neutrophil pheno-types and functions in cancer-bearing individuals.

Innate Immune Networks in the Promotion of Tumor Growth, Immune Suppression, and Metastasis

In the previous section, the origins, differentiation pathways, and diverse functions of innate myeloid cells were covered. During cancer, myeloid cells have the potential to provide robust and protective antitumor immune control, acting as sentinels against tumor growth. Here, we will focus on the mechanisms whereby inflammation and innate immune signaling increase cancer risk or promotion of tumor growth. Enhanced tumor progression is coordinated by innate im-mune cells, leading to immune evasion, increased angiogenesis, and metastasis. Tumors and the tumor microenvironment act on terminally differentiated myeloid cells or on immature precur-sors recently recruited into the tumor microenvironment, both of which transform myeloid cells into potent immune suppressive and protumorigenic innate immune subsets. Here, we will define key innate immune pathways that initiate cancer formation or that contribute to tumor progres-sion and metastasis.

INFLAMMATION IS A KEY MODULATOR OF TUMOR INITIATION

In the context of typical immune function, inflammation often is associated with host response against pathogens or sterile insults. Tumor promoting on the other hand, indicates nonspecific and unabated inflammation. In this context, inflammation itself can result in cancer development and progression. Inflammation is a hallmark of cancer,[97,98] with tumor-promoting inflammation affecting all aspects of tumorigenesis: driving oncogenic transformation, enhancing proliferation and survival of premalignant cells, facilitating tumor escape from the immune system, driving therapy failure and/or resistance, enhancing angiogenesis, and promoting metastasis. How inflammation is involved in cancer initiation and progression is summarized in Fig. 4.3.

The association between inflammation and cancer was first obtained by experimental evidence from preclinical animal models in addition to large-scale epidemiologic studies that identified a strong association between the use of nonsteroidal antiinflammatory drugs (NSAIDs) and reduced cancer incidence and/or cancer-associated mortality for multiple types of cancer.[99,100] However, caution should be observed when considering prescribing NSAIDs for prevention of

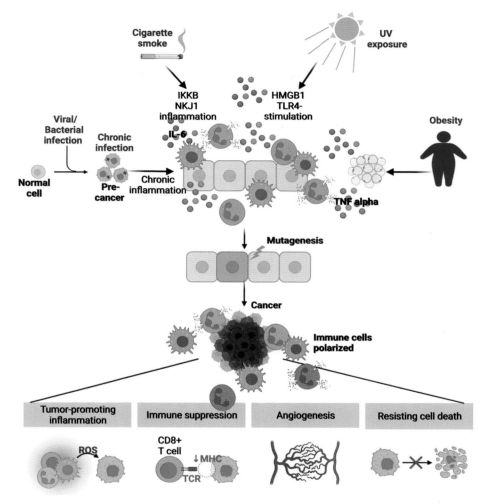

Fig. 4.3 Inflammation-induced tumor initiation and progression. Potential mechanisms of inflammation-initiated cellular transformation and tumor growth include infection, smoking, ultraviolet light exposure, and obesity. These initial events lead to chronic low-level inflammation, which initiates cellular transformation, myeloid cell polarization, tumor-promoting inflammation, avoidance of immune destruction, angiogenesis, and resistance of cell death. Inflammation is associated with each of these steps to further tumor growth. (Source: Figure generated in Biorender.)

or treatment of certain cancers, because the dose and cancer type could have negative effects. For example, a randomized clinical trial called ASPREE found that in individuals over 70 years of age, compared with the use of a placebo, low-dose aspirin was associated with an increased risk of advanced metastatic cancer.[101] On the other hand, there is evidence that chronic inflammatory diseases, such as inflammatory bowel disease[102] and systemic lupus erythematosus,[103] increase the risk of colorectal and gastric cancer, respectively.

A majority of cancers are caused by environmental factors, many of which are associated with inflammation. Cancer-causing inflammation can occur as a result of chronic exposure to

TABLE 4.2 ■ Inflammation-Mediated Mechanisms of Cancer Initiation and Progression

Stimulus	Type of Cancer	Inflammatory Mechanism	References
Smoking	Lung cancer	Pulmonary inflammation marked by IKKB and JNK1-induced inflammation. Increased IL-6 and TNF-α, accumulation of macrophages and neutrophils	106
Intermittent intense ultraviolet exposure	Metastatic melanoma	Ultraviolet-damaged keratinocytes release HMGB1, TLR4-dependent recruitment of neutrophils. Stimulation of angiogenesis	104, 105
Obesity	Pancreatic	Increased mitochondrial fatty acid B-oxidation, increased TNF-α signaling, adipose-derived IL-6 and TNF	107
	Colorectal cancer	Microbiome dysbiosis, reduced DC-mediated tissue homeostasis. Obesity and chemical carcinogens increase IL-6 and repolarize tissue macrophages	108
	Liver cancer	High-fat diet combined with fermented foods increased dysbiosis, cholestasis, hepatocyte death, and neutrophil influx	109

sunlight,[104,105] smoking,[106] and obesity,[107-109] the known inflammatory mechanisms of which are summarized in Table 4.2. Chronic infection can also lead to cancer. In the estimation of global burden of cancers attributable to infectious disease from the year 2018, 13% of all identified cancers arose because of infectious disease, with increased incidence in underdeveloped and developing countries.[110] Strikingly, 90% of the infection-associated cases worldwide were a result of infection with four pathogens: *Helicobacter pylori*, human papillomavirus (HPV), hepatitis B virus (HBV), and hepatitis C virus (HCV), all of which are either vaccine preventable (HPV, HBV) or treatable (*H. pylori*, HCV).[110] Infection with *Schistosoma* is linked with bladder cancer[111] and certain *Bacteroides* species are associated with colorectal cancer.[112] Unlike acute infection, where a robust inflammatory response leads to clearance of each pathogen, in these scenarios, the ability of the microorganism to evade the immune system results in a low level and chronic inflammation.

Depending on the tissue context, chronic inflammation can lead to cellular transformation because of recruitment of myeloid cells producing reactive oxygen species (ROS) and reactive nitrogen intermediates (RNIs) or the elevated production of proliferative and growth factors. For example, cytokines can activate STAT3 signaling, which in some instances can cause differentiated cells to loose their identity acquiring a non-differentiated stem cell phenotype capable of self-renewal.[113] Chronic signaling of nuclear factor kappa-light-chain-enhancer of activated B cells (NF-κB) can suppress cell death, activate genes related to cell proliferation, and enhance the expression of growth factors and protumorigenic cytokines in the tissue environment.[114] Tumor-promoting cytokines and growth factors, such as TNF-α, IL-1α, IL-1β, IL-6, IL-11, IL-23, and IL-17, initiate proinflammatory signaling networks resulting in enhanced cell proliferation and cell survival.[115] One of the most mutated pathways in cancer is loss of or mutation of *Tp53*, which encodes for the p53 protein, a critical regulator of cell homeostasis. Another critical role for p53 is control of NF-κB-mediated inflammation. In multiple contexts, loss of p53 leads to dysregulation of NF-κB expression, increasing the production of inflammatory cytokines and chemokines from mutant cells.[116,117] This signaling pathway further contributes to tumor growth via the establishment of a supportive immunologic niche that enables tumor growth and eventual metastasis.

INFLAMMATION-MEDIATED REPROGRAMMING OF MYELOID CELLS DURING CANCER

Multiple cytokine and chemokine networks have also been implicated as essential for the orchestration of tumor progression through the establishment of an immune suppressive environment that promotes angiogenesis and facilitates metastatic spread. The mechanisms outlined here are by no means comprehensive but are intended to provide general mechanistic insight into relevant inflammatory pathways and their effects on individual immune cells and the effects of these signaling pathways on tumor progression. Myeloid cells are exquisitely responsive to the multitude of inflammatory signals within the tumor microenvironment,[118-120] and as tumors progress, both lineage-committed[121,122] and immature myeloid precursors[123,124] are polarized into protumorigenic and suppressive phenotypes.

Monocytes

One of the major bottlenecks in defining how monocytes affect cancer is the lack of markers that differentiate monocyte-derived macrophages and dendritic cells from monocytes. This is because monocytes upregulate macrophage and dendritic cell markers such as F4/80, MHCII, and CD11c once they enter the tissue. These attributes, along with progenitor pathways that are distinct from those of other myeloid subsets during conditions of inflammation,[14] make tracking the trajectory that monocytes take from the bone marrow into the tumor environment more challenging. Despite these challenges, lineage tracing, specialized transgenic mice, and single-cell analysis technology have provided insight into the pro- and antitumor activity of monocytes during cancer.

Tumor- and stroma-associated expression of the chemokine CCL2 is one of the main signaling pathways involved in the recruitment of inflammatory monocytes into the tumor microenvironment. Once monocytes enter the tumor microenvironment, they are coopted to enhance tumor growth, enable immune evasion, or promote metastatic dissemination. Qian et al. demonstrated CCL2 signaling recruited Ly6C^{hi} CCR2-expressing monocytes into metastatic sites enhancing extravasation, tumor seeding, and growth in the lungs.[125] Once in the tumor microenvironment, inflammatory CCR2-expressing monocytes contribute to the pool of tumor-associated macrophages.[126] Other relevant signaling pathways associated with polarizing monocytes to acquire tumor-associated macrophage functions include CSF1 signaling. In a tumor setting, CSF1 enhances recruitment and polarization of monocytes into macrophages.[127] However, other pathways have been identified, indicating that there are multiple tissue and microenvironmental contexts in which monocytes can become polarized to become part of the tumor-associated macrophage pool. For example, expression of the receptor for IL-4 and IL-13 (IL-4R) results in polarization and enhanced tumor-promoting functions of monocytes recruited in the bone marrow, culminating in enhanced recruitment to and outgrowth of breast tumor cells in the bone marrow.[128] Another study identified that IL-6 and GM-CSF produced by cancer-associated fibroblasts induce polarization of monocytes into tumor-associated macrophages.[129] Inflammatory monocytes can also directly promote metastasis. In certain tumor models, inflammatory monocytes recruited into the tumor microenvironment via CCL2 express factor XIIIA, a transglutaminase that covalently crosslinks fibrin, creating a scaffold for tumor cells to invade and metastasize.[130] Monocytes also modulate the tumor microenvironment via production of IL-1β, IL-6, TNF-α, and CCL3, resulting in immune suppression and enhanced angiogenesis (see review by Olingy et al.[127]).

Nonclassical or patrolling monocytes are longer-lived than classic or inflammatory monocytes, constantly surveilling tissues and transporting antigen to draining lymph nodes. These attributes make patrolling monocytes well-suited for antitumor immune functions. Nonclassic monocytes patrol the lung environment for tumor cell debris and can activate NK cells to prevent metastatic seeding of the tissue.[131] Mechanistically, it was subsequently shown that patrolling monocytes are expanded by tumor-produced exosomes[132] and activated to produce IL-15, leading to subsequent activation of IFN-γ-producing NK cells that prevent metastatic colonization of the lungs.[133] Despite the tumor protective functions of patrolling monocytes, they are still susceptible to the signals within the tumor microenvironment and can be modulated or polarized to support tumor growth. For example, tumors treated with anti-VEGFR2 therapy acquire resistance. One of the mechanisms of resistance involves upregulation of CX3CR1 and recruitment of patrolling monocytes into the tumor microenvironment. Once recruited, the monocytes enhance angiogenesis and immune suppression through the production of chemokines that recruit suppressive neutrophils into the tumor microenvironment.[127]

Dendritic Cells

Dendritic cells are critical for the initiation of adaptive tumor immune responses. However, as tumors progress, conventional dendritic cells are coopted by tumors acquiring tolerogenic functions. These dendritic cells are termed *tumor-induced regulatory dendritic cells*. Although distinguishing dendritic cells from macrophages and other myeloid cells is more challenging under conditions of emergency myelopoiesis, bona fide dendritic cells can be identified by expression of the transcription factor *Zbtb46*[134,135] and the presence of DNGR1.[136] Using an approach to selectively deplete dendritic cells in an autochthonous model of ovarian cancer, Scarlett et al. demonstrated that during early stages of tumor progression, dendritic cells were instrumental for orchestrating antitumor CD8 T-cell immune responses. However, as tumors continued to evolve and the tumor microenvironment became more suppressive, tumor-produced transforming growth factor beta (TGF-β) and prostaglandin E2 (PGE2) polarized dendritic cells to suppress T-cell responses.[121] Mechanistically, dendritic cells became suppressive in response to sustained and elevated expression of the chromatin regulator Satb1. Although required for differentiation of conventional dendritic cells, unremitting Satb1 expression induces a phenotypic switch in conventional dendritic cells, leading to enhanced secretion of immune suppressive galectin 1 and tumor-promoting IL-6.[122]

Conventional dendritic cells can be polarized via additional suppressive pathways, including interactions with MDSCs, regulatory T cells, and metabolic stress. For an extensive review of mechanisms associated with dendritic cell polarization and suppression, see Veglia and Gabilovich,[137] Wculek et al.,[138] and Conejo-Garcia et al.[139] Herber et al. observed that dendritic cells in patients and in murine models of cancer were abnormally laden with oxidized lipids, a state termed *dyslipidemia*, resulting in endoplasmic reticulum (ER) stress, which is discussed later, and a reduced ability of dendritic cells to activate T cells.[140] Mechanistically, lipid accumulation was driven by expression of scavenger receptor A whereby oxidatively truncated lipids were bound to chaperone HSP70, effectively preventing transport of exogenous peptide-MHC class I complexes to the cell surface, limiting the ability of dendritic cells to stimulate CD8 T cells.[141]

Plasmacytoid dendritic cells represent a rare population within the tumor microenvironment. As such, evaluating the effects of pDCs on cancer progression has been challenging, and it is still unclear whether pDCs conclusively have pro- or antitumor functions. However, given the plasticity in the dendritic cell lineage, it is likely that pDCs have varied function depending on the signals that are present in the tumor microenvironment. Within the tumor microenvironment, pDCs were shown to enhance immune suppression by expanding regulatory T cells in an inducible T-cell costimulatory ligand (ICOSL)-dependent manner[142] while also inducing IL-10 in regulatory T cells[143] or initiating type 2 immune responses in CD4 T cells,[144] both of which are immune suppressive and protumorigenic. However, evidence also exists that plasmacytoid dendritic cells induce cytotoxic T-cell responses via production of IFN-α.[145] Additionally, when activated with ligands for TLR7, pDCs initiate substantial antitumor immune responses.[137]

Abnormal differentiation of myeloid cells and infiltration of tumors with immature dendritic cells are considered primary mediators of myeloid dysfunction within the tumor microenvironment.[146] Myeloid-derived dendritic cells are often referred to as *plastic* or *nonclassical monocytes*, rather than bona fide dendritic cells, and are thought to acquire dendritic cell–like attributes once they enter the tumor environment.[147] Myeloid-derived dendritic cells are associated with a negative prognostic outcome. Monocyte-derived dendritic cells arise from the differentiation of CCR2-expressing monocytes in response to inflammation, such as what would be found within the tumor microenvironment.[147] Myeloid-derived dendritic cells promote immune suppression within the ovarian tumor microenvironment[148] and are associated with poor outcome in other models of cancer.[149]

cDC1 dendritic cells, although a rare subpopulation within the tumor microenvironment, express CD103 and are dependent on IRF8 and Batf3 signaling. Importantly, cDC1 are one of the most capable cell subsets that stimulate CD8 T cells for tumor control.[150] In support of this, the abundance of cDC1 in tumors corresponds with positive cancer outcomes.[150] cDC1 can also produce IL-12 to potentiate adaptive antitumor immune responses. In situ expansion of cDC1 within tumors using systemic administration of FLT3L and intratumoral poly I:C resulted in activation and enhanced response to BRAF inhibition in combination with programmed death ligand 1 (PD-L1) blockade.[151] The response was so robust that mice were subsequently protected from tumor challenge,[151] demonstrating the potency of cDC1 in achieving protective antitumor immunity. NK cells recruit cDC1 into the tumor microenvironment via CCL5 and XCL1 expression,[152] identifying a key NK–dendritic cell–chemokine regulatory axis that is currently being explored as a potential cancer therapeutic. Mechanisms of tumor-induced dendritic cell dysfunction are summarized in Fig. 4.4.

Macrophages

In a tumor setting, macrophages are hijacked by tumors to promote malignant growth, invasion, metastasis, and outgrowth of tumors in distal organs. In general, the presence of macrophages associates with poor clinical outcomes for most cancer types.[153,154] Phenotypically, tumor-associated macrophages resemble M2-like macrophages, upregulating CD206 and acquiring a range of effector functions that enable the promotion of metastasis, angiogenesis, immune suppression, and tumor escape from therapy.

Aside from the surface expression of CD206, tumor-associated macrophages are functionally diverse and heterogenous in nature. Multiple signaling pathways have been identified that control macrophage polarization within the tumor microenvironment. One major mechanism involved in the polarization of macrophages is tumor hypoxia. Tumor hypoxia occurs because of aberrant growth of tumor cells and abnormal tumor vasculature, outpacing the limited oxygen and nutrient supply. Hypoxia forces tumors to adapt to new metabolic demands, initiating prosurvival, invasion, and inflammatory programs via upregulation of phosphoinositide 3-kinase (PI3K)/protein kinase b (Akt)/the mamalian target of rapamycin (mTOR), mitogen activated protein kinase (MAPK), and NF-κB signaling.[155] Heterogeneity of monocyte-derived macrophages has been demonstrated using murine models and single-cell phenotypic analysis. For example, in a murine model of breast cancer, seven functionally and molecularly distinct macrophage subsets were identified based upon Ly6C and MHC II expression levels.[156] The most suppressive macrophage populations resided adjacent to hypoxic tumor areas and had increased angiogenic and suppressive activities.[156] Tumor-derived lactic acid was also demonstrated to have similar effects on the polarization of macrophages.[157] Another contributor to macrophage heterogeneity is the nature of myeloid precursors that macrophages arise from. Macrophages that differentiate from M-MDSC are transcriptionally distinct and more immune suppressive compared with monocyte-derived tumor macrophages.[158] M-MDSC-derived tumor macrophages are dependent on S100A9 activity within the tumor microenvironment, a signaling pathway that induces C/EBPβ, a transcription factor associated with potent immune suppressive activity of M-MDSCs.[159] On the other hand, prostaglandin E2 (PGE2), a product of COX-1 or 2 activity, enhances the suppressive function of committed

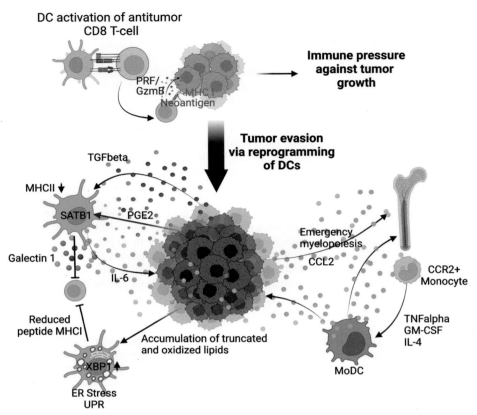

Fig. 4.4 Dendritic cell polarization in the tumor microenvironment. During early tumor progression, dendritic cells exert pressure against growing tumors through activation of cytotoxic CD8 T cells. As tumors progress, tumor-induced cytokines such as PGE2 and TGF-β upregulate the master regulator SATB1, downregulating MHC II and enhancing galectin 1 and IL-6 production from transformed dendritic cells. Dendritic cells undergo ER stress in response to accumulation of truncated oxidized lipids, diminishing processing and cross-presentation of antigen to CD8 T cells. Tumor-induced emergency myelopoiesis enhances accumulation of monocytes from the bone marrow, where some are differentiated into protumorigenic monocytic dendritic cells (MoDCs). (Source: Figure generated in Biorender.)

M2 macrophages,[160,161] and inhibition of PGE2 using COX-2 inhibitors restores efficacy of PD-L1 blockade in certain tumor models.[162]

Tumor-associated macrophages originating from tissue-resident macrophage pools complicate efforts to target tumor-associated macrophages. Tissue-resident macrophages self-renew locally, in the absence of input from the bone marrow. This establishes a scenario where tissue-resident macrophages can provide early and supportive signals to developing tumors to enhance growth, invasion, and avoidance of immune destruction. In non-small cell lung cancer, tissue-resident macrophages established a niche for developing tumors, facilitating epithelial to mesenchymal transition while also shielding developing tumors from adaptive immune pressure.[163] For pancreatic cancer, CSF1-polarized monocyte-derived macrophages[164] are more immune suppressive, and polarized tissue-resident macrophages have a profibrogenic phenotype.[165]

Depending on the signals present within the tumor microenvironment, a multitude of additional transcriptional and regulatory pathways influence the polarization of tumor-associated macrophages. Signaling through the aryl hydrocarbon receptor (AhR) can polarize multiple immune cell subsets in the tumor microenvironment, including dendritic cells and macrophages. AhR resides in the cytoplasm, and when AhR ligands enter the cytoplasm via passive diffusion, the AhR receptor complex translocates into the nucleus, binding target DNA sequences located in the promoter regions of multiple genes relevant to inflammation and procancer activities. AhR ligands include kynurenine pathway metabolites and arachidonic acid metabolites, both of which have tolerogenic effects on immune cells within the tumor microenvironment. AhR signaling in macrophages and dendritic cells within the tumor microenvironment increases expression of IL-1β, IL-6, TNF-α, IL-10, and NF-κB.[166] Hezaveh et al. added to this body of literature by demonstrating that indoles produced by certain *Lactobacilli* species from diet-derived tryptophan polarized tumor-associated macrophages overexpressing the AhR ligand in pancreatic cancer.[167] The effects of the gut microbiome on cancer progression and therapy response are covered in Chapter 11. These studies highlight the systemic effect of cancer and a cancer-affected gut microbiome on innate immune cells. Thus, potential therapies could involve dietary modifications such as consuming low-tryptophan diets. Indeed, for pancreatic cancer, provision of a diet low in tryptophan reversed macrophage-mediated immune suppression.[167]

Transcription factors associated with macrophage polarization into suppressive proangiogenic phenotypes include, but are not limited to, jumonji domain-containing protein 3 (JMJD3) and IRF4[168,169]; STAT1, 3, and 6 signaling[154]; and C/EBPβ.[159] Due to the underlying phenotypic plasticity of macrophages, protumor transcriptional changes can be triggered in response to multiple inflammatory cytokines and chemokines, PAMPs and DAMPs, metabolic changes, and changes in the vasculature and in the surrounding stroma. Other immune cells present within the tumor microenvironment can also polarize macrophages. For example, B-cell production of IL-10 leads to subsequent activation of TRIF/STAT1 signaling in macrophages, resulting in decreased proinflammatory functions; production of IL-10, IFN-β, CCL2; and upregulation of M2-like markers Ym1 and Fizz1.[170] Other studies have found that autoantibodies polarized macrophages by binding Fc receptors on macrophages.[171] Regulatory T cells and Th2 CD4 T cells are also able to polarize macrophages, through the production of IL-4, IL-13, and IL-10, as detailed in Gabrilovich et al.[154] Several reviews cover signaling pathways associated with macrophage polarization extensively.[154,172-174]

Mast Cells

Mast cells are potent innate immune cells whose role in inflammation extends beyond allergy and hypersensitivity reactions. As described previously, mast cells possess multiple effector functions that enable modulation of the tumor microenvironment. The effect of mast cells on cancer is variable and dependent on the types of cancer. For ovarian cancer[175] and esophageal cancer,[175] mast cells have been shown to be associated with a positive prognosis, whereas for melanoma,[176] breast cancer,[177] lung cancer,[178] and gastric cancer,[179] associations are either mixed or correspond with poor outcomes. Using a humanized model of melanoma, Somasundaram et al. demonstrated that mast cells are associated with immune suppression and failure of PD-1 blockade.[180]

Mast cells are potent immune effectors and are also highly sensitive to microenvironmental cues present in the tissues in which they are residing. As such, mast cells are functionally and phenotypically modulated by tumor-associated signals while having a reciprocal effect upon the inflammatory milieu of the tumor microenvironment. Mast cells can rearrange the tumor environment through release of metalloproteinases, serine proteases, and other factors that enhance angiogenesis and remodeling of the basement membrane. Cytokines such as IL-6, CCL2, and VEGF enhance angiogenesis and recruit cells into the tumor environment, whereas profibrogenic mediators such as PDGF-β activate fibroblasts. Mast cell–produced IL-6 and CCL2 can also enhance cell proliferation and polarization of other myeloid subsets. The chemokine IL-8 (CXCL1, a proposed homologue in mice) and histamine can chemoattract and induce proliferation of tumor cells.[181] Mast cells can also produce IL-13 and IL-4. Typically associated with an allergic response, these two cytokines have been associated with a fibrotic response, immune suppression, and tumor growth.[182] The alarmin IL-33, which is also produced by gastric tumor cells, has been shown to induce IL-13, CSF-2, CCL3 and IL-6 from mast cells.

Mast cells can accumulate in tumors and the tumor microenvironment through multiple chemotactic factors such as SCF, CCL2, VEGF, angiopoietin 1, IL-8, CXCL1, osteopontin, and CXCL10.[183] Activation and degranulation are also affected by signals in the tumor environment. For example, PGE2 produced by macrophages, other myeloid cells, and tumor cells can activate mast cells to degranulate via signaling through the PGE2 receptor EP3.[184,185] On the other hand, stimulation of EP2[184] and EP4[186] by PGE2 reduces activation of mast cells. Mast cells are also activated and phenotypically modulated by recognition of PAMPs and DAMPs. TLR4-mediated recognition of LPS can induce GM-CSF, IL-8, and IL-10 release without degranulation, whereas recognition of peptidoglycan via TLR2 signaling can trigger degranulation.[187]

Neutrophils

Neutrophils are often synonymous with antimicrobial defense; however, their recruitment into sterile tissues suggests that neutrophils also have a role in tissue defense or damage,[188] a process with high relevance to cancer. In patients with cancer, cancer-associated neutrophils sediment in the low-density fraction of blood gradients, along with myeloid-derived suppressor cells,[189] which are described later. Low-density neutrophils are derived from TGF-β signaling and have been shown to be highly immune suppressive, protumorigenic,[190] and prometastatic.[191] GM-CSF is also a potent chemokine produced by tumors that triggers emergency myelopoiesis and pathologic expansion of immature neutrophils from the bone marrow and other extramedullary sites.[192] CXCR1 and CXCR2 signaling on neutrophils, the ligands of which are induced by TGF-β and produced by tumor cells, are also involved in neutrophil exit from the bone marrow and into tumor-affected tissue. The ligands for these two pathways are produced in abundance by transformed cells, initiating the release of neutrophils from the bone marrow and into the tumor microenvironment.

Signaling through CXCR2 can culminate in the release of NETs into the tumor microenvironment.[193] Unlike their host-protective role during infectious disease, NETs in the tumor microenvironment protected tumors from T cell– and NK cell–mediated cytotoxicity.[193] NETs also have tumor metastasis effects, with studies demonstrating that NETs enhance extravasation from the primary tumor site[194,195] and recruit tumors into the premetastatic niche to facilitate metastatic colonization.[196] Thus, inhibitors limiting NET formation or neutrophil egress from the bone marrow have the potential to improve adaptive immune responses and reduce tumor growth and invasion. Several studies have identified multiple heterogenous neutrophil populations in cancer-bearing individuals, suggesting that host-intrinsic factors also affect neutrophil phenotype and abundance. Indeed, in a comprehensive outlook of neutrophils in cancer biology, Quail et al. outlined multiple factors, including but not limited to age, sex, circadian clocks, obesity, the microbiome, and smoking.[92]

INFLAMMATION AND TUMOR VASCULATURE

To sustain rapid growth and increased metabolic demand, tumors need to establish a blood supply. Cancer cells can initiate formation of tumor-supportive blood vessels from existing vessels, which is termed *sprouting angiogenesis*. Angiogenesis is facilitated via the coordination of multiple proangiogenic factors. Although the innate immune system is integral to this process, a consequence of angiogenesis is subsequently increased inflammation,[197] highlighting the reciprocal relationship between angiogenesis and a developing tumor.

Proinflammatory cytokines such as IL-1 family cytokines, IL-6, IL-17, TGF-β, TNF-α, and VEGF are upregulated in the evolving tumor microenvironment, leading to activation of NF-κB and STAT3 signaling in endothelial cells and pericytes. STAT3 upregulation in endothelial cells upregulates expression of adhesion molecules on endothelial cells, such as ICAM-1 and VCAM-1, to facilitate accumulation of immune cells into the tumor microenvironment. STAT3 acts upstream of HIF1 and VEGF, two potent angiogenic factors, while also increasing the expression of additional angiogenic factors such as FGF and Ang-2. STAT3 signaling also enhances synthesis of matrix metalloproteinases, which remodel the basement membrane and extracellular matrix, all part of the angiogenic pathway to support exponential tumor growth.[198] NF-κB activation also contributes to angiogenesis of multiple tumor types through upregulation of VEGF, enhancing expression of vascular adhesion molecules, subsequently amplifying the expression of multiple proangiogenic and inflammatory cytokines and chemokines.[198] Despite the known dependence of tumors on angiogenic signaling pathways, antiangiogenic agents have not yielded significant improvements in progression-free survival and overall survival for pancreatic adenocarcinoma, prostate cancer, breast cancer, or melanoma, with more mixed results for non-small cell lung cancer and glioblastoma.[199] Reasons for failures of antiangiogenic therapies are varied but could arise from tumors using non-angiogenic mechanisms to acquire vasculature, or vessel cooption. Vessel co-option is a process whereby tumor cells use existing tissue vasculature to meet their metabolic and growth needs.

The mechanisms of vessel cooption are not as well understood as angiogenesis. However, evidence has emerged to suggest that VEGF receptor blockade can initiate vessel cooption as a mechanism of tumor escape from antiangiogenic therapies.[199,200] Using a model of VEGF blockade–induced vessel cooption, single-cell RNA sequencing identified that coopted vessels were enriched in a population of macrophages with inflammatory potential—having an inflammatory M1-like phenotype, characterized by having high expression levels of IL-1β and IL-6, TNF-α, and IFN-γ[201]—all of which are capable of normalizing the abnormal tumor vasculature that arises during angiogenesis.[202] The question arises as to whether vessel cooption is an attempt to normalize the vasculature, once tumor cells co-opt it, or whether inflammatory macrophages are sufficient to drive the process. Several questions remain and more work is needed to develop models of tumor vessel cooption that would enable mechanistic understanding of the underlying process of vessel cooption and what role, if any, inflammation has during this process.

INFLAMMATION-MEDIATED EMERGENCY MYELOPOIESIS: MYELOID-DERIVED SUPPRESSOR CELLS

The hematopoietic system is capable of rapidly deploying immune cells from the bone marrow in response to systemic inflammation, referred to as *demand-adapted hematopoiesis*.[203] This can occur locally, in response to tissue-restricted infections or in response to systemic inflammatory signals. Emergency myelopoiesis is a state of pathologic immune activation, characterized by prolonged stimulation through release of cytokines, growth factors, and other tumor-associated mechanisms associated with chronic inflammation. Emergency myelopoiesis results in the systemic emergence of immature neutrophils and myelomonocytic cells from the bone marrow, where they become pathologically activated to become myeloid-derived suppressor cells (MDSCs, covered in the latter half of this chapter). MDSCs accumulate in distal sites of tumor spread and are programmed into suppressive cells in the presence of tumor-associated inflammatory factors.[204] Myeloid cells entering the tumor microenvironment are conditioned by the tumor to facilitate angiogenesis, promote metastasis, and aide tumor evasion from the immune system, all of which are hallmarks of cancer.[97,98] Thus, coordination between tumors and the hematopoietic compartment underlies a critical process of cancer-mediated cooption of host innate immune cells to support growth and invasion. Emergency myelopoiesis is a major node of this process, culminating in extensive efforts to define relevant pathways involved in tumor-associated myelopoiesis.

It is now well established that MDSCs become pathologically activated in two phases (Fig. 4.5) (for in-depth review, see Condamine et al.[205]). During phase 1, the bone marrow and

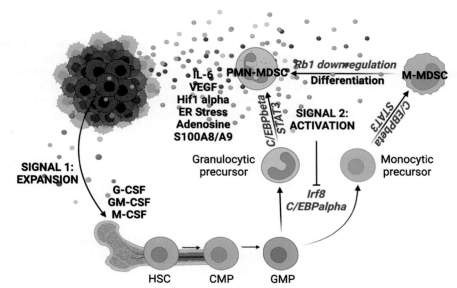

Fig. 4.5 Two step model for the generation of MDSCs. MDSCs are generated in two phases. The first phase occurs in response to chronic and systemic exposure to growth factors such as G-CSF, GM-CSF, and M-CSF. These growth factors lead to the expansion of granulocytic and monocytic precursors from the bone marrow. Once immature precursors are recruited into the tumor microenvironment, a variety of factors including IL-6, VEGFα, hypoxia and HIF1α, ER stress, adenosine signaling, and S100A8/A9 production inhibit the transcription factors IRF8 and C/EBPα, both of which are involved in the normal differentiation of myeloid precursors into dendritic cells and macrophages. Instead, C/EBPβ and STAT3, among other pathways, are induced in the precursors, retaining them in an immature and immune-suppressive state. M-MDSCs can also contribute to the pool of PMN-MDSCs through downregulation of Rb1. (Source: Figure generated in Biorender.)

spleen are conditioned by chronic low-level stimulation by cytokines and growth factors such GM-CSF, G-CSF, and M-CSF, resulting in expansion of granulocytic and monocytic precursor cells. During phase 2, pathologically expanded myeloid progenitors are exposed to inflammatory signals in the periphery, such as IL-6, IL-1β, VEGF, ER stress, adenosine signaling, and HIF1α. Myeloid cells derived in these conditions become unable to differentiate, have reduced phagocytic activity, produce antiinflammatory cytokines and signaling molecules, and produce ROS, NOS, MPO, and other suppressive factors, culminating in a significant inhibition of CD4 and CD8 T-cell effector activity in the tumor microenvironment.

MDSCs consist of two major populations in both humans and mice. One population consists of granulocytic/polymorphonuclear MDSCs (PMN-MDSCs) and the second population consists of mononuclear MDSCs (mMDSCs). Phenotypically, in mice, PMN-MDSCs and mMDSCs resemble neutrophils and monocytes, respectively, because there are no markers that distinguish between these subsets. In humans, although there is overlap in the markers used to identify these subsets from peripheral tissues, PMN-MDSCs in the blood are purified in the lower density gradient (1.077 g/mL) than neutrophils (1.1–1.2 g/mL).[206,207] Lectin-type oxidized LDL receptor 1 (LOX1) is an additional specific marker for PMN-MDSCs.[208] Although not an exclusive marker, mMDSCs are often distinguished from monocytes by expression of MHC II[207] or using a combination of CD14, CD66b, and either CXCR1 or CD84 wherein mMDSCs are CD14+ CD66b− and CXCR1+ (reviewed in Veglia et al.[207] and Bronte et al.[209]). Functionally, MDSCs are also distinct from neutrophils and monocytes. Neutrophil antimicrobial activity is dependent on degranulation and an intense respiratory burst. These functions are lost in PMN-MDSCs and tumor-associated neutrophils. On the other hand, genes associated with antigen presentation and inflammatory cytokine production can be upregulated in PMN-MDSCs.[210] RNA sequencing of PMN-MDSCs and neutrophils from patients with head and neck cancer or non-small cell lung cancer identified additional functional differences, including upregulation of genes associated with ER stress and the unfolded protein response, MAPK signaling, and a concurrent upregulation of M-CSF, IL-6, NF-κB, OLR1, and TGF-β in PMN-MDSC.[208] A similar approach was used to compare monocytes from mMDSC in patients with cancer, identifying that STAT3 signaling is involved in the reprogramming of monocytes into mMDSCs,[211] supporting in vitro studies using tumor-conditioned media.[124] Other notable differences between mMDSCs and monocytes included the expression of CXCR1, IL-10, CD14, and VEGFA. PMN-MDSC-specific immune suppressive mechanisms primarily involve the use of ROS, peroxynitrite, arginase 1, and PGE2. Immune suppression driven by mMDSC involves nitric oxide and immune-suppressive cytokines such as IL-10 and TGF-β and increased PD-L1 expression.

Deconvoluting the signaling cascades driving emergency myelopoiesis and emergence of MDSC into the tumor environment is a major focus in the field, complicated because of the lack of reliable MDSC markers. Cytokines and growth factors such as GM-CSF, G-CSF, IL-6, IL-1β, PGE2, TNF-α, VEGF, and S100A8/9 have been shown to enhance MDSC accumulation and differentiation. Seminal studies identified that GM-CSF + IL-6 polarize bone marrow–derived cultures into MDSCs because of the induction of STAT3 signaling.[124,212] Changes in metabolism also enhance MDSC suppressive function. Tumor-infiltrating MDSCs increase fatty acid uptake via upregulation of the scavenger receptor CD36, activating fatty acid oxidation and increasing mitochondrial mass, oxygen consumption, and immune inhibitory activity.[213] Uptake of fatty acids is mediated by the scavenger receptor CD36. Mohamed et al. identified that PKR-like endoplasmic reticulum (ER) kinase (PERK) signaling endows MDSCs with immune suppressive function. Inhibition of PERK in tumor MDSCs transformed MDSCs into myeloid cells capable of activating antitumor CD8 T-cell immunity.[214] Mechanistically, PERK activation led to phosphorylation of NRF2 and impaired mitochondrial capacity, resulting in immune suppressive functions of MDSCs.[214] Inhibition of PERK, on the other hand, enhanced accumulation of cytosolic mitochondrial DNA, triggering the stimulator of interferon genes (STING) and type I IFN signaling,[214] a major innate immune sensing pathway for the detection of tumor cells.[215] Fatty acid oxidation by PMN-MDSCs also results in indirect mechanisms of immune suppression. For example, PMN-MDSCs transfer oxidized lipids to dendritic cells, reducing the ability of dendritic cells to prime T cells or recall antigen.[216] The fatty acid transport protein 2 (FATP2) was an additional mechanism that has been identified to control PMN-MDSC suppressive function, whose expression enhances uptake of arachidonic acid, leading to increased synthesis of PGE2.[217] AMPKα1 was also demonstrated to control the suppressive activity of mMDSCs, whereas conditional deletion of the AMPKα1-coding gene Prkaa1 in myeloid cells reduced suppressive activity of mMDSCs and blunted mMDSCs to macrophage differentiation.[218]

Estrogen signaling, which has an important role in tumor progression, was demonstrated to enhance emergency myelopoiesis, accumulation of MDSCs into the TME, and their suppressive phenotype. Although many myeloid cell subsets present in the tumor microenvironment express the estrogen receptor ERα, and can thus be influenced by estrogen signaling, Svoronos et al. demonstrated that estrogen signaling was an underlying mechanism of pathologic myelopoiesis during ovarian cancer.[212] Estrogen signaling not only promoted the mobilization of MDSC accumulation in the tumor environment but estrogens also enhanced the immunosuppressive activity of myeloid cells in the tumor microenvironment.[212]

Innate Immune Sensing During Cancer Progression

Innate immune sensing pathways such as Toll-like receptors (TLRs), NOD-like receptors, AIM2-like receptors, and RIG-I-like receptors typically function to sense pathogens in addition to damaged or dying cells. In the context of cancer, these signaling pathways have critical roles in orchestrating innate immune defense against tumors. However, when innate immune sensing is chronic, this can lead to chronic inflammation which contributes to cellular transformation, tumor-promoting inflammation, and recruitment and polarization of suppressive myeloid cells in the tumor microenvironment. There are a significant number of studies summarizing the positive and negative attributes of innate immune signaling in the context of cancer progression. Here, we will summarize major findings within the field.

TLR signaling in myeloid cells is canonically associated with the induction of adaptive immunity.[219] The fact that TLR stimulation could have therapeutic benefits was established by the pioneering work of Coley in the early 1900s with his use of bacterial toxins as cancer therapeutics.[220] This has resulted in significant efforts to define combinations of TLR agonists and other immune adjuvants for use in anticancer vaccines[221] and anticancer therapies.[120,222] For example, DNA/RNA sensors such as RIG-1, TLR3, TLR4/TRAF endosomal signaling, TLR7, TLR8, and TLR9 in addition to STING signaling activate type I IFN signaling. Type I IFN signaling potently activates dendritic cells, upregulating costimulatory molecules such as CD40, CD80, CD86, and MHC class II complex, leading to an enhanced cross-presentation to CD8 T cells (reviewed in Fuertes et al.[223]). Other strategies to enhance antitumor immunity have involved the use of combinatorial therapies as vaccine adjuvants or anticancer therapies. Ahonen et al. demonstrated that using CD40 and TLR agonists as a vaccine platform resulted in substantial CD8 T-cell activation with corresponding tumor shrinkage, providing rationale for the use of adjuvants that trigger combined innate sensing pathways for cancer therapies and vaccines.[221] Other studies evaluating the use of the TLR3 agonist polyI:C have shown promising efficacy in activating dendritic cells and enhancing proinflammatory TH1-type cytokines, NK-cell activation, and dendritic cell cross-presentation to CD8 T cells.[224] Targeting TLR7/8 signaling using imiquimod has been approved for treatment of nonmelanoma skin cancers, with numerous other clinical trials ongoing to evaluate this therapeutic combination across a broad range of cancers.[225]

There is a growing body of evidence that chronic TLR engagement can tip the balance toward an environment favoring tumor progression via excessive inflammation.[226,227] For both ovarian cancer and soft tissue sarcoma, TLR5 recognition of host commensals was found to enhance immune dysfunction and tumor growth through amplification of the cytokine IL-6.[228] Mechanistically, TLR5 enhanced accumulation of suppressive myeloid cells into the TME by enhancing systemic IL-6 cytokine levels, resulting in sustained T-cell dysfunction. TLR5 signaling has been shown to synergize with TLR4 signaling[229,230] and the p53 signaling pathway,[231,232] both of which result in amplified production of the tumor-promoting cytokine IL-6. Whether the negative effects of TLR signaling on antitumor immune function are restricted solely to TLR5 or a general cell- and context-specific process, other studies have identified similar negative associations with TLR5 signaling and tumor growth and immune suppression. Studies in skin and pancreatic cancers support a role for TLR5 signaling in the induction of immune suppression and malignant growth.[233,234] Adding to the clinical relevance for TLR5 signaling is that approximately 7.5% of the general population contains a single nucleotide polymorphism (1174 C>T amino acid substitution) encoding a transcriptional termination site in place of arginine at codon 392 (referred to as *TLR5R392X*) within the flagellin binding domain of TLR5. This polymorphism acts in a dominant-negative fashion, reducing TLR5 signaling by 50% to 80%.[235] Heterozygous carriers are considered functionally deficient in TLR5 signaling. For ovarian cancer, patients who were identified to harbor this loss of function polymorphism experienced significantly increased long-term (> 6 years) survival and had reduced levels of IL-6 and immune suppression within tumors.[228] Similar outcomes have been identified for patients with polymorphisms in TLR5 for colorectal cancer.[236] On the other hand, having the polymorphism for breast cancer was associated with reduced survival[228] and increased susceptibility to developing breast cancer.[237]

High-mobility group box protein-1 (HMGB1), a damage-associated molecular pattern molecule that is associated with autophagy and prevention of apoptosis, enhances accumulation and survival of MDSCs in the tumor environment.[238] HMGB1 signaling activates inflammatory pathways such as NF-κB and PI3K signaling, resulting in increased inflammation within the tumor microenvironment. Other studies have demonstrated a link between HMGB1 signaling and cancer-associated metabolic changes. Exogenous or endogenous HMGB1 expression in necrotic cells increased production of adenosine triphosphate (ATP) to subsequently be used for energy in rapidly dividing tumor cell lines in vitro and in vivo.[239] Similar to TLR5 signaling, the effects of HMGB1 signaling are contextual and can also be associated with maturation of dendritic cells, increased antitumor immunity, and increased efficacy of chemotherapy (see review by Kang et al.[240]).

Cancer Therapies Targeting Innate Immunity

Research over the past several decades has indicated the outsized role that myeloid cells have on cancer progression, immune suppression, and metastasis. Paradoxically, myeloid cells are essential for the initiation of adaptive immune function, as described in **The cellular components of the innate immune response**. Given the divergent roles of myeloid cells on antitumor immunity and cancer progression, there has been significant effort to modulate the tumor immune environment through targeting and reprogramming myeloid cells. Although the therapies covered here are by no means comprehensive, we focus on pathways that are central to myeloid function and activities in the tumor environment, highlighting strategies to reprogram suppressive cells to promote antitumor immunity or to deplete suppressive cell subsets to alleviate immune suppression in tumor beds. The overarching goal is to enhance antitumor immune function and subsequent tumor clearance.

REPROGRAMMING MYELOID CELLS

Focused ultrasound has shown promise as a targeted modality for reprogramming the tumor microenvironment from one that is immune suppressed to one that favors the establishment of antitumor immunity. Focused ultrasound is a noninvasive means of delivering focused high-energy acoustic waves into targeted tumor regions. This nonionizing technique results in thermal ablation of the tumor. Multiple studies have indicated that this methodology reprograms the tumor microenvironment through the induction of thermal stress, mechanical perturbation, the release of antigen and damage-associated molecular patterns, breakdown of the tumor matrix, and modification of the tumor vasculature.[241] However, similar to radiation, the efficacy of focused ultrasound may be context dependent because of a multitude of factors, including the abundance of MDSCs infiltrating into the tumor microenvironment. In a preclinical model of triple-negative breast cancer (TNBC), high numbers of myeloid infiltrates prevented the efficacy of focused ultrasound therapy. To overcome this, MDSCs were depleted using the chemotherapy agent gemcitabine. Both gemcitabine alone or layered with PD-1 blockade enhanced efficacy of focused ultrasound to shrink established tumors.[242]

Targeted inhibitors modulating critical signaling pathways associated with inflammation, myelopoiesis, or regulation of suppressive function in myeloid cells have shown great promise in preclinical and clinical settings, the outcome of which is to boost antitumor immune function and reduce tumor growth and metastasis. The transcription factor CCAAT/enhancer-binding protein alpha (C/EBPα) regulates myelopoiesis, metabolism, proliferation, and the ability of myeloid cells to initiate adaptive immune responses.[243] It was found that MDSC in tumors and exposed to tumor-conditioned media significantly downregulated C/EBPα,[244] suggesting that the loss of this transcriptional regulator coincided with the acquisition of suppressive function. To target this pathway, Voutila et al. designed a small activating RNA that selectively increased transcription of C/EBPα packaged into liposomal nanoparticles,[245] a new therapeutic modality with high efficacy and safety in preclinical murine models and in a phase I trial for patients with hepatocellular carcinoma (HCC). When the C/EBPα nanoparticle mixture MTL-CEBPA was delivered in combination with sorafenib, the suppressive activity of M-MDSCs and tumor-associated macrophages, but not PMN-MDSCs, was prohibited.[246] When combined with lipofermata, an inhibitor of FATP2 to target PMN-MDSCs, or celecoxib, an inhibitor of PGE2 synthesis, and immune checkpoint blockade MTL-CEBPA had significant efficacy in a preclinical model of lung cancer.[246] CD40 activation can also reverse the suppressive potential of myeloid cells, restoring antitumor T-cell responses. Using an agonistic antibody against CD40 in combination with gemcitabine in patients with incurable pancreatic ductal adenocarcinoma led to tumor regression in some patients.[247] Interestingly, the beneficial effect of agonistic CD40 depended on macrophages.[247] Whether the immune benefit of CD40 agonism requires macrophages across multiple tumor types or is an effect of combining CD40 agonists with chemotherapy requires further study.

Epigenetically reprogramming myeloid cells is an additional strategy in the development of anticancer therapeutics. The chromatin organizer special AT-rich sequence binding protein 1 (Satb1) is a master regulator of suppressive tumor-associated dendritic cells.[122] Delivery of nanoparticles encapsulating siRNA against Satb1 restored antitumor immune function, effectively reducing tumor-associated dendritic cell secretion of immune suppressive IL-6 and galectin-1 in an aggressive orthotopic model of ovarian cancer.[122] Pharmacologic targeting of PI3Kγ, another master regulator that is highly expressed in myeloid cells from multiple tumor types, also synergizes with immune checkpoint blockade, a therapeutic strategy that is currently being tested in a phase I clinical trial.[248]

Histone deacetylase (HDAC) inhibitors have also shown promise clinically and in preclinical models because of their ability to prevent epigenetic changes associated with tumor immune evasion and immune suppression. In vitro, using HDAC inhibitors ITF-2357, MGCD-0103, and MS-275 increased tumor expression of the T-cell chemoattractant CCL5 in non-small cell lung cancer (NSCLC). In vivo, the use of these inhibitors reduced T-cell exhaustion and enhanced effective antitumor T-cell responses against tumor cells.[249] In a phase 2 expansion cohort of patients with NSCLC who have developed resistance to or are refractory to PD-1 blockade, the HDAC inhibitor entinostat was combined with anti-PD-L1 therapy, resulting in a slight but enhanced clinical benefit for patients with high levels of circulating monocytes.[250] The results from this clinical study indicate that broad clinical efficacy of specific HDAC inhibitors is dependent on multiple immunologic contexts, underscoring the need to further investigate mechanisms associated with positive and negative response while also working to identify combinations associated with broad clinical efficacy.

Mechanistic studies have provided more context to the efficacy of entinostat. Specifically, entinostat only reduced the immune suppressive activity of PMN-MDSCs, whereas no effect was observed on M-MDSCs or macrophage function. One possible reason why HDAC inhibitors were not effective in M-MDSCs is their high expression of HDAC6, which was amplified after treatment with entinostat. The team went on to demonstrate that targeting all MDSCs with entinostat and ricolinostat, a class IIb inhibitor against HDAC6, significantly delayed tumor growth through inhibition of both populations of MDSCs.[251] Treatment of breast tumors with class IIa inhibitor TMP195 against HDAC7 reprogrammed tumor-associated macrophages, reducing metastasis and enhancing antitumor T-cell function.[251] These studies highlight the distinct pathways involved in myeloid polarization and suppressive function in the tumor microenvironment. Whether these pathways are shared among the same cells and across multiple tumor types is an area of further investigation.

TARGETING TUMOR-MEDIATED CHANGES IN CELLULAR METABOLISM AND HYPOXIA

It is well known that the tumor microenvironment is a metabolically challenging environment. Alterations in tumor metabolism occur in response to oncogenic transformation, enabling tumor cells to quickly adapt to limited nutrient supply and increased bioenergetic demands. Metabolic constraints in the tumor microenvironment have tolerizing effects on infiltrating immune cells. These metabolic adaptations in infiltrating immune cells present challenges therapeutically, often undermining efficacy of chemotherapy, immunotherapy, and other targeted therapies. For these reasons, there has been an intense interest in understanding how changes in leukocyte metabolism affect cellular function and tumor control, with the goal of identifying therapeutics that reverse tolerogenic metabolic pathways.

Metabolic changes such as tumor hypoxia, nutrient starvation, increased levels of free radicals, and low pH can induce endoplasmic reticulum (ER) stress in infiltrating myeloid cells. In response to ER stress, unfolded proteins accumulate in myeloid cells, activating the unfolded protein response (UPR). This enables adaptation and survival of myeloid cells within the metabolically hostile tumor microenvironment. However, ER stress can enhance the expression of suppressive factors in myeloid cells, such as arginase I, PGE2, and protumor cytokines such as IL-6, IL-8, and TNF-α.[252] ER stress through the IRE1α-XBP1 pathway has been shown to impair the ability of dendritic cells to activate CD8 T cells, convert neutrophils into suppressive PMN-MDSCs, and polarize macrophages to promote invasion and metastasis.[253] Targeting of dendritic cell XBP1 in vivo using nanoparticles encapsulating siRNA against XBP1 effectively restored antitumor immunity and enhanced survival of mice bearing aggressive ovarian tumors.[254] CEB/P homologous protein (CHOP), downstream of the UPR, and PERK, also downstream of the UPR, have both been implicated in regulating MDSC suppressive function.[214,255] These studies support a rationale for reversing or inhibiting ER stress in myeloid cells as a novel immune therapeutic treatment strategy.

Additional metabolic adaptations in myeloid cells have been identified once they enter into the tumor microenvironment. Dendritic cells use glycolysis, which is controlled by HIF1α, whereas suppressive tumor-associated macrophages use the tricarboxylic acid (TCA) cycle and fatty acid oxidation and M1-like macrophages use glycolysis and amino acid metabolism.[256] This divergence in myeloid cell function reflects the heterogeneity within the myeloid compartment and suggests that tailored metabolic therapies can be designed to target specific myeloid cells or functional attributes. Targeting lactate has emerged as an additional strategy to modify immune cell phenotype within the tumor microenvironment. Enhanced glycolytic activity of cancer cells in hypoxic conditions increased the buildup of lactate. Lactate impairs dendritic cell differentiation[257] while promoting the polarization of tumor-associated macrophages.[157]

CELL-BASED THERAPIES

NK Cells

Imai et al. initiated a prospective study with an 11-year follow-up of individuals in Japan. The goal was to ask whether the abundance of naturally cytotoxic peripheral blood mononuclear cells affected cancer risk. In the follow-up phase of the study, the team identified that individuals with higher "natural" cytotoxicity in blood leukocytes also had reduced cancer risk.[258] Conversely, individuals with reduced NK cells peripherally had increased incidence of relapse and reduced survival.[258] Follow-up studies in mice[259] and humans[260] verified that in the absence of NK cells or in mice that that lacked the receptor NKG2D,[261] a stimulatory receptor expressed by NK cells, susceptibility to spontaneous formation of tumors increased. These were some of the earliest studies demonstrating that NK cells provided robust and spontaneous immune defense against tumor progression or metastasis.[262]

Given the potency and nonspecificity of NK-cell cytotoxicity against tumors, much work has gone toward developing NK-cell–based therapeutics for the treatment of cancer. Early phase I trials have demonstrated that unlike chimeric antigen receptor (CAR) T cells, NK-cell infusions are well tolerated and safe and achieve good engraftment in cancer-bearing adults[263,264] and children,[265] even if received in an allogenic setting.[266] Miller et al. established that preconditioning with cyclophosphamide to establish a lymphodepleted environment enabled more robust engraftment of NK cells, whereas subcutaneous administration of IL-2 enhanced expansion of engrafted NK cells.[264] There are other groups evaluating alternate methodologies to generate and expand NK cells ex vivo to enhance overall efficacy of NK-cell–based therapies. For example, expanding NK cells with combinations of IL-2 or IL-15 or the IL-15/IL-15Ra fusion complex ALT-803 enhanced NK functions in vitro and in vivo.[264,267] Others have found that preactivation of NK cells with a cocktail consisting of IL-12/IL-15/IL-18 enhanced antitumor effector activity and persistence in irradiated tumors after infusion.[268]

Engineering of NK cells is also being developed clinically, having numerous advantages over CAR T cells such as (1) an unlimited allogenic NK source without concern of graft versus host disease; (2) engineered NK cells or induced pluripotent stem cell (iPSC)-NK are more well tolerated, with cytokine release syndrome a rare occurrence (one case was reported[269]); (3) short production time and potential for "off-the-shelf" cell therapy NK or iPSC products; (4) recognition of tumors occurs via NK receptors, not antigens, enhancing potential tumor killing and minimizing tumor escape from T cells directed against dominant antigens, as has been documented for CAR T cells.[270] For an excellent review on NK cell–based therapies, see Liu et al.[271]

Dendritic Cells

Dendritic cells are professional antigen-presenting cells, potent inducers of robust T-cell responses against tumors. Given the potential of dendritic cells to induce therapeutic responses in patients with cancer through the stimulation of cytotoxic T-cell responses, there is intense interest in developing cell-based dendritic cell therapies. Approximately 41 phase I to III clinical trials based around dendritic cell–based vaccines are ongoing and recruiting until February 2022.[272] The only U.S. Food and Drug Administration (FDA)-approved dendritic cell vaccine is sipuleucel-T, or Provenge, for the treatment of castration-resistant prostate cancer. Dendritic cell vaccines are generated by isolating or using in vitro amplification of autologous dendritic cells, manipulating ex vivo (pulsing with tumor antigen or an antigen fused with GM-CSF), followed by reinfusion into patients. However, there are multiple factors that can attenuate the therapeutic effect of dendritic cell–based vaccines. For example, the type of dendritic cell isolated or expanded can have varying potency depending on whether it is differentiated in vitro or purified from patients,[273] lack of functionality of dendritic cells from the tumor microenvironment, and low frequency in the blood for cDC1.[138] To overcome these challenges, there are efforts to devise strategies that combine adjuvants (such as engineered viruses) with tumor antigens to reinvigorate isolated dendritic cells in addition to combining with approaches that expand dendritic cells ex vivo or in situ. Other strategies that are being proposed are to combine dendritic cell vaccines with immune checkpoint blockade.[272]

Activation and mobilization of endogenous dendritic cells is one strategy to enhance or restore function of dendritic cells using off-the-shelf therapeutics. One such strategy includes enhancing systemic or tumor-intrinsic GM-CSF levels, which stimulate dendritic differentiation, activation, and migration into the tumor microenvironment. Delivery of GM-CSF into the tumor microenvironment is being pursued using a few approaches. Talimogene laherparepvec (Imlygic, T-VEC), an attenuated oncolytic strain of herpes simplex virus that expresses human GM-CSF, has been approved for use in patients with advanced melanoma.[274] Other approaches include administration of irradiated syngeneic or autologous tumor cells overexpressing GM-CSF (GVAX vaccines), where clinical trials (including a phase III in prostate cancer) are ongoing to assess efficacy of GVAX as a cancer therapeutic.[275]

Key References

21. Wynn TA, Chawla A, Pollard JW. Macrophage biology in development, homeostasis and disease. *Nature*. 2013;496(7446):445-455.
34. Gordon S. Phagocytosis: the legacy of Metchnikoff. *Cell*. 2016;166(5):1065-1068.
46. Xue J, Schmidt SV, Sander J, et al. Transcriptome-based network analysis reveals a spectrum model of human macrophage activation. *Immunity*. 2014;40(2):274-288.
52. Chen B, Zhu L, Yang S, et al. Unraveling the heterogeneity and ontogeny of dendritic cells using Single-Cell RNA sequencing. *Front Immunol*. 2021;12:711329.
64. Yokoyama WM, Plougastel BF. Immune functions encoded by the natural killer gene complex. *Nat Rev Immunol*. 2003;3(4):304-316.
92. Quail DF, Amulic B, Aziz M, et al. Neutrophil phenotypes and functions in cancer: a consensus statement. *J Exp Med*. 2022;219(6):e20220011.
127. Olingy CE, Dinh HQ, Hedrick CC. Monocyte heterogeneity and functions in cancer. *J Leukoc Biol*. 2019;106(2):309-322.
137. Veglia F, Gabrilovich DI. Dendritic cells in cancer: the role revisited. *Curr Opin Immunol*. 2017;45:43-51.
138. Wculek SK, Cueto FJ, Mujal AM, et al. Dendritic cells in cancer immunology and immunotherapy. *Nat Rev Immunol*. 2020;20(1):7-24.
139. Conejo-Garcia JR, Rutkowski MR, Cubillos-Ruiz JR. State-of-the-art of regulatory dendritic cells in cancer. *Pharmacol Ther*. 2016;164:97-104.
154. Gabrilovich DI, Ostrand-Rosenberg S, Bronte V. Coordinated regulation of myeloid cells by tumours. *Nat Rev Immunol*. 2012;12(4):253-268.
172. Larionova I, Kazakova E, Patysheva M, et al. Transcriptional, epigenetic and metabolic programming of tumor-associated macrophages. *Cancers (Basel)*. 2020;12(6):1411.
173. Niu Y, Chen J, Qiao Y. Epigenetic modifications in tumor-associated macrophages: a new perspective for an old foe. *Front Immunol*. 2022;13:836223.
174. Noy R, Pollard JW. Tumor-associated macrophages: from mechanisms to therapy. *Immunity*. 2014;41(1):49-61.
205. Condamine T, Mastio J, Gabrilovich DI. Transcriptional regulation of myeloid-derived suppressor cells. *J Leukoc Biol*. 2015;98(6):913-922.
206. Bronte V, Brandau S, Chen SH, et al. Recommendations for myeloid-derived suppressor cell nomenclature and characterization standards. *Nat Commun*. 2016;7:12150.
207. Veglia F, Sanseviero E, Gabrilovich DI. Myeloid-derived suppressor cells in the era of increasing myeloid cell diversity. *Nat Rev Immunol*. 2021;21(8):485-498.
209. Bronte V, Brandau S, Chen SH, et al. Recommendations for myeloid-derived suppressor cell nomenclature and characterization standards. *Nat Commun*. 2016;7:12150.
240. Kang R, Zhang Q, Zeh HJ III, et al. HMGB1 in cancer: good, bad, or both? *Clin Cancer Res*. 2013;19(15):4046-4057.
271. Liu S, Galat V, Galat Y, et al. NK cell-based cancer immunotherapy: from basic biology to clinical development. *J Hematol Oncol*. 2021;14(1):7.

Visit Elsevier eBooks+ (eBooks.Health.Elsevier.com) for complete set of references.

CHAPTER 5

Tumor Antigenicity and Cancer as Non-Self

John E. Niederhuber

SUMMARY OF KEY FACTS

- Professor Paul Ehrlich is credited with introducing the concept of cancers as non-self and proposing the concept of tumor immune surveillance in 1909.
- Evidence for tumor immunity was suggested by early animal tumor transplantation experiments carried out in nonhomogeneous mouse strains.
- The development of congenic inbred murine strains was an essential contribution that enabled the study of human tumor immunogenicity.
- TSTAs (tumor transplantation antigens) was the initial term to define tumor antigens. This term was later refined to be TSAs (tumor-specific antigens).
- Similarly, tumor-associated transplantation antigens (TATAs) are now called TAAs (tumor-associated antigens).
- The human immune system comprises B cells, T cells, and antigen-presenting cells. B cells are the cells responsible for interacting with T cells and antigen-presenting cells to produce highly specific antibodies against antigens.
- T cells have subsets; for example, cytotoxic $CD8^+$ T cells (CTLs) and $CD4^+$ T cells.
- In 1973, Steinman and Cohen identified a class of antigen-presenting cells termed *dendritic cells* that function to present antigen in association with MHC class II molecules to CTLs, other T cells, and B cells.
- Tumor cells are genetically unstable and a source of altered genes and altered proteins that may become recognized by the host's immune system as non-self TSAs.
- Though SNVs are most common variant occurring in tumor cells, they have not proved to be a very good source of neoantigens. Indels (insertions and deletions) are the second most common type of variant occurring in tumor cells.
- Studies indicate that TSAs originating from genomic variants occurring in noncoding regions of the tumor genome (alternative reading frames, antisense coding segments, variants altering splicing in formation of mRNA, 5′ untranslated regions, and long noncoding RNAs) are proving to be a more important source of actionable TSAs.
- TAAs actually represent a form of wt peptide but are found in much greater abundance (overexpression) as a result of epigenetic alterations in tumor cell DNA methylation and/or alterations of chromatin structure resulting in shifts in gene expression. TAAs also include cancer germline antigens.
- The proteasome and its chamber located in the cytosol function as site of proteolysis to generate short antigenic peptides from the altered proteins suitable for restricted MHC class I presentation. The proteasome can ligate distal peptides together (transpeptidation).

Continued on following page

Introduction

One of the great experiences in my career was the time spent at the famous Karolinska Institute, Stockholm, Sweden. I arrived there in 1970 during a break in my surgery training and with very little experience as a student of immunology. One of the special benefits of joining the Möller laboratory on the Karolinska campus was the proximity to the laboratory of the famous immunologist and cancer researcher Professor George Klein, who headed the Karolinska Institute's Department of Tumor Biology. My mentors, Erna and Göran Möller, had both trained under Professor Klein, so there were lots of opportunities for cross-lab interactions. This was the very early days of tumor immunology and just the beginning of the recognition that the immune system involved two major, functionally unique, immune cells, T cells and B cells. Of course, this was long before the identification of T-cell subtypes such as tumor-directed cytotoxic T lymphocytes (CD8[+] CTLs) and the defining of the unique functions of these cells in the adaptive antitumor immune response. The exciting story of immuno-oncology today is very much the history of our evolving understanding of the intricacies of the human immune system and its response to foreign "antigens."

The primacy concept underpinning the development of our newest weapon against cancer—immunotherapy—is the understanding that when normal cells undergo genetic transformation to the cancer phenotype and acquire their unique capacity for uncontrolled division, the invasion of normal tissues, and the spread to distant sites, they have also acquired non-self-antigens. Tumor cells are, by their very nature, quite genetically unstable and have been shown to express between 50 and 1000 missense mutations. Theoretically, this array of genetic alterations should result in numerous antigenic differences from self and be adequate to trigger a reaction within the host's immune system to destroy these abnormal cancer cells in their earliest state of development. A process often referred to as immunosurveillance.

The initial introduction of the hypothesis of immune surveillance is most often credited to the German Professor Paul Ehrlich. As early as 1909, Professor Ehrlich reasoned that without the host's immune system monitoring the development of abnormal cancerous cells, "so konnte man vermuten, dass das Karzinom in einer geradezu ungeheurlichen Frequenz aufteten wurde," which translates as "one could therefore suspect that the carcinoma would occur with an almost unbelievable frequency."[1,2] However, the state of our knowledge at that time regarding the intricacies of the immune system, as well as the limitations of available scientific tools, made it difficult to validate his hypothesis. Thus, over the years the concept of "host immune surveillance" remained controversial and in fact, does so even today. (See also Chapter 6, Tumor Immune Surveillance.)

Early experiments involved the simple grafting of fresh pieces of animal tumor tissue into mice or rats in an effort to immunize the animal to a subsequent tumor challenge. Beginning in the early years of the 20th century, scientists repeatedly observed what appeared to be immuno-logic differences between tumor tissues and normal tissues. Much of this early work involved the use of experimental tumors occurring spontaneously as well as those induced by chemicals such as methylcholanthrene and tumors produced by DNA and RNA oncogenic viruses. Despite somewhat variable findings, there was general recognition that tumor antigens, to be defined as such, needed to be present only in the tumor cells and not present in normal cells. Further, immunity to this tumor antigen brings with it the ability to destroy the tumor cell.

Lumsden is most often given credit for being the first to use an early attempt at developing an inbred mouse strain in his experiments to study the immune response to tumor tissue. He used an "inbred" strain of mice obtained from Lashoploeb's laboratory in Buffalo that were more than 32 generations. For his experiments, Lumsden used a mouse tumor that had developed spontaneously. Unfortunately, of 170 mice tested, only 3 proved resistant to the tumor.[3]

In 1935, Besredka and Gross reported a series of mouse experiments in which a small amount of a tumor cell suspension was injected intradermally. This resulted in tumor growth which soon regressed and appeared to make the mice resistant to subsequent inoculation of the tumor.[4] Gross later reported a similar set of experiments but using the inbred mouse strain C3H developed by over 20 years of brother–sister mating. Gross used a methylcholanthrene tumor that had been induced originally in C3H mice. In these experiments, the immunized group was resistant to tumor challenge but, interestingly, Gross noted that this resistance to tumor challenge could be overcome by using a larger challenge dose of tumor cells.[5,6]

Sjögren is most often credited with proposing that the antigens unique to tumor cells be desig-nated as tumor-specific transplantation antigens (TSTAs).[7,8] This was based on the observation that tumors in mice induced by a small DNA virus contained a common immune response-inducing antigen. TSTAs were capable of being identified on the surface of tumor cells by antibodies they induced in the host. Though they were capable of killing tumor cells in a complement-dependent fashion in vitro, it soon became apparent that such antibodies directed at the surface TSTAs of carcinomas and sarcomas did not protect the host animal from tumor challenge.

The majority of these reported efforts to demonstrate tumor immunogenicity or the existence of TSTAs, dating from the turn of the century and through the 1940s and early 1950s, were carried out in genetically nonhomogeneous mouse strains. Therefore in almost all instances they were most often the result of normal tissue transplantation antigens also present on tumor cells rather than any unique tumor antigen. These observations by the early "giants of immunology"— R. T. Prehn, G. Klein, H. O. Sjögren, K. E. Hellström, and others—demonstrated to varying degrees evidence that cancers possessed non-self unique antigens. Much of this early work to demonstrate TSTAs, however, was rewritten once immunologists, perhaps influenced by *Drosophila* geneticists of the time, recognized the necessity of developing truly inbred strains of mice to study mammalian genetics and immunology.[9]

In the early 1970s after returning from the Karolinska Institute, I was also privileged to be mentored by Donald C. Shreffler, an immunogeneticist and professor in the Department of Human Genetics at the University of Michigan. Shreffler was a recognized pioneer in researching the genes, including their functional roles, that comprised the murine major histocompatibility and the human leukocyte antigen (HLA) system. Don and his lab were especially recognized for develop-ing numerous, very precious inbred congenic and recombinant H2 complex murine strains as well as strain-specific antisera to the proteins of the H2 locus.[9-13] It was during these years that the time invested in developing truly isogenic mouse strains began to bear fruit and define the critically dominant genes governing tissue transplantation termed the *major histocompatibility complex* (MHC) and the processes of antigen recognition. Understanding the role of MHC in antigen presentation was a crucial step in beginning to define and characterize true tumor-specific antigens (TSAs).

During this time, immunology evolved to the point at which it was evident that there existed two principal immunologically competent cell types, the antibody-producing B lymphocytes and the thymus-derived lymphocytes termed T cells.[13,14] As a result, experiments demonstrated that T cells could be sensitized to TSTA and alone, in either in vitro or in vivo experimental models, could be shown to destroy targeted tumor cells by a process known as *cell-mediated killing*.[15-17] Thus, there was beginning to be ample evidence to support the presence of TSTAs in animal models, but it remained to demonstrate their presence in human tumors. Because tumor transplantation experiments were limited to animals, the analogous antigenic proteins in humans were more appropriately termed *tumor-specific antigens*. TSAs are defined as being specific to the tumor and, as a result, are not proteins or oligopeptides normally present in the nontumor tissues of the body.

TSAs can result from somatically mutated genes and structural genomic variants occurring during tumor evolution and, as such, produce structurally novel tumor proteins. They can also arise secondary to exposure of the cell's DNA to viral genomes and to carcinogens. A second class of tumor antigens have been classified as being tumor-associated transplantation antigens (TATAs). TATAs, later termed simply tumor-associated antigens (TAAs), are normal cellular proteins that, when overexpressed by growing tumors, become antigenic in terms of immune recognition and no longer elicit complete immunologic tolerance in the patient.[18] Several examples of the presence of human TAAs can be found in breast cancer, ovarian cancer, and prostate cancer, as well as proteins normally present in skin melanocytes at low levels. Melanoma has been the most intensely studied human tumor in terms of TSAs and TAAs, perhaps because it is an example of a human malignancy that can undergo spontaneous remission (see **Tumor-associated antigens**).

Identification of Human Tumor Antigens

I have often thought that it was the surgeons' feverish efforts to successfully replace diseased human organs with transplanted heterologous tissues that, in many ways, drove a new generation of young scientists to enter the field of immunology. Renal transplantation presented the human model for developing the needed methods of immune suppression and thus the need to understand the mechanisms underlying the complex processes of tissue rejection. I still recall my excitement as a young surgeon seeing the newly transplanted kidney produce urine even before completing the implantation of the ureter into the bladder and, as a result, markedly changing the life of the recipient. Organ transplantation and the challenges of immunosuppression really opened up the field of immunology and attracted many young scientists to study immunology.

As a result, advances in the field of immunology, driven by organ transplantation, had a tremendous effect on the study of the immune system's interaction with a progressing human cancer. Today, the central efforts in this new era of cancer immunotherapy are directed at generating an enhanced adaptive immune response, the end result of which is a focused destruction of the cancer cells by cytolytic T lymphocytes (CTLs), while avoiding significant unwanted immune-based toxicities. This adaptive response, whether CTL-based, antibody-directed immune checkpoint inhibition, vaccines, oncolytic viruses, or some combination of these, requires the recognition of unique TSAs/TAAs and a process for their presentation that stimulates an adaptive immune response against the cancer.

A BRIEF REFLECTION ON IMPORTANT HISTORIC EVENTS REGARDING TSAS AND TAAS

It is important perhaps to pause a moment and reflect on the tools of the field and our historical understanding of the immune response to a foreign antigen, whether of an infectious origin, an evolving tumor, or a transplanted organ. As noted earlier, the demonstration of the presence of the T lymphocyte as a critical cellular component of the immune system was a landmark step forward in the mid-1960s.[19] I remember very clearly the ability to use "antitheta" antibodies to separate mouse T cells from B lymphocytes for use in our in vitro antigen presentation experiments, as well as the challenge purifying a rabbit anti-B cell antibody during my days in the Möller lab.[20-22]

It soon became clear that the TSAs were recognized by the T cells often to be found in the tumor itself and in the tumor-draining lymph nodes. The recognition that it was T cells interacting with antigenic determinants on the tumor cells and the resultant tumor cell destruction marked the beginning of characterizing the subclasses of T lymphocytes, including CD8[+] cytolytic T cells (CTLs) and eventually CD4[+] T cells.[23]

In 1973, Ralph Steinman and Zanvil Cohn reported on the identification of a novel "glass and plastic" adherent cell found in the skin and peripheral lymphoid tissues termed *dendritic cells* (DCs).[24] These cells soon became recognized as a critical cellular component of the immune system response to foreign antigen. Today, a number of morphologically similar cells have been defined as DCs with a diversity of functions. The classic DC has the ability to be an immunostimulatory cell in response to specific stimuli and in this higher state of differentiation to express high levels of peptide-bound MHC class II molecules that can interact directly with T cells. DCs are capable of recognizing foreign antigen materials—bacteria, viruses, toxins, and TSAs (tumor-derived peptides and lipids)—and through their own proteosome converting them to small peptide fragments to be presented in association with MHC class II molecules for adaptive immune response presentation. The classic DC, we now know, is also capable of interacting with and transmitting information to B cells, as well as other immune system cells such as CD4[+] T cells and natural killer (NK) cells[25] (for an in-depth review, see Cabeza-Cabrerizo et al.[25]). Another important advance was the development by Kohler and Milstein in 1975 of the ability to generate immortalized B cells and to create hybridoma cell lines that would produce an abundance of specific monoclonal antibodies.[26] These murine monoclonal antibodies were used early on to identify TSAs on mouse tumors and eventually on some human cancers. The evolution of this discovery has today become a central feature of immuno-oncology.

In 1989, Lurquin and colleagues reported a series of experiments demonstrating that a peptide derived from a normal self-protein that had become mutated in cancer cells could be recognized by CTLs.[27] This observation has been expanded experimentally over the years to define the process of antigen presentation and T-cell receptor recognition. Recognition of the antigenic peptide begins in the cytosol of the tumor cell where genetically altered self-proteins occur as part of the tumor cell's cancerous progression. These altered proteins are cleaved into small peptides that are presented at the surface of the tumor cell, complexed in the binding cleft of the MHC class I molecules where they can be presented and recognized by the T-cell receptors (TCRs).[28]

These MHC class I–associated peptides, often referred to as MAPs, are key to the process of CD8[+] T-cell maturation and their ability to functionally discriminate between normal cells (self) and those cells that are infected or cancerous (non-self). Thus, the vast majority of TSAs are products of normal cellular proteins that have been genetically altered during tumor initiation and progression and subsequently processed to be non-self-MAPs. This intracellular process of the presentation of MAPs on the cell surface can occur in virtually all cells of the body and is often referred to as the *immunopeptidome* processing mechanism.[29,30] It should be remembered that MHC class I alleles are highly polymorphic and, therefore, each allotype has a unique MAP peptide-binding motif.[31] It is important to note that in contrast to MAPs, the process of antigen presentation by MHC class II determinants is the special activity of the classical antigen-presenting cells: the macrophages, dendritic cells, and B cells.

Two caveats appear worth noting. First, though much of the search for TSAs has naturally focused on the genetic alterations occurring in the exome of the gene, it is increasingly apparent that a much more common occurrence is MAPs derived from the unmutated peptides of cancer-specific epigenetic and splicing alterations.[32,33] The existence of MAPs derived from noncoding regions of the genome greatly increases the number of TSAs potentially recognizable by CD8[+] T cells from roughly 2% to perhaps as great as 75%.[34] Secondly, cancer cells have proven to be rather poor antigen-presenting cells and therefore the response to TSAs is significantly dependent on cross-presentation by DCs. If this DC presentation does not occur in sufficient robustness, then many potential TSAs are not immunologically active.[35,36]

As indicated earlier in this chapter, antigenic neoepitopes as in TSAs unique to the tumor (or a class of tumors such as melanoma) must be recognized by T cells through the T-cell surface receptor (TCR). What makes this MHC class I peptide complex a valuable therapeutic tool in cancer immunotherapy is the tremendous antigenic epitope binding diversity of these T-cell receptors—a receptor-binding diversity similar to that of B cell–produced antibodies. The generation of the immunogenic neoepitope has its origin in the cytosol, where in the case of a cancer cell, altered self-proteins are cleaved by the proteasome and aminopeptidases into peptide fragments.[34] The peptides are then translocated in the endoplasmic reticulum (ER) via a transporter associated with antigen processing and further resolved by enzymes (ER aminopeptidases) to reach a size of ~8 to 10 amino acids. These neoepitope peptides are then loaded into the specific peptide cleft of an MHC class I molecule, and if the complex is stable, it is exported as a MAP complex to the tumor cell surface where it can be recognized by TCRs of the T cell.[37] A more detailed description of the intracellular processes operative in creating the short neoantigen peptides for MHC class I binding is presented later in this chapter in the section **Tumor antigens—Intracellular processing and MHC presentation**.

The Origins of Targetable Tumor-Specific Antigens—Today's Science

The rapid evolution of affordable high-throughput sequencing—based assays, advances in mass spectroscopy, the National Cancer Institute's Cancer Genome Atlas (TCGA) project, the accumulating number of critical databases, and advances in computational biology have resulted in exciting advances in the field of tumor biology. These tools of science are providing new insights into tumor-specific antigenicity and the potential for developing novel immunotherapies. This rapid progress since 2005 has led to some confusion in the field regarding the true definition of tumor antigens and their actual potential as useful targets. This section is designed to add some definition and clarity to our understanding of the various sources of tumor antigens arising in the genetically unstable cancer cell.

TSAs can be subdivided broadly into two groups: those derived from exon or nonexon mutated/altered DNA gene sequences (mTSAs) and those derived from aberrant expression of transcripts not expressed in nonmalignant tissues, including in medullary thymic epithelial cells, which provide a source of antigen tolerance. A second group of TSAs are derived from human endogenous retroelements (EREs) that comprise approximately 42% of our genome. Much of this part of our genomic DNA results from the integration of transposable elements into the genome millions of years ago (retroviruses) that, through genetic evolution, have lost their ability to be expressed. Aberrantly expressed EREs, however, can occur in the genomically unstable cancer cell via epigenetic dysregulation of the cancer genome such as H3K27me3 loss. You will see these latter TSAs frequently denoted as aeTSA.[37,38]

SINGLE NUCLEOTIDE VARIANT NEOANTIGENS

Tumor cells as altered self are by their very nature genetically unstable and undergo a series of genetic and epigenetic alterations during tumor growth and metastasis. Single nucleotide variants (SNVs) are the most common genetic alteration even in normal cells and, as such, have long been considered an excellent initiator of novel tumor TSAs. These neoantigens and their resultant MAPs have been considered a source of potential antitumor T-cell targets. Nonsynonymous SNVs are most commonly the result of simple DNA replication errors during abnormal tumor cell division and are sometimes positively selected. SNVs can also result from genetic alterations in the tumor cell that damage critical enzymes essential for faithful DNA damage repair. SNVs can, of course, result from ongoing exposure to external mutagens during cancer treatment.

As therapeutically promising as SNV-generated TSAs may appear, it has proved much more difficult to identify suitable targets for the development of novel immunotherapies. As pointed out by Minati and colleagues at the Université de Montreal, Canada,[37] in their excellent review, except perhaps for highly mutated tumors such as melanoma and lung, "all studies based on whole-exome or ribonucleic acid sequencing (WES and RNAseq respectively) combined or not with mass spectrometry (MS) analysis, could only identify a very limited number of SNV-derived MAPs."[37,39]

It appears, therefore, that sources of neoantigens other than those originating from exome SNVs will be more critical to the design of future immunotherapies.[37] In fact, in mass spectroscopy studies by Laumont and colleagues, some 90% of the identified TSAs in two mouse cancer cell lines and seven primary human tumors were unexpectedly found to be derived from noncoding regions of the genome. These potentially more important sources for actionable TSAs will be discussed in later sections of this chapter.[40,41]

INSERTIONS AND DELETIONS (INDELS)

Insertions and deletions (indels), small nucleotide (nt) insertions or deletions, represent the second most common type of genomic alteration found in cancer cells but, as will be discussed, are by their nature more likely to prove immunogenetic than the more common SNVs. Single nt insertions or deletions are most common and are estimated to account for ~68% of indels. When nt insertions or deletions occur as in-frame indels, they are, as expected, less likely to be significantly immunogenic. In contrast, those that result in frameshift variants cause the protein produced to be truncated or to be otherwise significantly altered. This can generate peptide fragments and eventual MAPs that are highly immunogenic. Frameshift indels create a novel open reading frame with the potential of producing a large number of peptide fragments that are highly distinct from self and therefore potentially attractive tumor neoantigens.[41-43]

Studies by Turajlic and colleagues searched TCGA for whole-exome sequence data of 5777 solid tumors across 19 cancer organ sites. They found, for example, that the pattern of indel mutations across the various subclasses of kidney cancer had the highest pan-cancer burden of indel mutations and were enriched for frameshift-based mutant-specific neoantigens. They also reported that in their studies the indel mutation number in cutaneous melanoma was significantly associated with the presence of an effective response to checkpoint inhibitors.[42] Renal cell cancers and melanoma, interestingly, have historically been recognized as immunologically responsive and to have a significance occurrence of spontaneous regression and are known to have a more abundant presence of tumor-infiltrating lymphocytes (TILs). TILs are often seen as a predictor of tumor immune responsiveness. Frameshift-based mutations have also been reported to be more abundant in tumors harboring impaired functions of homologous recombination and DNA mismatch repair.[44-48]

TSAS DERIVED FROM ALTERED MRNA SPLICING

In discussing the tumor cell's dysregulation of the normal processes involved in the generation of cellular proteins, it is relatively easy to understand how the instability of such a complex intracellular process as messenger RNA (mRNA) splicing could become an important source of TSAs. In order for a gene to be correctly translated into protein, the mRNA transcribed by RNA polymerase must first be processed and spliced together to remove all noncoding regions (introns). In this multistep nuclear process, the splicing together of the exons requires many highly regulated enzymatic proteins and small RNA molecules. Taken together, the machinery for this process is termed the *spliceosome*. Thus, the mRNA splicing process involves the formation of a highly dynamic and complex spliceosome and a catalytic process to accomplish the required sequence rearrangements. Any dysregulation of these complex mechanisms within the transformed tumor cell is a potential origin for TSAs.

As the intricacies of transcription and translation have been increasingly defined, anticancer therapeutic efforts have been initiated that are directed at correcting or inhibiting core components of the spliceosome in the cancer cell. The future holds great promise that research into the dysregulation of the mRNA splicing mechanisms in malignancy will provide not only potential new TSAs but opportunities for the development of future anticancer therapeutics[49] (for an in-depth review, see Blijlevens et al.[49]). In addition to targeting abnormalities of the spliceosome itself, alterations in the splicing process of the tumor cell have the potential to result in novel transcripts not found in the patient's normal cells. These cancer-specific transcripts can be translated by the tumor cell into new isoforms of the protein, resulting in immunogenic TSAs. Aberrantly spliced mRNAs, whether arising from *cis*-acting splice junction mutations or transacting spliceosome dysregulation, have the potential to result in cancer-specific neojunctions.[37,50-52] The nature of the cancer-specific messenger neo junction can significantly affect the function and structural formation of the resultant protein and its potential immunogenicity as a suitable TSA. It is believed that altered splicing events—whether *cis*-acting or *trans*-acting—are more likely to result in antigenic peptides capable of binding to MHC class I molecules for antigen presentation than those TSAs resulting from SNVs. Beyond a potentially novel TSA as a result of aberrant splicing, the resultant protein isoforms with altered function may also affect the tumor in a variety of ways. For example, the resultant proteins may make the tumor more resistant to therapies—both immunotherapies and chemotherapy.

ABERRANT TRANSCRIPTION TSAS (PRE-MRNA ALTERNATIVE SPLICING)

We have discussed at some length the generation of actionable TSAs as a result of altered splicing events in the genomically unstable tumor cell. Our discussion focused largely on the *trans*-acting splicing mutations that target the enzymatic proteins and small RNA factors of the spliceosome as a source for generating altered tumor-specific antigenic peptides with potential for T-cell recognition. The pre-mRNA stage in the nucleus can also be a source for the formation of TSAs. The pre-mRNA stage involves alternative choices of exon assembly secondary to mutated splice sites, which result in multiple (mRNA) isoforms being produced from a single gene.

The process of alternative splicing in a normal cell is the major way in which a single gene can create protein diversity. Alternative splicing, in general, occurs as a result of one of five basic actions: (1) exon skipping, (2) use of different options at the 5′ splice site, (3) alternatives at the 3′ splice site, (4) as the result of mutually exclusive exons; and (5) as the result of intron sequence retention. In addition, the family of a specific gene's mRNA isoforms can be further expanded by a process termed *RNA editing*. RNA editing is the mechanism by which an RNA transcript can undergo site-specific nt change. An example of the most common mRNA editing is when adenosine deaminase catalyzes the conversion of adenosine to inosine (A to I).[53-56] A to I RNA editing is associated with cancer progression and impaired patient survival (Fig. 5.1).

As discussed previously, the transcriptomes of cancer cells are highly vulnerable to dysregulation, which can also occur in the pre-mRNA stage on the path to gene transcription and final protein production. Dysregulation within the tumor cell at the pre-mRNA stage occurs via *cis*-acting mutations targeting the actual splicing of the exons. The highly regulated process of mRNA splicing in the pre-mRNA stage is a function of specific sequence of elements present on the pre-mRNA template, as well as many RNA processing proteins. This is often referred to as the *supraspliceosome*, and genetic alterations of the many factors involved in mRNA splicing may also provide a rich and expanding source of cancer-unique immunogenic proteins/peptides. Research reported by Seiler and colleagues demonstrated that 119 splice factor genes had significantly elevated rates of nonsynonymous mutations in a group of 33 different tumor types examined.[52] There is increasing validation for aberrant splice factor genes as a rich source

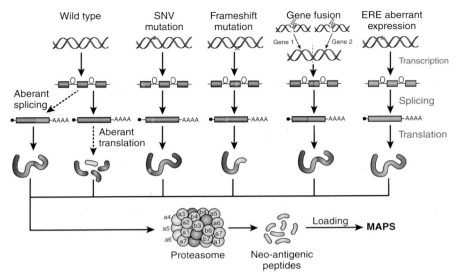

Fig. 5.1 The schematic provides an overview of potential mechanisms for TSA development in the genomically unstable cancer cell. Though SNVs and indels have been a prime source of neoantigen discovery in the past, there is increasing evidence that variants occurring in the noncoding regions of the gene and in the genes coding for factors operative in gene splicing, proteasome processing, and other steps in the cytosol such as within the endoplasmic reticulum may represent more important sources of TSAs and TSAs of more value as therapeutic targets in the future. The proteasome is depicted in this figure as the "standard" 20S subtype. There are variations on this model to form other subtypes to meet differing functional needs. Basically, the proteasome consists of four heptameric rings to form a cylindrical structure with an inner chamber. The outer rings at each end control the entry of proteins into the chamber where the proteins are catalytically broken down into peptides of a size suitable for placement in the groove of the MHC molecule.[37,94]

of highly antigenic epitopes capable, in animal models, of eliciting strong T cell–mediated antitumor responses. These observations are generating an interest in the induction of "forced" aberrant genetic alterations of highly selected splice factor genes as a novel therapeutic approach for augmenting immune checkpoint inhibition. The search for and characterization of these novel cancer-specific genetically altered splice factor genes has been greatly enhanced by new technologies such as high-throughput screening, Whole Genome Sequencing (WGS), RNAseq of both bulk tumor and single cells, and computational tools applicable for mining multiomic, publicly available cancer databases.

RNA DYSREGULATION

Genetic instability and high mutation rates in progressing cancers provide an ideal opportunity for RNA screening dysregulation as a source of neoantigens capable of being targetable TSAs. These have been broadly subdivided into five categories as follows:

(1) *Altered RNA expression* in which overexpression is most common. In case of overexpression, the mRNA alteration in the tumor cells consistently causes the overproduction of a normal protein in the cancer cell compared with the noncancer cell. Examples include CD19 and GPC2.[56-58]

(2) *Alternative splicing* is the process normal cells commonly use for creating diversity in the protein family of a single gene. In the genetically unstable cancer cell, mechanisms regulating alternative splicing are significantly enhanced and more open to mutation, including actual mutation events at splice junction sites. The resultant protein isoforms often

function to enhance tumor cell proliferation and the processes of invasion through metastasis. These protein isoforms may also alter the tumor's response to therapy. Of course, some of the alternatively spliced exons and altered splice junctions can also be a source of highly cancer-specific antigenic peptides.[50,56,59] This source of peptides is felt to be seen by the host as more antigenically foreign than TSAs arising from SNVs. Non-sense-mediated mRNA decay is a normal cellular process that degrades mRNA transcripts that contain premature stop codons.[56,60] However, mutations in the non-sense-mediated mRNA decay pathway may alter this process, resulting in neoantigens being formed.[56,61]

(3) *Noncanonical splicing* can occur in tumor cells producing unusual chimeric mRNA transcripts and, therefore, potentially novel tumor-specific proteins that are foreign to the host.[56] These fusion transcripts may occur between segments of distant genes or through splicing of segments of adjacent genes. It should be noted that chimeric RNAs have also been found in embryonic stem cells and other noncancer tissues.[62] Though the potential exists for the products of chimeric RNAs to be biomarkers of the cancer and potential antigenic targets, this is very preliminary work and will require considerable future studies for validation. Another class of RNAs also found in normal cells are RNAs that have formed a covalently linked closed loop. These closed-loop RNAs have been shown to also occur at the time of pre-mRNA splicing. Although circular RNAs lack a 5′ cap, they can use other methods for actual translation.[56,63] This certainly raises the possibility that such cancer-specific circular RNAs may be sufficiently genetically altered to be a source of antigenic peptides. To support such research, investigators have developed a database for circular RNAs found in cancer (MiOncoCirc).[63,64]

(4) *RNA editing* has been noted earlier as a posttranscriptional editing process in normal cells and is another important contributor to protein diversity. There exist many opportunities in the genomically unstable cancer cell for genetic alterations to occur at the level of the enzymes operative in the editing process.[65] RNA editing–derived peptides have been found to generate antigenic peptides that could combine with MHC class I molecules and be recognized by tumor-infiltrating T cells.[66] Nevertheless, though an intriguing possibility, much future work is required to show that such antigenic peptides are suitable for development as therapeutic targets.

(5) A discussion of expressed *transposable elements* (TEs) seems appropriate for this section on aberrant transcription.[56] TEs are DNA sequences that possess the ability to move from one location in the genome to another.[67] TEs represent close to half the human genome and were first identified by Barbara McClintock of Cold Spring Harbor over 50 years ago.[68] TEs can be divided into two major classes (although there are many subgroups in each class) based on the method used for transposition. Class I TEs require reverse transcription of an RNA intermediate into a cDNA copy in order to transpose. Class II TEs are complete in that they encode the protein transposase, allowing them to move and never use RNA intermediates. Dysregulation of TEs secondary to loss of DNA methylation is common in malignancy and permits reexpression of previously silenced TEs. Thus, apparently expressed TEs in cancer may result in proteins and their derived peptides that are antigenic to the host's immune system.[37,53,69,70]

NEOANTIGENS RESULTING FROM CODING SEQUENCE REARRANGEMENTS (GENE FUSION TSAS)

These potential TSAs are relatively uncommon in cancer and result from the chromosomal rearrangement and juxtaposition of two independent DNA coding regions. These gene fusions may occur in nontumor cells, but many have been identified in a variety of cancers; for example, leukemias, sarcomas, breast cancer, and colon cancer. The most famous, of course, is the translocation that resulted in the formation of the BCR-ABL gene on chromosome 22 known as the *Philadelphia chromosome* in chronic myelogenous leukemia (CML) and other leukemias.[71] Gene fusions occur by (1) chromosomal translocation, (2) transcriptional read-through of adjacent genes, or (3) *trans-* and *cis*-splicing of pre-mRNAs. The resultant fusion transcript can be translated into a novel fusion protein. Often these fusion or chimeric proteins are used clinically as biomarkers in diagnosis, response to therapy, and prognosis.[37,72-76]

Recent evidence seems to highlight the importance of fusion peptides as effective tumor regression antigens. Investigators at Memorial Sloan Kettering Cancer Center identified a patient with metastatic head and neck cancer that had a complete response to immune checkpoint inhibitor therapy despite a tumor with a relatively low mutational load and minimal tumor-infiltrating T cells. Using whole-genome sequencing and RNA sequencing, they identified a novel gene fusion and showed that the resultant peptide neoantigen could elicit a host T-cell response. Using this approach, they identified a series of gene fusion–derived neoantigens that generated CTL responses.[77]

Other fusion-driven cancers include *EWS-FLI1* in Ewing sarcoma, *EML4-ALK* in lung adenocarcinoma, *TMPRSS2-ERG* in prostate cancer, *ETV6-RUNX1*, *FGFR3-TACC3*, *TEL-AML1*, and others, including driver fusions, have been reported.[78] Fusion proteins that function as oncogenic drivers appear to be highly clonal and thus it would not be advantageous to the tumor to reduce their expression. Clonality, however, they may occur only during the early initiation stages of the tumor process, becoming more heterogeneous during later stages, especially during metastatic development. In thinking about the future of research to identify oncogenic fusions, it would appear that fusions with breakpoints shared across tumor types and across patients would be highly relevant to developing vaccine and chimeric antigen receptor (CAR) T-cell therapies. There is evidence that these oncogenic fusions may be more relevant for tumors that have a relatively low tumor somatic mutational burden and a minimal immunocyte infiltration.

ENDOGENOUS NONMUTATED ANTIGENS

Endogenous retroviruses (ERVs) are a significant proportion of the human genome. The reference genome is reported to contain some 450,000 ERV-derived sequences. ERVs resulted from the integration into our genome of transposable elements more than 30 million years ago. As a result of this long evolutionary process, the vast majority of endogenous retroelements (EREs) in our genome are now truncated or mutated and can no longer transpose. It should be noted that ERVs are a major source of millions of gene regulatory elements as seen in pluripotent cells of early embryogenesis.[79]

During the progression of cancer and the accompanying genomic instability, previous studies have found that dysregulation of certain EREs can lead to transcription and translation of aberrantly expressed EREs (aeEREs) generating viral-like neoantigenic peptides. It is possible that such nonmutated neoantigens could be shared TSAs across tumor types and hosts.[37] During the early stages of cancer initiation and progression, induction of the viral mimicry response may occur, causing peptides translated from repeat-derived RNAs to be generated. These have been found to comprise the majority of the ERE-derived neoantigens processed and presented for immune recognition.[80]

NEOANTIGENS RESULTING FROM MUTATIONS IN TUMOR HLA

Mutations that actually occur in the genes coding for the tumor MHC molecule, though apparently relatively uncommon, have become more readily identified. It is not unreasonable to accept that these somatically mutated MHC molecules could, in themselves, be a recognizable TSA. This occurrence was first described by Brandel et al. in 1996.[81] A similar finding was also reported

---

BOX 5.1 ■ The Origins of Targetable Tumor-Specific Antigens

SNPs: Single nucleotide variants; that is, mutated peptide causing non-self TSA
Indels: Insertions and deletions
Altered mRNA splicing
Pre-mRNA alternative splicing—Aberrant transcription
  ■ altered RNA expression
  ■ alternative splicing
  ■ noncanonical splicing
  ■ RNA editing
  ■ transposable elements
Coding sequence rearrangements (gene fusions)
Endogenous nonmutated peptides
Mutations in tumor HLA molecules
Posttranslational alterations

---

for melanoma, showing evidence that tumor-specific T cells could recognize antigens (polypeptide fragments of potential tumor antigens) presented in association with somatically mutated tumor HLA-A11.[82]

It is possible that this form of TSA neoantigen is more common than initially thought because a number of new software tools have emerged that can identify HLA somatic mutations with a high degree of sensitivity (sensitivity 94.1%, specificity 53.3%). Using software tools such as NetMHCpan, it now appears possible to predict the sets of tumor antigenic peptides that would actually bind to the mutated MHC class I molecule and be recognized by the T-cell antigen receptor.[83]

POSTTRANSLATIONAL TSAS

Posttranslational modification of proteins within the cytoplasm is a biochemical process that adds specific biochemical moieties to specific protein residues. The most common biochemical posttranslational modification is phosphorylation. Others include sumoylation, acetylation, and ubiquitination. Studies have demonstrated that these modifications of proteins contribute to the malignant phenotype, including alterations in cell signaling, apoptosis, and transcriptional regulation.[84] Though it is logical to assume that such posttranslation modified proteins can be recognized as foreign antigens and result in peptides suitable for binding to the cleft of MHC class I molecules, it has been challenging to confidently confirm such and to establish these as viable therapeutic antigen targets (Box 5.1).

Tumor-Associated Antigens

TAAs represent a form of tumor neoantigen MHC class I associated peptides (MAPs). An important characteristic is that TAAs actually represent wild-type (wt) sequence and therefore normal peptides that are found to be in much greater abundance (overexpression) on the surface of tumor cells than on the surface of nonmalignant cells. The varying degrees of genetic instability in tumors also manifest in alterations of tumor cell DNA methylation and in alterations of chromatin structure, both of which can result in significant shifts in gene expression and, as a result, are a potential source for TAAs.[85,86] The peptide products of overexpressed genes can be attractive TAA targets for antibody-based therapies and cell-based immunotherapies. An example is the MUC-1 antigen.[87] Their identification is generally based on the ability to compare the transcriptomes of cancer cells of a specific tumor with their normal cell counterparts. Mesothelin, for example, is highly expressed in almost all pancreatic cancers, mesotheliomas, and ovarian tumors. It is not expressed in normal tissues of these organs and only has low expression in the pleural mesothelium.[88] In addition to comparing transcriptomes, mass spectroscopy plays a contributing role in identifying TAA MAPs and quantifying their specificity for malignant vs nonmalignant cells. Their presence on normal cells, even minimally, may, of course, induce central immune tolerance, making TAAs more challenging targets for use in immunotherapies. An exception may occur when TAAs are presented on the surface of cells considered less essential to host survival such as reproductive tissues or B cells, for example. In the end, the accurate identification of a true wt-based TAA that has immunotherapeutic potential requires a rigorous laboratory effort to ensure confidence that the proposed TAA MAP has significant tumor exclusivity to be useable.[35,38,89-91]

There is another group of tumor antigens that perhaps best fits in the group termed TAAs. These are the cancer germline (testis) antigens (CGAs). These antigens and their MAPs are coded by the protein-coding exons normally only expressed in germ cells and therefore are completely absent in normal tissues. Their unusual presence in cancer cells is the result of epigenetic alterations.[92] Examples of CGAs are melanoma-associated antigens A-1, A-3 (MAGE A family); synovial sarcoma X-2 (SSX-2); and New York esophageal squamous cell carcinoma-1 (NY-ESO-1).[93]

Tumor Antigens: Intracellular Processing and MHC Presentation

As stated earlier in this chapter, aberrant genetically altered malignant cells can only be detected by the TCR on $CD8^+$ T cells in the context of antigenic non-self-peptides complexed to MHC class I molecules—the so-called MAPs. The intracellular processes generating the antigenic peptides underpin the eventual direct interaction between the progressing malignancy and the host's adaptive immune response system. The MAP complexes are presented on the cell surface of viable malignant cells but can also be presented by the host's classic antigen-presenting cells (APCs) as well.

The process of generating a recognizable tumor rejection antigen begins with the genetic diversity of the transformed malignant cell and the accumulation of nonsynonymous somatic genome alterations; for example, missense mutations, silent mutations, formation of indels, splice variants, and copy number variants. Alterations within the tumor, defined as the tumor mutation burden, correlate with the likelihood of generating new strictly tumor-specific peptide sequences (neoantigens). The processing and production of these potential neoantigens is a multistep pathway that begins in the cytoplasm where intracellular structurally aberrant or misfolded proteins unique to the malignant cell are ubiquitinated and fragmented into small peptides by the proteasome.

The proteasome is a 20S cylindrical structure within the cytoplasm. This particle is composed of four stacked heptameric rings that create a chamber where proteins are degraded into small peptide fragments. The two inner rings of the cylinder are composed of seven subunits, with three types of β subunits (β1, β2, and β5) being catalytically active (chymotrypsin, trypsin, and caspase-like activities), and cause cleavage of the peptide bonds in the protein captured within the proteasome chamber. It should be noted that entry into the proteasome chamber through the outer ring is tightly regulated, as would be expected, to prohibit the normal and properly folded proteins from entry, protecting them from protein degradation that would be detrimental to the cell. The entry pores in the two outer α-rings responsible for regulating protein entry are associated with the 19S regulatory cap particle, creating the actual 26S proteasome. The ubiquitin-tagged abnormal proteins formed in the malignant cell are recruited to the 19S regulatory particle at the entry pore. The 19S complex recognizes the ubiquitin tag and removes the tag and unfolds and translocates the abnormal tumor cell–generated protein into the main catalytic chamber[94,95] (for an in-depth review, see Mpakali and Stratikos[95]).

Research concerning the steps occurring within the proteasome of the malignant cell has shown that new catalytic subunits transition the protein-loaded proteasome to become what has been termed the *immunoproteasome*, which acts to enhance cleavage specificity and optimize the peptide fragment for efficiency of final MHC class I ligand generation. Cleavage within the immunoproteasome generates peptides of 2 to 26 residues with a C-terminus residue anchor compatible with the binding groove in the MHC class I molecule. Peptides are then released from the immunoproteasome into the cytosol of the malignant cell.

During their presence in the cytosol, they are at risk of further degradation by peptidases prior to being assisted by a heterodimer transporter molecule. This transporter functions to form a transmembrane entrance pore in the cell's endoplasmic reticulum membrane. This pore has a greater efficiency for the transfer of shorter 9 to 16 residues in contrast to longer peptides. Once inside the endoplasmic reticulum, a multisubunit complex, termed the *peptide loading complex*, is involved in the final placement of the peptide into the binding groove of a nascent MHC class I molecule. It should be noted that endoplasmic reticulum aminopeptidases ERAP1 and ERAP2 have tumor-specific levels of expression, often being downregulated or upregulated and on occasion suffering function-altering mutations. These aminopeptidases have been shown on occasion to alter the peptide, destroying its capacity for MHC I binding.

Once the peptide in the endoplasmic reticulum is placed in the MHC class I molecule's special binding groove, another transporter binding protein, TAPBPR, functions to ensure that the peptide is of suitable structure and that peptide binding in the groove is stable. The loaded MHC class I molecule then exits the endoplasmic reticulum and traffics through the cell's cytoplasmic Golgi network to be displayed on the tumor cell surface as a TSA capable of presentation to the host's adaptive immune system, specifically the CD8[+] T cell. Experiments using MAP-stimulated CTLs suggested that some number of the presented neoantigenic peptides actually show evidence of peptide splicing. More work is required to understand where this occurs in the process: only in the proteasome or perhaps post proteasome (Fig. 5.2).[96,97]

THE STRUCTURE OF MHC CLASS I AND II ANTIGEN PRESENTATION PROTEINS

MHC class I and class II are essential protein components of the human adaptive immune system. Both molecules are responsible for presenting antigenic peptides (MAPs) on the cell surface for T-cell recognition. MHC class I antigenic MAPs are presented on the surface of nucleated cells and, in the case of cancer, on the surface of the malignant cells. The neoantigenic peptides derived from the tumor cells can also be cross-presented using the MHC class II molecule on the surface of the professional antigen-presenting cells (APCs) such as dendritic cells, macrophages, or B cells. In all cases of antigen presentation by the two classes of MHC molecules, T-cell recognition/activation occurs via a clonotypic TCR.

At any step in this complex process—such as the synthesis of critical enzymes and transporter molecules, molecular assembly of the MAP and surface expression—there is ample opportunity for genetic alterations. Such alterations of the processing "machinery components" not only affect the opportunity for generating the neoantigen MHC class I complex capable of stimulating the host's adaptive immune response but can further compromise the host's response to other therapeutic approaches using other immunotherapies and chemotherapies. Such alterations of the malignant cell's protein generation and processing machinery can, of course, directly affect the stability of the tumor, the functions of the tumor microenvironment, the tumor's susceptibility to therapy, and, therefore, the overall progression of the malignancy.

The first crystallization experiments of MHC class I molecules occurred in 1989.[98] This determined that MHC class I molecules are heterodimers with a polymorphic α-subunit heavy chain coded for in the MHC locus and an invariant β_2 microglobulin subunit coded outside the

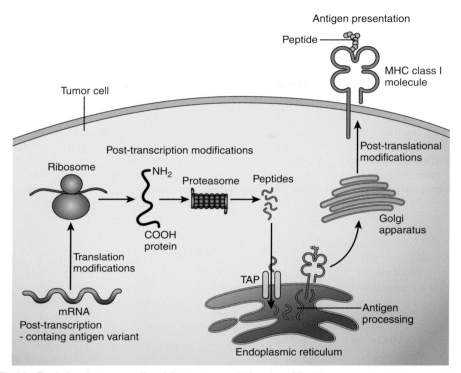

Fig. 5.2 Depicting the tumor cell and the posttranscriptional modifications occurring in the generation of and processing of a neoantigenic peptide for placement in the MHC class I binding groove and for presentation to the TCR of the T cell. The schematic illustrates multiple steps required to develop a suitable TSA peptide for MHC presentation. The figure illustrates the many protein factors involved at each step in the process and thus the increased opportunities for further posttranscriptional and posttranslational modifications of the original tumor cell gene variant encoding the neoantigen peptide. The proteasome has factors that select for shorter peptides. The proteasome cavity into which the peptides enter contains three major catalytic activities, the caspase-like activity, the chymotrypsin-like activity, and the trypsin-like activity. The original peptide thus exits the cavity of the proteasome as short peptides. The transporter for antigen processing (TAP) is involved in the entrance of the peptides into the endoplasmic reticulum for further processing, followed by entrance to the Golgi apparatus for eventual loading into the groove of the MHC class I molecule.[35]

MHC locus on a different chromosome. The heavy chain of MHC class I molecules contains an N-terminal extracellular region with $\alpha 1$, $\alpha 2$, and $\alpha 3$ domains; a transmembrane helix; and a cytoplasmic tail. The $\alpha 1$ and $\alpha 2$ domains form the peptide-holding groove. The floor of this groove consists of eight β strands. The immunoglobulin-like $\alpha 3$ domain is involved in the interaction with the TCR of the CD8$^+$ T cell.

Recall that the antigenic peptide is noncovalently bound in the MHC molecular groove. The MHC class I structural peptide-binding groove is closed at both ends by tyrosine residues, which limits the size of the bound peptide generally to 8 to 10 residues (amino acids). The MHC class I and MHC class II protein structures known as human leukocyte antigens are coded for by three gene regions in the major histocompatibility complex located on chromosome 6p. MHC class I is derived from HLA regions A, B, C and MHC class II is derived from HLA regions DR, DP, DQ, all of which are highly polymorphic and, as such, affect the character of the binding capacity of the groove and modulate the potential peptide repertoire that can be presented. MHC class I peptide loading is facilitated by the catalyst tapasin and is facilitated by the catalyst HLA-DM for MHC class II. Human leukocyte antigen DM (HLA-DM) is an intracellular chaperone protein operating in APCs to protect the integrity of MHC class II molecules and determines which antigenic peptides are appropriate for binding and subsequent T-cell presentation. The direct neoantigen T-cell presentation by tumor cells is recognized to be generally poor or weak in nature compared with APC presentation of pMHC class II molecules. pMHC class I molecules tend to present peptide fragments that are unstable and, thus, short-lived (Fig. 5.3).

This cross-presentation of exogenous antigenic peptides by MHC class II molecules on APCs relies on the ability of the APC to actually acquire the genetically altered protein from the cancer cell where it is generated. This process favors tumor cell antigenic proteins that are longer-lived and more stable. These antigenic proteins are transferred by endocytosis to the APC. The most efficient endocytic process for this transfer is simply phagocytosis. The internalized antigenic

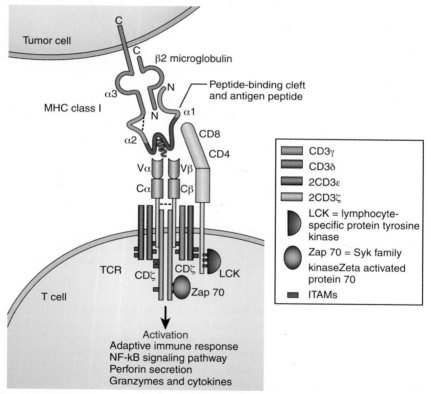

Fig. 5.3 Showing the T cell (CD8⁺) and its T-cell receptor (TCR) interacting with the neoantigen–peptide MHC class I complex displayed on the tumor cell surface. The TCR–neoantigen–peptide interaction triggers the T cell–adaptive immune response. Approximately 95% of T cells express a TCR composed of α and β chains coupled with six CD3 chains (see figure). Each CD3 chain contains one to three immunoreceptor tyrosine-based activation motifs (ITAMS). The schematic depicts the MHC class I molecule presented on the tumor cell surface containing the neoantigenic peptide in the MHC binding groove being presented to the TCR on the T cell. The MHC class I molecule has a polymorphic α-chain noncovalently attached to a nonpolymorphic β₂-microglobulin.

> ## BOX 5.2 ■ Important Observations Regarding Neoantigen Presentation
>
> Increasing evidence that the more immunogenic tumor-derived antigenic peptides for CD8[+] T-cell recognition are derived from noncoding sequences, alternative reading frames, and antisense coding segments.
>
> Evidence supports the observation that CD4[+] T-cell responses focus mainly on antigenic peptides that have a high affinity binding to MHC class II molecules.
>
> Antitumor vaccine strategies require linked recognition of B-cell and CD4[+] T-cell antigenic epitopes.

protein undergoes a similar degradation process in the APC as occurs in the tumor cell being degraded by the APC proteasome into small peptides for coupling with the MHC class II molecule. Cross-presentation by APCs therefore introduces some bias into TSA T-cell presentation because the APCs can only present to the T cell a small fraction of the neoantigenic peptides generated within the tumor (Box 5.2).[99,100]

Though in theory MHC class II peptide-loaded molecules can be presented by all cell types, in general they are only significantly present on the surface of classic antigen-presenting cells, especially dendritic cells. On the antigen-presenting cell surface the presented antigen can be recognized by receptors of helper CD4[+] T cells via their TCRs[101-103] (for an in-depth review, see Sant[103]).

Bioinformatic Strategies for Neoantigen Discovery and Validation. Tumor-specific neoantigenic epitopes derived from malignant cells that demonstrate a capacity for T-cell recognition and stimulation of an adaptive immune response can be identified and characterized today with a variety of bioinformatic options. In fact, the current TSA discovery processes and the exciting new tools available for validating novel tumor antigens comprise a very rapidly expanding field of cancer biology and are key to new immunotherapy development. It is certainly a time of great scientific opportunity in cancer immuno-oncology. The goal of this section of the chapter is to build on the prior sections where an effort was made to comprehensively define all potential sources of malignant cell TSAs. This section highlights new databases and bioinformatic approaches available for neoantigen identification, validation, and prioritization for potential clinical application such as vaccine development. It is hoped that the reader will have a reasonable understanding of sequencing analysis and the computational tools comprising the discovery pipeline supporting today's research.

First and foremost, the advent of massively parallel next-generation sequencing (NGS) that replaced the labor-intensive technique of cDNA library screening has proved to be transformative at every step of neoantigen/neoepitope discovery, immunoproteasome processing, and the validation path. The high-throughput technologies of WGS and whole-exon sequencing (WES) not only identify somatic mutations such as SNVs but also perhaps even more critical to the identification of potential neoantigens is the identification of large structural genomic variants. In genetically unstable malignant cells, structural variants may be even more common and more valuable than SNVs in leading to the appearance of altered malignant cell proteins and potential highly efficacious antigenic peptides.[104]

RNAseq, used in conjunction with deep WGS or WES, adds the critical gene expression information to identify the proteins or protein isoforms of the altered tumor cell most likely to produce a clinically useful antigenic epitope. RNAseq extends the ability to identify potential neoantigens beyond small variants to include antigenic peptides derived from the more common structural variants: gene fusions, copy number variants, alternate splicing isoform variants, translocations, and mRNA editing. Of course, it is well established that not all produced mRNAs are actually translated into proteins with an identical efficiency, and some mRNA isoforms are not translated at all. This potential information gap can be addressed by applying high-throughput sequencing of those mRNA fragments that are ribosome protected. The addition of this sequence data along with proteomics data provides a complete profile of all translated messages.[105] Data generated from deep DNA sequencing and RNAseq provide the basis for the application of bioinformatics tools to eventually identify and even rank the tumor neoantigenic peptides most likely to successfully navigate the proteasome processes and be successfully bound to the MHC molecule (Fig. 5.4).[106,107]

The ability to predict and rank the likely successful binding of an antigenic peptide to the MHC class I molecule is also strongly dependent on HLA typing to identify the HLA allotype

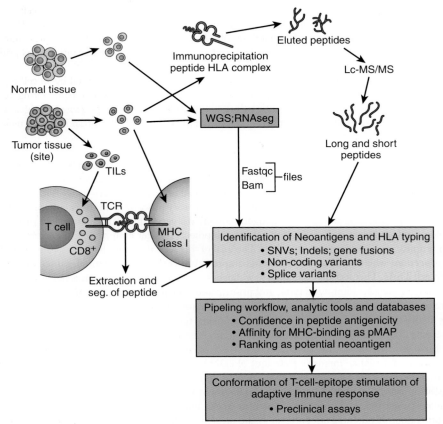

Fig. 5.4 A schematic showing all potential sources of information for a genomics-based analytic pipeline designed to optimize the identification of and ranking of tumor-generated neoantigens. As illustrated, DNA and RNA are extracted from tumor and normal tissue for high-throughput sequencing comparing germline and tumor sequence to identify high-quality somatic variant calling. Initial analysis generates high-quality curated sequence files. Additional data may be generated from immunoprecipitation and eluted neoantigenic peptides bound to MHC on tumor cells and tumor-infiltrating T cells using LC-MS/MS and additional sequencing. These data, when available, are integrated with the tumor and germline sequence data. Bioinformatics analysis uses the identified potential neoantigens in a variety of analytic pipelines and publicly available data sets to predict altered peptide suitability for intracellular proteasomal processing, the potential for further antigenic modifications, a ranking in terms of antigenicity with therapeutic potential, affinity for MHC binding/stability, TCR affinity/recognition, and ability to trigger a significant adaptive immune response.

> **BOX 5.3 ■ Characteristics of the Ideal Cancer Antigen**
>
> A defined therapeutic function
> Demonstrated immunogenicity
> A role in oncogenicity
> Demonstrated tumor specificity
> Presence on a high percentage of the tumor's cells and in high numbers
> Expression on cancer stem cells
> Expression in a significant number of patients with cancer
> Significant number of antigenic epitopes
> Expression in a critical cellular location

and the use of algorithms to characterize the potential HLA peptide T cell–binding affinity. The end result still remains predictive in nature. True validation, however, requires further study to demonstrate the presence of the MHC class I peptide complex expression on the actual tumor cell surface, the ability of the CD8$^+$ T-cell TCR to effectively recognize and bind to the neoantigen being presented, and finally evidence for this reaction to produce an adaptive immune response.

High-throughput liquid chromatography–tandem mass spectroscopy (LC-MS/MS) has become an important tool when used in conjunction with deep sequencing data to directly identify the actual presence of MHC peptide complexes on the cell surface. LC-MS/MS is capable of revealing the entire peptidome that is MHC bound. As a result, LC-MS/MS provides addition insights into any immunoproteasome-generated neopeptide alterations, as well as posttranslational modifications of the tumor-specific neoantigen (Box 5.3).[108,109]

The tools of deep DNA sequencing, WGS and WES, and mRNAseq result in very large files of raw data. The interpretation of these data has been enabled by the progressive development of computational tools and specific bioinformatics analysis pipelines used in processing the raw sequencing data to perform quality checking and filtering and mapping of the sequence to the reference genome. The resultant BAM files (BAM files are compressed binary format of a SAM file used for storing aligned sequence data) provide the basis for variant calling of somatic mutations, including SNVs, indels, and structural variants, for the purpose of identifying all malignant cell sources for potential tumor-specific neoantigens. In addition, the sequenced reads provide the information to accomplish HLA typing. Most important, the creation of high-quality BAM files is essential to all further bioinformatics analysis and interpretation of tumor genomic variants.

Using the BAM files, high-priority genetically altered tumor protein/peptide sequences can be selected and subjected to further bioinformatics pipeline analysis in order to rank these peptides in terms of their potential as actionable tumor neoantigens. Computational analysis can be used to identify/predict the potential immunoproteasome specificity limits for generating the peptide, predict peptide–MHC affinity, and even predict pMHCs' affinity to TCR. This process requires the implementation of specially designed bioinformatics software. An in-depth discussion of all of the published and validated tools available is beyond the scope of this chapter. However, a summary-style overview should provide the reader with an understanding of the analytic process and the importance of critical databases that have been built in support of the different analysis tasks.[110]

In previous sections of this chapter, an attempt has been made to review all of the potential ways in which the genetically unstable malignant cell can produce genetically altered antigenic peptides suitable for presentation on the tumor cell surface. The shear variety of the potential mutational origins of neoantigenic peptides requires a variety of computational tools and databases to clarify/define the antigenic epitope, its tumor specificity, and its relevance as a potential cancer therapy target. Today's computational tools are being expanded by the addition and integration of machine learning and the application of artificial neural networks to the analytic pipeline. Examples of machine learning software used in developing epitope prediction tools are NetMHCpan, NetMHCIIpan, MHCflurry, ConvMHC, PLAtEAU, and NetCTLpan.[108,111-115]

These and other epitope prediction algorithms rely significantly on existing knowledge of the HLA allotype and ligand–MHC affinity. Machine learning tools are only as good as the quality and size/scale of the data sets available for training and tool validation. In this case, data sets of MHC class I peptide binding affinity data from actual biochemical physical measurements and high-throughput mass spectroscopy–eluted ligand data from a significant number of study subjects have contributed to the data set.

As might be expected, experience indicates variation in performance of the various software depending on HLA type and length of the bound peptide. For example, O'Donnell et al. reported achieving better epitope prediction with the addition to the MHCflurry 2.0 tool of an antigen processing predictor based on MHC ligands identified by LC-MS/MS. There are advantages, as well, to using more than one MHC binding predictor tool in tackling the challenge of predicting and scoring the value of potential tumor antigenic peptides.[116] Other tools that have been published are Epitope Discovery in cancer Genomics (EDGE), MuPeXI, EpitopeHunter, and Neopepsee. Each of these brings its own set of values to the search and priority rating process.[117-122]

It is critical, of course, not only to identify the ability of an altered tumor protein to navigate proteasomal processing and MHC–peptide binding but to identify those antigenic peptides that will optimally interact with the TCR and stimulate T cell–mediated adaptive immunity. The development of tools designed to predict MHC–antigenic peptide epitope binding efficiency to the CD8$^+$ TCRs are still in the early phase of development and highlight the need for adequate training data sets. Several such tools include TCRex, NetTCR, Repitope, ERGO, and Deepwalk.[123-129]

Of interest are several databases built around information concerning tumor neoantigens, experimentally defined antigenic epitopes, HLA typing information, and MHC binding data. In some instances, building these tools also used existing resources of the TCGA and The Cancer Immune Atlas (TCIA). These databases include TSNAdb (http://biopharm.zju.edu.cn/tsnadb/),[130,142] NeoPeptide (https://github.com/lyotvincent/NeoPeptide),[131,143] and dbPepNeo (http://www.biostatistics.online/dbPepNeo/).[132,133,144] Tools generated from experimentally derived data are now key to helping researchers identify potential neoantigenic peptides and their critical epitopes. These tools are used in the ranking of such peptides likely to be bound into the MHC class I molecule binding groove, the HLA molecule type best suited to developing the restricted pMHC, the stability of the pMHC molecular complex, and, finally, predicting pMHC-TCR binding.[130-138]

Each of these database resources has weaknesses, including either sparse information in certain areas or an actual absence of critical neoantigen-related information, including antigen sequence, level of expression, level of pMHC presentation, the corresponding TCR sequence, and evidence for actual clinical activity. In an effort to address these database gaps, Xia and colleagues undertook the construction of a database NeoEPitope (NEPdp) by conducting an extensive literature search. NEPdb is a publicly available reference database of actual reported, experimentally validated immunogenic neoepitopes, ineffective neopeptides, and computationally predicted HLA antigenic peptides validated for clinical relevance.[135-139] NEPdb is supported by a user-friendly online interface. The top genes in their database include *MUC4, KRAS, PABPC3, MUC16, MAGEC1, MUC12, ZNF737, FGFR1, CRCP,* and *MUC2* in descending order. Their search of published and validated data concerning the distribution of HLA alleles found the respective allele frequencies to be HLA-A 25.67%, HLA-B 22.37%, HLA-C 21.7%, HLA-DRB 10.11%, HLA-DQB 10.06%, and HLA-DQA 10.05%.[135-139] An in-depth review by Gopanenko and colleagues on the strategies for identifying neoantigens provides a very comprehensive table (table I) that provides currently available computational pipelines suitable for tumor neoantigen prediction(s).[140]

THE CANCER GENOME ATLAS

I take special pride in being involved in the decision to make the federal investment in this landmark National Cancer Institute (NCI) and National Human Genome Research Institute (NHGRI) project, initially as chair of President Bush's National Cancer Advisory Board, which voted to direct the NCI to partner with the NHGRI to establish a pilot study of WGS of tumors. TCGA was initiated by the NCI in collaboration with the NHGRI in 2005 to 2006 at a time when I served as director of NCI. NCI developed a project leadership team of scientists to build the initial pilot study. Much credit for the success of TCGA goes to NCI Deputy Director Dr. Anna Barker for recruitment of an outstanding team of scientists and for leading the collaboration with the NHGRI, led at that time by Director Dr. Francis Collins.

The initial pilot study began in 2006 and was planned for 3 years. The pilot focused on three tumor types: glioblastoma multiforme, lung, and ovarian cancer. The pilot program involved setting up and coordinating a number of extramural academic centers to provide high-quality tumor specimens, sequencing centers, and bioinformatics analysis centers. The pilot proved highly successful and, as a result, in 2009 TCGA was greatly expanded and eventually curated data on 33 cancer types.

Today, TCGA is the largest resource in the field of cancer biology that is aimed at the discovery of the molecular features of various cancer types (https://cancergenome.nih.gov/).[141,145] TCGA includes genomic, transcriptomic, and epigenetic data for 33 human cancer types (including 10 rare types) represented with more than 11,000 individual tumor samples and supports the TCGA pan-cancer data portal (http://tcga-data.nci.nih.gov/tcga).[137-143] These advances in the development of high-throughput microarray, sequencing technologies, and LC-MS/MS applications have provided opportunities to generate public cancer transcriptomic databases, including TCGA and Gene Expression Omnibus, and, as a result, have dramatically affected the opportunities for future TSA and TAA discovery and the development of immune-based cancer therapeutics.

In an effort to provide a degree of guidance to the evaluation and selection of potential therapeutic targets, in 2019 the NCI asked its Translational Research Working Group to establish a set of criteria to be used for evaluating the suitability of a specific, appropriately characterized TSA to be a therapeutic target. The working group defined the "ideal cancer antigen" for potential therapeutic application as (1) having therapeutic function, (2) having immunogenicity, (3) the role of the antigen in oncogenicity, (4) specificity, (5) expression level and percentage of antigen-positive cells, (6) stem cell expression, (7) number of patients with antigen-positive cancers, (8) number of antigenic epitopes, and (9) cellular location of antigen expression (Box 5.3). Forty-six of the 75 TSAs reviewed were deemed immunogenic in clinical trials and 20 appeared efficacious in the first criterion of "therapeutic function."[143,144]

What the Future Holds—Integrating Immune Response and Network Biology

As noted, TCGA has provided insights into the genetic alterations occurring in thousands of human cancers. TCGA has confirmed our understanding of cancer as a highly heterogeneous disease even for tumors of the same organ site and further, that cancers are highly complex, often having more than 1000 genes showing some form of genetic alteration. Though most of these genetic variants are rare, it is increasingly apparent that specific signaling pathway alterations ultimately define an individual patient's cancer, including the tumor's relationship to the inflammatory environment of the Tumor Microenvironment (TME) and to the patient's immune system. Despite our ability to identify and catalog these genetic variants, it remains extremely challenging to translate this information into changes at the level of protein–protein interactions involved in molecular pathways and into therapeutic clinical opportunities.

In efforts to build on the accumulating data detailing genetic variants in cancer, investigators are starting to apply network biology approaches in an effort to tie genetic variants to protein–protein interactions and altered molecular communication pathways. Integrating the information of genetic variations with that of mass spectroscopy is enabling researchers to build the necessary multidimensional protein–protein interaction maps and the internal systems of altered signaling pathways of a specific cancer. By building maps of critical molecular pathways operative in cancer, new therapeutic targets will be identified and potential therapeutic toxicities will be made more visible.[145,146]

From all of these efforts it seems quite clear that future advances in the field of immuno-oncology will be even more dependent on powerful computational methodologies for multisource data integration and analysis. The power of computing and computational biology will be enhanced by the validating capabilities of sequencing, especially RNAseq, and of protein characterization by mass spectroscopy. The evolving application of computational biology, our growing reservoir of information in highly curated databases, and the potential of machine learning and applications of artificial intelligence provide a rich future for identification of patient-specific therapies. This will greatly expand the power of predicting those neoantigens and their actual epitopes most likely to be priority therapeutic targets. These computational tools will also enhance our capability to expand the TSAs that are commonly shared across the population for a specific tumor or perhaps several tumor types, enabling "off-the-shelf" antitumor immuno-therapies. Perhaps even more important will be the opportunity to integrate therapies directed at enhancing antitumor adaptive immune responses with novel therapies targeting the altered molecular cell signaling pathways of the tumor and the TME.

Key References

2. Klein G. Tumor immunology. In: Bach FH, Good RA, eds. *Clinical Immunology*. Vol 1. New York, London: Academic Press; 1972:219-240.
7. Sjögren HO, Helstrom I, Klein G. Resistance of polyoma virus immunized mice against transplantation of established polyoma tumors. *Exp Cell Res*. 1961;23:204.
8. Hellsröm KE, Hellström I, Sjögren HO, Warner GA. Cell-mediated immunity to human tumor antigens. In: Amos B, ed. *Progress in Immunology*. Academic Press, Elsevier; 1971:939-949. doi:10.1016/B978-0-12-057550-3.50075-2.
10. Klein J, Shreffler DC. Evidence supporting a two-gene model for the H-2 major histocompatibility system of the mouse. *J Exp Med*. 1972;135:929-937.
23. Waldman AD, Fritz JM, Lenardo MJ. A guide to cancer immunotherapy: from T cell basic science to clinical practice. *Nat Rev Immunol*. 2020;20:651-668. doi:10.1058/s41577-020-0306-5.
25. Cabeza-Cabrerizo M, Cardoso A, Minutti CM, Pereira da Costa M, Reis e Sousa R. Dendritic cells revisited. *Annu Rev Immunol*. 2021;39:131-166.
29. Caron E, Vincent K, Fortier MH, et al. The MHC I immunopeptidome conveys to the cell surface an integrative view of cellular regulation. *Mol Syst Biol*. 2011;7:533. doi:10.1038/msb.2011.68.
33. Wei LH, Guo JU. Coding functions of "non-coding" RNAs. *Science*. 2020;367:1074-1075.
36. Apavaloaei A, Hardy M-P, Thibault P, Perreault C. The origin and Immune recognition of tumor-specific antigens. *Cancers*. 2020;12:2607. doi:10.3390/cancers12092607.
37. Minati R, Perreault C, Thibault P. A roadmap toward the definition of actionable tumor-specific antigens. *Front Immunol*. 2020;11:583287. doi:10.3389/fimmu.2020.583287.
49. Blijlevens M, Li J, van Beusechem VW. Biology of the mRNA splicing machinery and its dysregulation in cancer providing therapeutic opportunities. *Int J Mol Sci*. 2021;22:5110. doi:10.3390/ijms22105110.
53. Obeng EA, Stewart C, Abdel-Nahebo O. Altered RNA processing in cancer pathogenesis and therapy. *Cancer Discov*. 2019;9:1493-1510. doi:10.1158/2159-8290.CD-19-0399.
56. Pan Y, Kadash-Edmonson KE, Wang R, et al. RNA dysregulation: an expanding source of cancer immunotherapy targets. *Trends Pharmacol Sci*. 2021;42(4):268-282.

64. Li J, Sun D, Pu W, Wang J, Peng Y. Circular RNAs in Cancer: biogenesis, function, and clinical significance. *Trends Cancer*. 2020;6(4):319-336. doi:10.1016/jtrecan.2020.01.012.

67. Burns KH. Transposable elements in cancer. *Nat Rev Cancer*. 2017;17:415-424. doi:10.1038/nrc.2017.35.

95. Mpakali A, Stratikos E. The role of antigen processing and presentation in cancer and the efficacy of immune checkpoint inhibitor immunotherapy. *Cancers*. 2021;13:134-164. doi:10.3390/cancers13010134.

103. Sant AJ. Overview of T-cell recognition: making pathogens visible to the immune system. In: Rich RR, Fleisher TA, Shearer WT, et al., eds. *Clinical Immunology: Principles and Practice*. 5th ed. New York, NY: Elsevier Pub; 2019:93-106.

133. Zhou WJ, Qu Z, Song CY, et al. NeoPeptide: an immunoinformatic database of T-cell-defined neoantigens. *Database (Oxford)*. 2019;2019:baz128. doi:10.1093/database/baz128.

134. Tan X, Li D, Huang P, et al. dbPepNeo: a manually curated database for human tumor neoantigen peptides. *Database*. 2020;2020:baaa004. doi:10.1093/database/baaa004.

135. Xia J, Bai P, Fan W, et al. NEPdb: a database of T-cell experimentally-validated neoantigens and pan-cancer predicted neoepitopes for cancer immunotherapy. *Front Immunol*. 2021;12:644637. doi:10.3389/fimmu.2021.644637.

Visit Elsevier eBooks+ (eBooks.Health.Elsevier.com) for complete set of references.

CHAPTER 6

Tumor Immune Surveillance

Daniel Delitto

SUMMARY OF KEY FACTS

- The concept of tumor immunosurveillance can be traced back to the early 1900s in association with observations that a potentially overwhelming frequency of carcinomas must be repressed by the immune system.
- The cancer immunosurveillance hypothesis was formally proposed in 1970 by Burnet and Thomas,[6-7], describing the immune contribution to tumor control as an "evolutionary necessity" given the lifetime accumulation of genetic changes in somatic cells.
- Despite setbacks from preliminary observations in the athymic nude mouse, a host of mouse models and epidemiologic data in the 1990s overwhelmingly supported the concept of cancer immunosurveillance.
- The cancer immunosurveillance hypothesis has evolved into the three Es of immune editing: elimination, equilibrium, and escape.
- Tumor-associated antigens can be recognized by the immune system and arise from multiple different processes, including mutation-associated neoantigens, reexpression or overexpression of antigens associated with immune privileged tissue, and posttranslational modifications, such as alternative splicing.
- Oncogene-induced senescence in the setting of intact tumor suppressor pathways can lead to antigen-specific immune responses that may contribute efficacy to tumor immunosurveillance and elimination.
- The microbiome can influence the function of innate and adaptive immune cells. In addition, given the genetic diversity of the microbiota, it is likely that resultant peptides will mimic neoantigens from tumors, representing a promising avenue to further understand the complexity of tumor immunosurveillance.
- Data from populations of transplant recipients and those with HIV infection demonstrate higher rates of cancer in individuals who are immunocompromised, supporting a role for the immune system in cancer prevention.

The Concept of Immune Surveillance in Cancer

Tumor immunology is grounded on the central principle that cancer can be controlled and even eliminated by an intact host immune response. Thus a resulting corollary is that cancer development and progression represent a failure, to some extent, of the immune system to perform one of its primary functions. This is a hotly debated topic historically, with large swings within the scientific community over the past few decades. In this manner, the history of tumor immunology highlights the importance of incorporating new insights into established concepts.

The concept of immune regulation in cancer development can be traced back to the works of Elie Metchnikoff and Paul Ehrlich, who received the Nobel Prize in 1908. Metchnikoff described the process of phagocytosis, laying the foundation for innate immunity. Ehrlich pioneered the idea of humoral immunity, and both scientists proposed that the immune system might control tumors. Ehrlich specifically suggested a potentially overwhelming frequency of carcinomas that must be repressed by the immune system. He hypothesized that this occurred via mechanisms outlined in the side-chain theory to describe soluble mediators and their receptors, analogous to side chains in dyes that determine coloring properties.[1,2]

The contribution of cell-mediated immunity was expanded by Peter Medawar in the 1950s. The context of this advance was allograft rejection in transplantation. In fact, tumors transplanted within inbred strains of mice were not typically rejected, arguing against an immune-mediated antitumor response. However, certain tumor-associated antigens were confirmed to exist because these mice could be immunized against transplanted tumors, lending some support to the idea behind cancer immunosurveillance.[3-5] The concept of cancer immunosurveillance was then formally proposed by Macfarlane Burnet and Lewis Thomas in 1970, which suggested that it was an "evolutionary necessity" for the immune system to control the lifetime accumulation of genetic changes in somatic cells.[6-8]

The cancer immunosurveillance hypothesis underwent major setbacks over the following 2 decades because of a faulty assumption that *any* immune suppression would lead to higher rates of cancer. Experimental induction of an immunocompromised state was primitive at this time and typically involved thymectomy or antilymphocyte serum. Indeed, an increase was seen in these models in lymphomas and viral-associated tumors, but this was assumed to be because of infectious susceptibility rather than faulty immune surveillance against tumors.[9,10] The athymic nude mouse exploded onto the scientific scene during this time, bearing a spontaneous deletion in the *Foxn1* gene that leads to thymic absence and a loss of mature T cells. These mice were first described by Flanagan[13] in 1966 after their discovery within a group of albino mice in Glasgow. Nude mice became a commonly used strain because of their capacity to accept allografts and even xenografts without rejection.

A common model for spontaneous tumor induction at the time was 3-methylcholanthrene (MCA)-induced sarcomas. It was reasoned that if the cancer immunosurveillance hypothesis were true, then nude mice should develop more tumors with earlier onset after exposure to MCA. This was not the case in landmark experiments from Stutman and others, which led many investigators to conclude that the immune system does not affect cancer development.[11-14] Rygaard and Povlsen went as far as performing necropsies on 10,800 nude mice between 3 to 7 months of age, with no detectable difference in tumor formation compared with immunocompromised mice, again concluding that the immune system did not play a role in cancer development.[15] As an aside, nude mice have underdeveloped mammary glands and are unable to nurse their offspring, necessitating breeding with heterozygous females, lending some perspective to the scale of the work from these authors. Taking it a step further, Prehn uncovered inflammatory pathways that led to more aggressive tumors, ultimately proposing the immunostimulation theory to explain tumor-promoting inflammation.[16] Taken together, these findings led many to believe that the immune system could not target spontaneously developing tumors and may even fuel tumor progression.

Mouse Models Stimulate Resurgence of Cancer Immunosurveillance

To understand the gap between our current understanding of tumor immunology and the views held in the 1980s, it is worth examining the experimental limitations of this time. This is perhaps most evident in subsequent studies focusing on the biology of the athymic nude mouse. Not only do these mice have functional populations of T cells but they also produce a full complement of natural killer (NK) cells, about which little was known at the time.[17-20] It has been subsequently shown that a completely functional innate immune system can maintain some degree of cancer immunosurveillance in conjunction with the incomplete adaptive immune system present in the nude mouse. It is worth noting that toxin metabolism also contributed to discrepancies between expected and observed MCA-induced tumor formation. The strain of control mice used by Stutman[14] metabolized MCA into its carcinogenic form at a much higher rate than the nude mice, which predisposed these mice to higher rates of tumor formation.[21,22] Knowing these limitations, we can understand how the stage might be set for future insights to conflict with findings from the nude mouse.

Indeed, experiments incorporating MCA-induced tumor formation in mice on a different background (BALB/c) demonstrated increased tumor formation in athymic nude mice.[23-25] The introduction of severe combined immunodeficiency (SCID) mice further supported the resurrection of the cancer immunosurveillance concept. These mice lack functional DNA-dependent protein kinase (DNA-PK) and are unable to undergo somatic recombination, resulting in a lack of functional B and T cells. SCID mice also demonstrated increased MCA-induced tumor formation, although critics at the time attributed increased tumorigenicity to global defects in DNA repair.[26,27]

Definitive findings supporting tumor immunosurveillance are often attributed to a few sets of landmark tumor transplantation findings. The central concept here can be boiled down to this: If a tumor must evolve in response to cancer immunosurveillance to progress, these immune-evading adaptations may not be present in immunocompromised mice. Thus transplantation into an immunocompetent host may trigger immediate recognition and rejection. The field of cancer immunology would soon be inundated with investigations confirming this effect.

The effects of interferon gamma (IFN-γ) on immune stimulation and tumor immunosurveillance were soon confirmed. Mice with defects in IFN-γ signaling demonstrated enhanced MCA-induced tumorigenicity, and many of these tumors were rejected when transplanted into immune-competent hosts.[28-30] A prominent role for cytotoxic T cells was confirmed with perforin$^{-/-}$ mice displaying enhanced susceptibility to tumor formation.[31] The importance of lymphocytes was further confirmed with the development of recombination activating gene (*RAG) 1* or *RAG2* knockout mice, genes required for somatic recombination *and* only expressed in lymphoid tissue.[32] Thus the counterargument that global DNA repair defects led to cancer development no longer applied.

Schreiber et al.[25] incorporated these concepts in a groundbreaking investigation that anchored support in the scientific community for the cancer immunosurveillance hypothesis. A key finding from these experiments is displayed in Fig. 6.1. To summarize, mice with defects in *RAG2*, *IFNGR1*, *STAT1*, or both *RAG2* and *STAT1* (RkSk) were all more susceptible to tumor formation from MCA treatment. Of note, STAT1 signaling is part of the IFN-γ pathway. Both *RAG2*$^{-/-}$ and *RkSk* mice developed spontaneous tumors at a higher rate than controls in pathogen-free environments. Finally, approximately 40% of MCA-induced tumors transplanted from *RAG2*$^{-/-}$ mice into immunocompetent controls were rejected. No tumors were rejected by *RAG2*$^{-/-}$ mice transplanted from controls.[25] A host of similar investigations supporting tumor immunosurveillance ensued, which are summarized in Table 6.1.[25,30,33-38] Thus advances in our understanding of mouse models effectively rejuvenated scientific enthusiasm for the tumor immunosurveillance hypothesis.

Current Experimental Evidence Supporting Tumor Immune Surveillance

The development of organ transplantation heralded a series of clinical observations confirming that patients who are immunocompromised are at higher risk for the development of cancer. Early epidemiologic studies examining this population did demonstrate an increase in cancers of

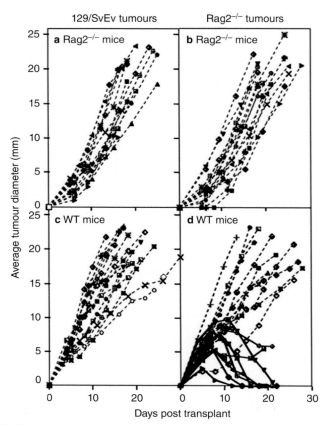

Fig. 6.1   (a) Cells derived from MCA-induced tumors in *RAG2⁻ᐟ⁻* mice or (b) wild-type (WT) mice were inoculated into *RAG2⁻ᐟ⁻* mice. Similarly, cells derived from MCA-induced tumors in (c) WT mice or (d) *RAG2⁻ᐟ⁻* mice were inoculated into WT mice. Solid lines represent rejected tumors.[25] (Adapted from Shankaran V, Ikeda H, Bruce AT, et al. IFNgamma and lymphocytes prevent primary tumour development and shape tumour immunogenicity. *Nature.* 2001;410(6832):1107–1111, figure 3.)

viral etiology, such as lymphoma, Kaposi sarcoma, and anogenital carcinomas.[39-41] Thus it was initially difficult to tease out whether viral susceptibility drove the increased rate of cancer, rather than defects in immunosurveillance. However, subsequent studies over longer periods of time confirmed significantly increased rates of malignant melanoma, particularly in the pediatric population.[42] Investigations also demonstrated elevated rates of colon, pancreatic, lung, bladder, kidney, ureter, and endocrine tumors.[39,43] There is currently a wealth of data supporting increased rates of non-viral-associated malignancies in patients who are immunocompromised, lending further support to the cancer immunosurveillance hypothesis.

In addition to observations in individuals who are immunocompromised, the composition of immune cells within solid tumors has consistently demonstrated prognostic value, particularly with respect to cytotoxic T-cell presence.[44-53] The concept of cancer immunosurveillance is perhaps most compellingly supported by the development of immune checkpoint blockade. Agents such as ipilimumab and nivolumab antagonize inhibitory receptors on T cells that accumulate with prolonged activation. These agents have met with unprecedented success in treating numerous types of tumors, confirming the idea that the immune system is capable of targeting tumors.

TABLE 6.1 ■ **Effects of Immune-Related Factors on Tumor Formation**

Phenotype	Tumor Susceptibility
RAG2$^{-/-}$	MCA-induced sarcomas (Shankaran et al, Nature, 2001) Spontaneous intestinal neoplasia (Shankaran et al, Nature, 2001)
RkSk	MCA-induced sarcomas (Shankaran et al, Nature, 2001) Spontaneous intestinal and mammary neoplasia (Shankaran et al, Nature, 2001)
BALB/c SCID	MCA-induced sarcomas (Smyth et al, Int Immunol, 2001)
Perforn$^{-/-}$	MCA-induced sarcomas (Street et al, Blood, 2001), (Smyth et al, J Exp Med, 2000), (van den Broek et al, J Exp Med, 1996) Spontaneous disseminated lymphomas (Street et al, J Exp Med, 2002), (Smyth et al, J Exp Med, 2000)
TCR Jα281$^{-/-}$	MCA-induced sarcomas (Shankaran et al, Nature, 2001), (Street et al, Blood, 2001), (Smyth et al, J Exp Med, 2000)
Anti-asialo-GM1 antibody	MCA-induced sarcomas (Shankaran et al, Nature, 2001)
Anti-NK1.1 antibody	MCA-induced sarcomas (Shankaran et al, Nature, 2001), (Smyth et al, J Exp Med, 2000)
Anti-Thy1 antibody	MCA-induced sarcomas (Shankaran et al, Nature, 2001), (Smyth et al, J Exp Med, 2000)
αβ T cell$^{-/-}$	MCA-induced sarcomas (Girardi et al, Science, 2001)
γδ T cell$^{-/-}$	MCA-induced sarcomas (Girardi et al, Science, 2001) DMBA/TPA-induced skin tumors (Girardi et al, Science, 2001)
STAT1$^{-/-}$	MCA-induced sarcomas (Shankaran et al, Nature, 2001), (Kaplan et al, PNAS, 1998)
IFNGR1$^{-/-}$	MCA-induced sarcomas (Shankaran et al, Nature, 2001), (Kaplan et al, PNAS, 1998)
IFN-γ$^{-/-}$	MCA-induced sarcomas (Street et al, Blood, 2001) Spontaneous disseminated lymphomas (Street et al, J Exp Med, 2002) Spontaneous lung adenocarcinoma (Street et al, J Exp Med, 2002)
Perforin$^{-/-}$ x IFN-γ$^{-/-}$	MCA-induced sarcomas (Street et al, Blood, 2001) Spontaneous disseminated lymphomas (Street et al, J Exp Med, 2002)
IL-12$^{-/-}$	MCA-induced sarcomas (Smyth et al, J Exp Med, 2000)
Exogenous IL-12	Lower incidence of MCA-induced sarcomas (Noguchi et al, PNAS, 1996)

Adapted from Dunn GP, Bruce AT, Ikeda H, Old LJ, Schreiber RD. Cancer immunoediting: from immunosurveillance to tumor escape. *Nat Immunol.* 2002;3(11):991–998, table I.

Immune Editing in Cancer

The concept of cancer immunoediting has evolved from the original hypothesis of cancer immunosurveillance to account for immune activity at later stages of cancer development. We can again draw on the experiments of Shankaran et al. for evidence of immune editing, which demonstrated that tumors formed in immunocompromised mice were more immunogenic that tumors formed in immunocompetent mice.[25] A series of tumor transplantation experiments confirmed these findings. Clinical correlates supporting the concept of immune editing include frequent observations that tumors lack antigen presentation components or mediators of the IFN-γ signaling pathway.[54]

The current model of cancer immune editing encompasses three processes: elimination, equilibrium, and escape. Elimination is thought to include early alarm signals to the presence of a tumor, IFN-γ production, chemotaxis and activation of innate immune cells, limited tumor cell killing with antigen processing by dendritic cells, and, finally, T-cell activation and chemotaxis to eliminate the remaining tumor.[55-64] In agreement with many of the experiments discussed in this chapter, IFN-γ is central to the process of early tumor elimination. However, the coordination of the innate and adaptive immune systems is also critical.

Equilibrium refers to a state of tumor development that has survived the elimination phase. Like the name implies, equilibrium can be likened to a stalemate between the immune system and the tumor. Lymphocytes and NK cells continue to exert selection pressure on the entrenched tumor as it continues to accumulate mutations and evolve in response to this pressure. The immune system is unable to eliminate the tumor, but the tumor is unable to progress. Equilibrium is thought to be the longest of the three processes, occurring over a period of years. One can imagine how this phase provides a perfect environment for tumors to evolve mechanisms to evade detection and/or killing by the immune system.

The escape process refers to the malignancies diagnosed clinically. By this point, the tumor has evaded constraints from the immune system and progresses at a largely unchecked pace. Until the 2000s, we had no reliable methods to stimulate the immune system and challenge this process. Immune checkpoint blockade has provided a way to even the balance again and confirm observations from a prolonged equilibrium phase, such as T-cell exhaustion with chronic stimulation. A summary of immune editing is presented in Fig. 6.2. For further reading, the evolution of tumor immunosurveillance and current framework of immune editing is summarized well in Dunn et al.[65]

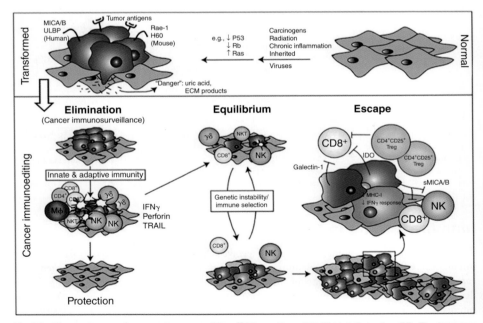

Fig. 6.2 Three phases of cancer immunoediting.[85] (From: Dunn GP, Old LJ, Schreiber RD. The immunobiology of cancer immunosurveillance and immunoediting. *Immunity.* 2004;21(2):137–148, figure 1.)

Tumor-Associated Antigens

The idea of conserved tumor-associated antigens that provide targets for antitumor immune responses has been posited for some time. Early experiments in the 1960s demonstrated that irradiated tumor cells could induce sustained immunity to future tumor challenges.[66,67] Modern approaches have allowed us to identify many of these antigens at the molecular level.

The development of hybridomas in the 1970s allowed for B-cell immortalization to expand rare clones. With this approach, mice could be immunized with tumor cells and tumor-specific targets could be identified (Fig. 6.3).[68] In the late 1980s and early 1990s, several investigators were able to isolate T cells reactive to mucin antigens from patients with epithelial cancers.[69-75] A major advance came with the identification of the cancer testis antigens, with expression normally restricted to germ cells. Many tumors express these genes, particularly melanoma. Cancer testis antigens include MAGEA1, NY-ESO-1, SSX, and many others. MAGEA1 was first cloned in 1991 and found to be recognized by T cells in a human leukocyte antigen (HLA)-dependent manner.

Discovery of these agents was a long, laborious, and, in many cases, quite fortuitous process. The capacity to elute peptides from HLA class I molecules and characterize the products with mass spectrometry provided a high-throughput modality to identify potential T-cell targets.[75] This methodology led to years of experiments eluting peptides from cancer HLA class I molecules and testing T-cell reactivity to these peptides, ultimately leading to a small library of known tumor-associated antigens.

Current methods to identify tumor-associated antigens largely revolve around whole exome sequencing, which allows rapid identification of personalized targets. Candidate mutations are typically analyzed with an algorithm to predict binding affinity to the patient's HLA molecules (i.e., NetMHCpan). This is a common approach, and efforts have compiled an extensive library of tumor neoantigens from The Cancer Genome Atlas (TCGA) database, which can be accessed as

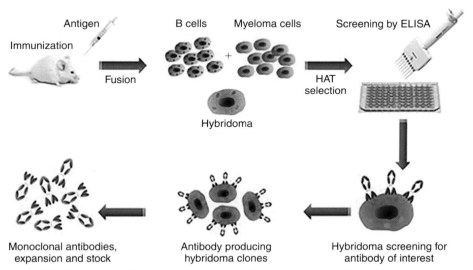

Fig. 6.3 Hybridoma technology to isolate clonal antibodies against new targets. B cells from mice immunized against tumor antigens are isolated and fused with myeloma cells, generating hybridomas that can be further analyzed and used for antibody production.[86] (From: Saeed AF, Wang R, Ling S, Wang S. Antibody engineering for pursuing a healthier future. *Front Microbiol.* 2017;8:495, figure 2.)

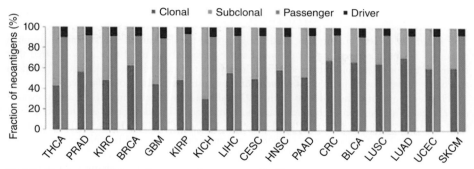

Fig. 6.4   Data compiled from the cancer immunome atlas[76]. The fraction of neoantigens representing driver mutations across solid tumors is displayed in purple, representing an average of 7.6%. Factoring in tumor heterogeneity, clonal neoantigens are displayed in blue and subclonal neoantigens are displayed in yellow. On average, 56% of neoantigens were clonal in origin.[76] *BLCA,* Bladder urothelial carcinoma; *BRCA,* breast invasive carcinoma; *CESC,* cervical squamous cell carcinoma; *CRC,* colorectal adenocarcinoma; *GBM,* glioblastoma multiforme; *HNSC,* head and neck squamous cell carcinoma; *KICH,* kidney chromophobe; *KIRC,* kidney renal clear cell carcinoma; *KIRP,* kidney renal papillary cell carcinoma; *LIHC,* liver hepatocellular carcinoma; *LUAD,* lung adenocarcinoma; *LUSC,* lung squamous cell carcinoma; *PAAD,* pancreatic adenocarcinoma; *PRAD,* prostate adenocarcinoma; *SKCM,* skin cutaneous melanoma; *THCA,* thyroid carcinoma; *UCEC,* uterine corpus endometrial carcinoma. (From: Charoentong P, Finotello F, Angelova M, et al. Pan-cancer immunogenomic analyses reveal genotype-immunophenotype relationships and predictors of response to checkpoint blockade. *Cell Rep.* 2017;18(1):248–262, figure 3F.)

The Cancer Immunome Atlas (https://tcia.at).[76] Antigens predicted to bind a patient's HLA molecules may then be evaluated by generating the corresponding peptides and testing recognition by autologous T cells. In some cases, identification of neoantigens from common driver mutations has led to extraordinary clinical responses when these neoantigen-specific T cells are expanded and reinfused. However, as may be seen in Fig. 6.4, the fraction of neoantigens involving driver mutations is uniformly low across tumor types. Additionally, analysis of the cancer immunome atlas identified 911,548 unique neoantigens, of which only 24 were shared in at least 5% of patients, suggesting that an "off-the-shelf" neoantigen therapy may not be feasible at this time.

In addition to libraries of neoantigens from these analyses, it is important to note that tumor-associated antigens can arise from processes other than mutation-associated peptides and expression of cancer testis antigens. Data suggest that alternative splicing of RNA sequences may account for more tumor-associated antigens than somatic mutations.[77] Resultant proteins are now being evaluated for therapeutic potential as vaccines and T-cell targets in adoptive cellular therapies. This remains a novel and exciting avenue of research. Taken together with our current understanding of tumor-associated antigens, we have come a long way in identifying personalized targets. However, therapeutic application of these vast libraries of peptides remains in its infancy.

Antigen-Specific Immune Surveillance of Oncogene-Induced Premalignant Senescent Cells

Though cellular senescence was initially thought to be limited to cells with terminal telomere erosion and no further replication potential, we now know that this genetic program is incorporated by cells undergoing a variety of stressors. Oncogene activation can paradoxically trigger senescence under certain conditions, termed *oncogene-induced senescence,* which typically involves intact tumor suppressor pathways.[78] Senescent cells in the microenvironment were often considered a tumor-promoting entity, because the senescence-associated secretory profile involves a number of growth factors. However, contemporary analyses repeatedly demonstrate a chemokine

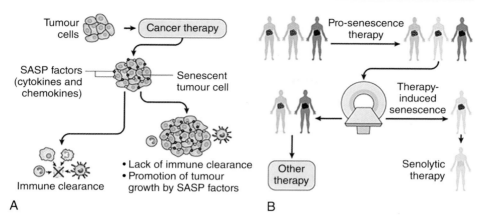

Fig. 6.5 Therapy-induced senescence (TIS) in cancer. (A) Senescence-associated secretory phenotype (SASP) results in immune clearance or, in some cases, fuels tumor growth. (B) Therapies promoting senescence must be selectively delivered to patients with cancers undergoing an appropriate TIS.[87] (From: Wolter K, Zender L. Therapy-induced senescence—an induced synthetic lethality in liver cancer? *Nat Rev Gastroenterol Hepatol.* 2020;17(3):135–136, figure 1.)

response that attracts innate immune cells. This can lead to a cascade of events described in the tumor elimination process described in the section **Immune editing in cancer**, leading to sustained antitumor immunity.

Experimental evidence of antigen-specific immune surveillance targeting senescent cells is exemplified by experiments from Kang et al.[79] examining premalignant senescent hepatocytes. Genetic ablation of CD4 T cells impaired clearance of $Nras^{G12V}$-expressing senescent hepatocytes, resulting in increased susceptibility to the development of hepatocellular carcinoma. Similar findings were demonstrated in SCID mice. Accordingly, CD4 T cells reactive against $Nras^{G12V}$-mutated hepatocytes were found in mice with senescent $Nras^{G12V}$ hepatocytes but not in mice with impaired tumor suppressor pathways and $Nras^{G12V}$ hepatocytes, in which senescence induction was blunted. The authors concluded that senescence induction in premalignant cells leads to an antigen-specific immune response.[78] Cancer immunosurveillance may therefore be fueled, at least in part, by oncogene-induced senescence in premalignant cells.

Subsequent data from Brenner et al. demonstrated that deletion of senescence-inducing cell cycle regulators CDKN2A or CDKN1A conferred resistance to immune checkpoint blockade in tumors that were previously susceptible. The group further demonstrated that melanoma lesions progressing rapidly through immunotherapy were associated with loss of senescence-inducing genes.[80] These findings are summarized in Fig. 6.5, demonstrating a potential role for directed senolytic therapies in cancer.

Microbiome and Microbial Proteins

The microbiome will be covered in detail in Chapter 11 of this text, but it is worth noting certain relationships between microbial proteins and tumor immunosurveillance. The gastrointestinal tract is colonized by trillions of organisms; any compositional and functional alteration in this microbiota is termed *dysbiosis*. Chronic inflammation from dysbiosis has been linked to accumulation of suppressive myeloid phenotypes, such as the M2 macrophage and the myeloid-derived suppressor cell (MDSC). Bacterial proteins can target inhibitory receptors on lymphocytes and NK cells. Alternatively, certain bacterial species, such as *Bacteroides fragilis* and *Bifidobacterium*, are associated with positive effects on dendritic cell (DC) maturation. Accordingly, antibiotic treatments can blunt the efficacy of antigen presentation and costimulatory signals in DCs.[81] These findings that aid our understanding of this very complex relationship are encouraging. However, given the density and diversity of bacterial species, more work is needed to deconvolute effects on innate immunity.

Effects of the microbiome on T-cell function are also important to discuss, although effects on innate immunity in these cases are often difficult to exclude. Certain bacterial species have been shown to predispose T cells to IFN-γ-associated T helper (Th) 1 cell responses, an effect that was abrogated with antibiotic treatment. The microbiome has also been associated with regulatory T-cell function, which may contribute to immune escape in early tumors. B cells have also been implicated in microbiome effects on tumor development, as certain bacterial species have been associated with interleukin (IL)-10 production in B cells. Taken together, our knowledge regarding microbiome effects on tumor immunosurveillance remains incompletely described. However, a number of promising translational avenues are being pursued, as summarized in Fig. 6.6. For further reading, a review of current data regarding the microbiome in cancer immunology was provided by Liu et al.[81]

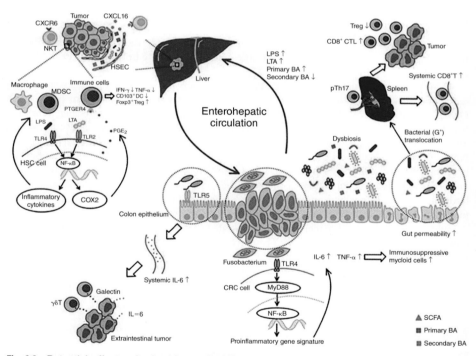

Fig. 6.6 **Potential effects of microbiome alterations on tumor immunosurveillance.** Many of these effects are centered around innate immune pathogen detection pathways, with subsequent production of cytokines and further innate immune cell recruitment.[81] *BA,* Bile acid; *CRC,* colorectal cancer; *HCC,* hepatocellular carcinoma; *HSC,* hepatic stellate cell; *HSEC,* hepatic sinusoidal endothelial cell; *LPS,* lipopolysaccharide; *LTA,* lipoteichoic acid; *MDSC,* myeloid-derived suppressor cell; *PAMP,* pathogen-associated molecule pattern; *SCFA,* short-chain fatty acids; *TLR,* Toll-like receptor; *TME,* tumor microenvironment. (From: Liu X, Chen Y, Zhang S, Dong L. Gut microbiota-mediated immunomodulation in tumor. *J Exp Clin Cancer Res.* 2021;40(1):221, figure 2.)

In addition to direct effects on immune cell signaling, the concept of antigen mimicry has been studied in the context of the microbiome. By the numbers, it is estimated that the cumulative microbiota contain roughly 10,000 times the DNA content of the human body. Statistically, the likelihood of some of the resulting peptides to mimic tumor-associated antigens is high.[82] However, this remains a complex area of investigation and observations remain largely correlative. Fig. 6.7 displays a schematic describing a bioinformatic approach to elucidate the relevance of microbial neoantigen mimicry in cancer. This remains an exciting investigative direction that may considerably advance our understanding of tumor immunosurveillance.

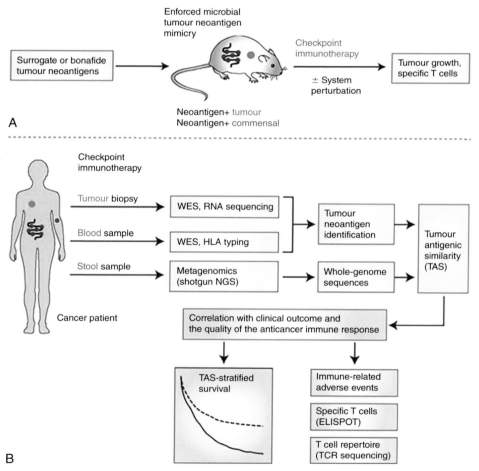

Fig. 6.7   Strategies to assess the relevance of microbial neoantigen mimicry in cancer. (A) Tumors with validated neoantigens and engineered microbial contents can be evaluated as a model of "enforced" mimicry. (B) Clinical correlates of microbial neoantigen mimicry, culminating in a tumor antigenic similarity (TAS) score that may be correlated with antitumor immune responses.[82] *ELISPOT,* Enzyme-linked immunospot assay; *NGS,* next-generation sequencing; *TAS,* tumor antigenic similarity; *TCR,* T-cell receptor; *WES,* whole exome sequencing. (From: Boesch M, Baty F, Rothschild SI, et al. Tumour neoantigen mimicry by microbial species in cancer immunotherapy. *Br J Cancer.* 2021;125(3):313–323, figure 2.)

Cancer in the Immunocompromised Host

As discussed briefly in the section **Current experimental evidence supporting tumor immune surveillance**, the widespread use of organ transplantation has led to a plethora of insights regarding tumor immunosurveillance in individuals who are immunocompromised. The elevated incidence of cancer in the human immunodeficiency virus (HIV)-infected population has prompted similar insights. A consistent finding in both of these populations is that viral-mediated cancers tend have the highest standardized incidence ratio (Fig. 6.8).[83,84] However, the incidence of nonviral solid tumors remains elevated in both populations, suggesting defects in tumor immunosurveillance. A comprehensive summary of current epidemiologic data regarding cancer in the immunocompromised host may be found in Engels.[83]

Interestingly, with the exception of cutaneous squamous cell carcinomas, the prognosis of cancer in individuals who are immunocompromised is not worse when outcomes are narrowed to

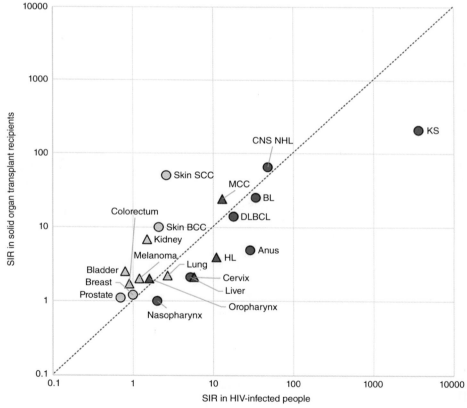

Fig. 6.8 **Standardized incidence ratios (SIRs) of cancer types in solid organ transplant recipients versus individuals with HIV infection.** Cancers in red are associated with a viral etiology. Triangles signify susceptibility to immune checkpoint blockade and subsequent U.S. Food and Drug Administration (FDA) approval as of 2019.[83] *BCC,* Basal cell carcinoma; *BL,* Burkitt lymphoma; *DLBCL,* diffuse large B-cell lymphoma; *HL,* Hodgkin lymphoma; *KS,* Kaposi sarcoma; *MCC,* Merkel cell carcinoma; *SCC,* squamous cell carcinoma. (From: Engels EA. Epidemiologic perspectives on immunosuppressed populations and the immunosurveillance and immunocontainment of cancer. *Am J Transplant.* 2019;19(12):3223–3232, figure 1.)

cancer-specific mortality. This is an important distinction, because all-cause mortality in patients who are immunocompromised remains higher than that among nonimmunocompromised populations. It is also logical to assume that cancers with higher mutational burdens would be more common in patients who are immunocompromised. Again, with the exception of cutaneous squamous cell carcinoma, patients who are immunocompromised demonstrate little to no differences in tumor mutational burden compared with the general population.[83] In summary, epidemiologic studies in immunocompromised populations generally support the concept of tumor immunosurveillance, but more work is needed to understand this process in clinically relevant immunocompromised environments.

Key References

6. Burnet M. Immunological factors in the process of carcinogenesis. *Br Med Bull.* 1964;20:154-158.
14. Stutman O. Tumor development after 3-methylcholanthrene in immunologically deficient athymic-nude mice. *Science.* 1974;183(4124):534-536.
15. Rygaard J, Povlsen CO. The mouse mutant nude does not develop spontaneous tumours. An argument against immunological surveillance. *Acta Pathol Microbiol Scand B Microbiol Immunol.* 1974;82.
16. Prehn RT. Perspectives on oncogenesis: does immunity stimulate or inhibit neoplasia? *J Reticuloendothel Soc.* 1970;10.
25. Shankaran V, Ikeda H, Bruce AT, et al. IFNgamma and lymphocytes prevent primary tumour development and shape tumour immunogenicity. *Nature.* 2001;410(6832):1107-1111.
28. Dighe AS, Richards E, Old LJ, Schreiber RD. Enhanced in vivo growth and resistance to rejection of tumor cells expressing dominant negative IFN gamma receptors. *Immunity.* 1994;1(6):447-456.
30. Street SE, Trapani JA, MacGregor D, Smyth MJ. Suppression of lymphoma and epithelial malignancies effected by interferon gamma. *J Exp Med.* 2002;196(1):129-134.
31. Street SE, Cretney E, Smyth MJ. Perforin and interferon-gamma activities independently control tumor initiation, growth, and metastasis. *Blood.* 2001;97(1):192-197.
32. Shinkai Y, Rathbun G, Lam KP, et al. RAG-2-deficient mice lack mature lymphocytes owing to inability to initiate V(D)J rearrangement. *Cell.* 1992;68(5):855-867.
34. Girardi M, Oppenheim DE, Steele CR, et al. Regulation of cutaneous malignancy by gammadelta T cells. *Science.* 2001;294(5542):605-609.
35. Smyth MJ, Thia KY, Street SE, MacGregor D, Godfrey DI, Trapani JA. Perforin-mediated cytotoxicity is critical for surveillance of spontaneous lymphoma. *J Exp Med.* 2000;192(5):755-760.
37. van den Broek ME, Kagi D, Ossendorp F, et al. Decreased tumor surveillance in perforin-deficient mice. *J Exp Med.* 1996;184(5):1781-1790.
38. Noguchi Y, Jungbluth A, Richards EC, Old LJ. Effect of interleukin 12 on tumor induction by 3-methylcholanthrene. *Proc Natl Acad Sci U S A.* 1996;93(21):11798-11801.
41. Gatti RA, Good RA. Occurrence of malignancy in immunodeficiency diseases. A literature review. *Cancer.* 1971;28(1):89-98.
42. Penn I. Malignant melanoma in organ allograft recipients. *Transplantation.* 1996;61(2):274-278.
44. Clemente CG, Mihm MC Jr, Bufalino R, Zurrida S, Collini P, Cascinelli N. Prognostic value of tumor infiltrating lymphocytes in the vertical growth phase of primary cutaneous melanoma. *Cancer.* 1996;77(7):1303-1310.
54. Khong HT, Restifo NP. Natural selection of tumor variants in the generation of "tumor escape" phenotypes. *Nat Immunol.* 2002;3(11):999-1005.
78. Hoenicke L, Zender L. Immune surveillance of senescent cells-biological significance in cancer- and non-cancer pathologies. *Carcinogenesis.* 2012;33(6):1123-1126.

Visit Elsevier eBooks+ (eBooks.Health.Elsevier.com) for complete set of references.

CHAPTER 7

The Essential Elements of Adaptive Immunity and Their Relevance to Cancer Immunology

Timothy N.J. Bullock

SUMMARY OF KEY FACTS

- Receptors of adaptive immune cells and the ensuing signaling networks are exquisitely specific and sensitive to new or altered antigens and thus poised to respond to tumors.
- The capacity of adaptive immune cells to traffic to sites of inflammation is programmed during initial priming and allows them to seek and destroy metastatic deposits throughout the body.
- The ability to form self-renewing memory cells that can reside in strategically important locations in the body can promote rapid responses to reexposure to antigen.
- Dendritic cells serve as conduits of both antigenic and inflammatory information between innate and adaptive immune systems.
- Dendritic cells exist in several maturation and differentiation states that have different capacities to acquire and present antigen in different costimulatory contexts.
- Cytokine production during antigen presentation by dendritic cells influences how T cells differentiate into effector and memory cell populations.
- Both T and B cells undergo metabolic alterations that provide the building blocks for their expansion and subsequent differentiation to either effector or memory populations.
- Chemokine receptors and integrins regulate the recruitment and trafficking of T and B cells both in secondary lymphoid organs and in inflamed peripheral tissues.
- Diversity in the differentiation state of helper CD4$^+$ T cells promotes their ability to interact with and influence both innate immune populations such as macrophages and other adaptive immune cells including cytotoxic CD8$^+$ T cells and antibody-producing B cells.
- The absence of inflammation within tumors limits dendritic cell activation and the quality of the ensuing immune response.
- Tumors and the tumor microenvironment contain molecules that are designed to limit adaptive immune responses and can limit immune-mediated destruction of tumors.
- Understanding the composition and function of adaptive immune receptors has allowed their development as therapeutic and diagnostic tools for cancer therapy.
- Biologic variations such as age and sex can have important influences on the quantity and quality of adaptive immune responses.

Introduction

Overwhelming evidence, both experimental and observational, indicates that cells of the adaptive immune system can limit the ability of tumors to grow and spread throughout the body. Mice with genetic lesions in molecules critical for the development or regulation of adaptive immune responses have a dramatically increased level of tumor formation and more advanced tumors than their wild-type counterparts.[1] Transfer of lymphocytes from mice that have eradicated tumors can provide protection against tumor challenge in naïve, unexposed mice.[2] The presence of lymphocytes, particularly T cells, within patients' tumors is commonly a positive prognostic indicator.[3-6]

To fulfill these functions, cells of the adaptive immune system must have mechanisms to sense and respond to subtle changes in antigens expressed by transformed cells and the ability to traffic to the site of tumor growth and perform functions that limit tumor growth. This is achieved by the transfer of antigen from transformed cells to diverse populations of professional antigen-presenting cells (APCs), primarily dendritic cells. These cells traffic from the periphery to lymph nodes, the hubs of interactions between APCs and lymphocytes, or acquire free antigen in the lymph node via lymphatic drainage and present antigen in the context of major histocompatability complex (MHC) molecules to T cells. Soluble antigen follows the lymphatics and diffuses into the subcapsular sinus where it can be recognized by B cells. Larger antigens are presented to B cells by trafficking dendritic cells, macrophages, or follicular dendritic cells.

If the T cells express a cognate receptor that can bind MHC–antigen complexes and the APC is expressing critical costimulatory molecules, T cells will expand, differentiate, and traffic back to the site of antigen origin. Once in the tissue, T cells reencounter antigen on MHC molecules expressed by tumor cells, or local APCs, and are triggered to perform effector functions such as cytolysis and cytokine release. These effector molecules can either directly eliminate tumor cells or induce innate immune cells within the tumor microenvironment to release further effector molecules and induce tumoricidal activity that constrains tumor growth. Some of the expanded T cells differentiate to long-lived memory cells that can reside in tissue, recirculate, or take up long-term residence in lymph nodes, poised to respond to further exposure to antigen.

B cells, once activated by their cognate antigen, differentiate either into extrafollicular antibody-producing cells, called *plasmablasts*; traffic to germinal centers to become plasma cells whose antibody is modified by affinity maturation; or become long-lived memory B cells that are also capable of reexpanding into antibody-producing cells. The role of tumor antigen-specific antibodies in adaptive immune responses is not well defined. In addition, B cells can help promote nests of immune cells, known as *tertiary lymph node structures*, that can serve as local hubs that support and sustain both T- and B-cell responses to tumors.

Recognition of Tumor Antigens: Specificity Engendered by the T-Cell and B-Cell Receptors

A considerable advantage of immunotherapy compared with standard of care chemotherapies or radiation therapy is the exquisite specificity of the T-cell receptor (TCR) and the B-cell receptor (BCR)/antibodies for their cognate ligand. There are important differences in the nature of the ligand recognized by these two antigen receptors: the TCR binds to a complex of MHC and peptide derived from an independent protein, whereas antibodies, and thus the BCRs, bind to regions of free antigens without the involvement of other molecules (Fig. 7.1). Further, TCRs generally recognize ligands that are formed from antigens that are produced either from within the cell (MHC class I) or from extracellular sources (MHC class II), whereas antibodies and the BCRs primarily recognize extracellular antigen (because antibodies cannot naturally penetrate the cell membrane). In this chapter we will explore the basis of this specificity and delineate the signaling events initiated by these receptors because this knowledge has a direct effect on not only

Antibodies bind to unproccessed
segments of antigens

T cells recognize peptides from
antigen from inside cells,
presented on MHC molecules

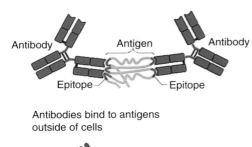

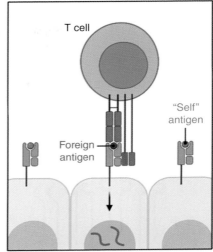

Fig. 7.1 Antibodies and T cells recognize different forms of antigen. Antibodies bind to either linear or discontinuous regions of their target antigen, known as *epitopes*. These antigens are almost exclusively extracellular. The T-cell receptor responds to small proteolytic fragments of antigens that are bound by MHC molecules within cells and then transported to the cell surface. (Created with BioRender.com.)

understanding checkpoint inhibition therapy but also the differences in the iterations of chimeric antigen receptor (CAR)-T generations currently in therapy.

STRUCTURE OF αβ T-CELL RECEPTOR

The TCR consists of two polypeptide chains, α and β, that are composed of variable (V) and junction (J) domains for the α chain (VJ) and an additional diversity (D) region for the β chain (VDJ) (Fig. 7.2). These chains result from somatic DNA recombination of germline genes during T-cell development in the thymus. Because gene rearrangement occurs at the somatic level, each T cell expresses thousands of copies of an identical single receptor after the recombination process is complete. This gene rearrangement is driven by recombinase-activating genes (*RAG1* and *RAG2*). The TCR α V locus comprises ~80 gene segments and ~60 J gene segments. The TCR β locus contains 52 V gene segments, 13 J gene segments, and 2 D segments. A single constant domain links the αβ TCR chains to signaling components of the CD3 complex that are responsible for initiating the signaling cascade within the T cell. Rearrangement of gene segments continues until the T cell receives a positive signal from self-MHC peptide complexes in the thymus or until the cell dies because of a lack of instructive signal from a successful rearrangement. The consequence of having two interacting chains that are derived from such a tremendous diversity of gene segments is the production of T cells each with a unique, highly specific TCRs capable of productively interacting with only a few MHC–peptide complexes. This notion is reinforced by evaluating crystal structures of the TCR, which show that the V region gene segments are clustered at the N-terminus of both the α and β chains, generating an antigen-binding domain that will contact the MHC–peptide complex.

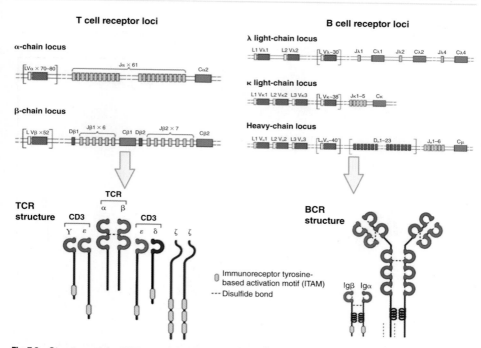

Fig. 7.2 **Structure of the TCR and BCR locus and encoded proteins.** Both the TCR and BCR loci consist of gene segments that are recombined to make α and β chains (for the TCR) or heavy and light chains (for the BCR). Both receptors interact with coreceptor molecules that contain signaling domains that initiate the lymphocyte's response to receptor engagement. Hypervariable regions in the membrane-distal regions of the receptors account for the majority of the binding specificity of these molecules. (Created with BioRender.com.)

A critical element in adaptive immunity is the ability to discriminate self-derived antigens from foreign or altered self-antigens. On the one hand, this is achieved with the incredible diversity and specificity of the TCR. However, an excessive T-cell pool is energetically demanding and raises the possibility of responding to self-antigens and the initiation of autoimmunity. One part of this puzzle is solved by survival signals in the thymus only being delivered to T cells whose TCR has an ability to engage the host MHC molecules. Those whose TCRs do not "match" the MHC of the host die by neglect. This process is referred to as *positive selection*.[7-9] If the resulting TCR has too high an affinity for MHC-self peptide complexes, the bearing T cell will subsequently undergo activation-induced apoptosis, known as *negative selection*.[10,11] This process is required to limit autoreactive T cells from transiting to the periphery. Together, these selection events sculpt the T-cell repertoire such that it is focused on discerning alterations in the proteome of the host cells. Interestingly, some of the first identified tumor antigens were shown to be normal melanocyte proteins,[12-14] suggesting that the selection process is not absolute.

STRUCTURE OF THE B-CELL IMMUNOGLOBULINS

Significant similarities are present in the construction of antibodies and their receptor counterparts to the processes that occur with TCR construction. The BCR is composed of heavy and light chains, which together generate the antigen-binding domain (Fig. 7.2). As with T cells, B-cell development and selection is a function of successful steps in the assembly of antigen receptor genes.[15] Progenitor B cells begin by rearranging the heavy chain locus containing V, D, and J gene segments. D-J recombination occurs first, followed by recombination with V genes, and finally the constant (C) region is added. In humans, the heavy chain locus contains 38 to 46 V gene segments, 23 D gene segments, 6 J segments, and 9 C segments. Two light chains, k and l, are available to pair with the heavy chain, and each of these has a high number (~29–38) of V genes and 5 J genes but no D genes. As with the TCR, this diversity results in a tremendous number of possible sequences encoded in the antigen-binding region and thus the repertoire of antigens that can be bound. Further variability is generated in antibody segments by two additional steps: (1) imprecise joining of gene segments, resulting in junctional diversity, and (2) DNA repair enzymes and terminal deoxynucleotidyl transferase activity removing and adding nucleotides randomly to the single-strand ends.[16]

Whereas the antigen binding fragment (Fab) is responsible for the neutralizing and absorptive activities of antibodies, for immunoglobulins, the addition of different constant regions (M, D, G, E, and A) to the heavy chain, thus defining their *isotype*, imbues different functional activity on the molecule.[17] These include different efficiencies in activating complement, binding to Fc receptors, and ability to cross the placenta. Immunoglobulin (Ig) D and IgM are translated from the same pre-mRNA transcript and are coexpressed on the surface of naïve, mature B cells. These heavy chains undergo instructional class-switching after first engagement with antigen, under the guidance of T cells. Importantly, transmembrane (B-cell receptor) and secreted (antibody) forms of these immunoglobulins are generated from the same mRNA transcript by differential splicing of mRNA to replace exons encoding a membrane anchor with exons encoding secretion sequences. These concepts are more thoroughly described in Chapter 2. The secreted forms of antibodies have been extensively exploited in therapeutic settings, particularly once the development of monoclonal antibody *hybridoma* technology (where an immortalized B cell secretes large quantities of a single antibody) allowed the production of large quantities of homogeneous, highly defined antibody product.[18] Some of the uses of monoclonal antibodies in cancer therapy are described in Table 7.1.

Understanding the proteomic and genetic makeup of antibodies has allowed the further development of this resource beyond the initial hybridoma approaches to those that include isolation and expression of antibodies from individual B-cell clones and approaches that limit the inherent immunogenicity of murine proteins injected into humans. Note that exploration of synthetic TCRs as potential therapeutics,[19,20] targeting MHC–peptide complexes presented at the surface of tumor cells, is an ongoing and expanding field of research.

TABLE 7.1 ■ Uses of Monoclonal Antibodies

Type	Intent	Example
Antagonist	Blocks receptor–ligand interactions	Impeding checkpoint molecules; e.g., PD-1 or CD73; CSF-1
Agonist	Cross-linking activating receptors	Stimulating costimulatory molecules; e.g., CD134 (OX40), CD40
Antibody–drug conjugate	Tumoricidal activity	HER2-neu; ado-trastuzumab emtansine (T-DM1)
Imaging	Detection of metastases	Indium-111 satumomab, colorectal and ovarian cancer
Antigen capture	Monitoring tumor burden	CA-125; PSA
Antigen capture	Immune function assays	Cytokine ELISA; ELISPOTs

ELISA, Enyzme-linked immunoabsorbance assay; *ELIspot,* enzyme-linked immunospot; *HER-2,* human epidermal growth factor receptor 2; *PD-1,* programmed death 1; *CSF-1,* colony stimulating factor 1; *PSA,* prostate specific antigen

Antigen Receptor Signaling

SIGNALING FROM T-CELL RECEPTOR

For naïve T cells to proliferate and differentiate after engagement of the TCR by MHC–peptide complexes presented by dendritic cells (DCs), or for effector T cells to perform their functions upon reencountering their cognate antigen, signals must by propagated within the T cell, generally via the induction of enzymatic activity. Many of the common principles of receptor signaling were originally determined in the study of T cells. Knowledge of the mechanistic basis of TCR signaling has been critically important for understanding how checkpoint molecules such as Cytotoxic T lymphocyte Antigen -4 (CTLA-4) and Programmed Death 1 (PD1) work,[21] and how the construction of more effective chimeric antigen receptor T cells (CAR-T) can be achieved.[22]

Antigen-binding αβ T-cell receptor chains have no signaling capacity on their own. Rather, they associate with other molecules at the cell surface, CD3γ, CD3δ, CD3ε, and a ζ chain, which together form the CD3 complex (see Fig. 7.3).[23,24] The CD3 molecules are composed of immunoglobulin-like structures that have extracellular domains, and the ζ chain is primarily composed of a longer intracellular domain with only a short extracellular addition to the transmembrane domain. Critical to the ability to propagate signals, the intracellular domains of the CD3 proteins and the ζ protein contain immunoreceptor tyrosine-based activation motifs (ITAMs).[25,26] These ITAMs become

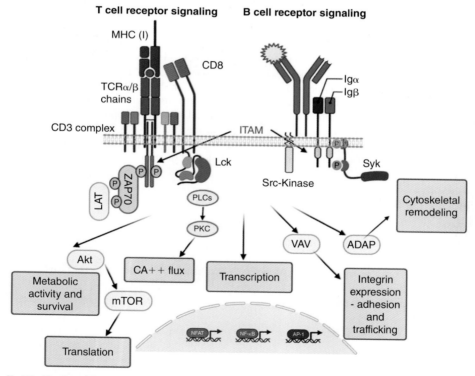

Fig. 7.3 **T-cell and B-cell receptor signaling share many common elements.** Signal transduction from TCR involves the recruitment and accumulation of phosphotyrosine kinases and SH-containing scaffold proteins that result in the coordinated activation of a variety of downstream enzymes that initiate the cellular modifications needed for further engagement, activation, and proliferation. Though molecules used in BCR signaling are slightly different, they are highly related and result in similar activation events. (Created with BioRender.com.)

phosphorylated by protein tyrosine kinases (PTKs) when the receptor complex engages its ligand. PTKs exist in two forms: as either intrinsic components of receptors (receptor tyrosine kinases [RTKs], such as the Fms-like tyrosine kinase 3 ligand (FLT3L) receptor) or as non-RTKs.[27] An example of non-RTKs would be Janus Kinases (JAK) associated with cytokine receptors or Lymphocyte-specific protein tyrosine kinase (Lck) associated with the TCR.[28] Non-RTKs are either constitutively associated with their receptors or are recruited after ligand binding. RTKs often multimerize to activate or are kept in inactive states by posttranslational modifications, as is the case with Lck.

Initial Signals

Charge interactions lead to the assembly of the TCR complex, which occurs in the endoplasmic reticulum and is required for export to the plasma membrane. ITAMs found in the invariant chains of the TCR drive phosphotyrosine signaling. In the case of the TCR, this function is performed in both $CD4^+$ and $CD8^+$ T cells by Lck. In naïve T cells, Lck is normally kept in a nonfunctional confirmation by autophosphorylation and phosphorylation by Csk[29]; it is released to function in the activation of TCRs by the CD45 phosphatase.[30] The initial phosphorylation of CD3 ITAMs is performed by Lck, allowing the recruitment of Src homology 2 (SH2)-containing scaffold proteins, including Linker for Activation of T cells (LAT) and SH2 domain containing leukocyte protein of 76kDa (SLP76) to the TCR complex (see Fig. 7.3). Antigen receptor ITAMs have two phosphorylation motifs, and the signaling intermediary ZAP70 has tandem SH2 domains that match these phosphorylation sites.[31-34] This stoichiometry enhances the specificity and interactivity of ZAP70 with the ε and ζ chains of the TCR. It is worth remembering that the ability of the TCR to recognize antigen must be very sensitive (because of the low copy numbers of MHC–peptide on APCs) and very specific (must not respond to similar ligands).[35,36] The arrangement and interactivity of the TCR signaling complex likely contributes to making it relatively difficult to activate, limiting nonspecific activation, but the presence of multiple enzymes also strongly enhances the signal once activated. It is currently unclear how antigen binding affects the stoichiometry/confirmation of the TCR complex to initiate signaling, and clustering of TCRs is difficult when antigen (i.e., infrequent MHC–peptide complexes on APCs) density is low. Microclusters of TCRs may form, changing the apparent concentration of TCRs and the ratio of activating and inactivating enzymes.[37,38]

The intensity, and thus effectiveness, of the signal varies with the affinity of the ligand (interestingly, the TCR has relatively low affinity for MHC–peptide complexes compared with antibody/BCR for their antigen; it is thought that this is necessary to allow sustained T-cell activation), the concentration of the ligand, the activity of phosphatases, and the concentration and availability of intracellular signaling components. Thus TCR signaling can by tunable and dynamic, and the signal strength has qualitative effects on downstream T-cell activity. The system is reset by a combination of phosphatases and ubiquitination and degradation of recycling receptors.

The signaling complex formed after initial TCR engagement is responsible for activating the enzymes that work downstream of TCR signaling to promote the functional activities of T cells (Fig. 7.3). These include Phospholipase C γ (PLCγ), which activates transcription factors via the production of Inositol trisphospate (IP3) and the initiation of Ca^{++} flux, which in turn serves as critical amplifier of post-TCR signals.[39] The transcription factors for full T-cell activation include nuclear factor of activated T cells (NFAT), activator protein 1 (AP-1) (for interleukin [IL]-2 production), and nuclear factor kappa B (NF-κB).[40,41] Activation of protein kinase B (AKT) (a serine/threonine kinase) promotes metabolic changes and initiates mammalian target of rapamycin (mTOR) activation, which is critical for protein translation.[42-44] Further pathways of activation include Vav, which controls cytoskeletal remodeling necessary, and adhesion and degranulation promoting adaptor protein (ADAP), which instigates the expression of integrins needed for cellular adhesion and trafficking. This remodeling drives the accumulation of the appropriate molecules into the contact site between the T cell and the antigen-presenting cell, known as the *supramolecular activation complex* (SMAC).

Many forms of severe combined immunodeficiency (SCID) result from defects in Lck, ZAP70, and other RTK involved in regulating T-cell activation.

B-CELL RECEPTOR SIGNALING

The BCR serves both as a signaling receptor, inducing the propagation of events that lead to functional changes within the B cell, and as an antigen-binding receptor for the purposes of antigen processing and presentation. Though in some instances, B cells can respond to antigen directly (T-independent antigens), these antigens tend to be associated with pathogenic infections and their allied adjuvant effects. Most B-cell responses require support of T cells, and the antigenic targets of these responses are referred to as T cell-dependent. Many aspects of BCR signaling are analogous to TCR signaling, because the antigen-binding domains of the BCR are associated with ITAM-containing components (Igα and Igβ) that transmute the signal.[45] In place of Lck, B cells use the protein tyrosine kinases Fyn, B lymphoycte kinase (Blk) and Lyn to phosphorylate ITAMs after BCR multimerization. Spleen tyrosine kinase (Syk) serves as the ZAP-70 equivalent in B cells and it contains two SH2 domains that allow recruitment to the phosphorylated BCR. In each case, the primary proliferative signal from the BCR is communicated via PI-3 kinase-mediated activation of RAS/MAPK (mitogen activated protein kinase) pathway, inducing the activation of the transcription factors AP-1 and NFAT. The coreceptor functions of CD4 and CD8, and to a certain extent CD28 costimulation, are replaced in B cells by the CD19–CD21–CD81 complex. CD21 binds complement CD3dg–decorated antigen and the ensuing activation results in the activation of Src family tyrosine kinase. This promotes further Syk activation and the recruitment of the scaffolding protein SLP-65 (a LAT-SLP76 equivalent) to the BCR,[33] and phosphorylation of CD19 permits the recruitment of phosphatidylinositol 3-kinase (PI3K). As a consequence of these activation events, the B cell can initiate remodeling events very similar to that seen in T cells, with phosphatidylinositol (3,4,5)-trisphosphase (PIP$_3$)/3-phosphoinositide-dependent kinase 1 (PDK1) leading to the activation of AKT, Bruton's tyrosine kinase (BtK) leading to the activation of phospholipase C-gamma (PLC-γ) to make diacylglyceride (DAG) and inositol trisphosphate (IP3),[46] and Vav activating Wiskott-Aldrich Syndrom Protein (WASP) and actin polymerization that precedes synapse formation that is necessary for antigen uptake and subsequent engagement of T helper cells. Targeting BtK is a therapeutic option for some B-cell malignancies.

Costimulation

CD28-SIGNAL 2

Antigen receptor binding (Signal 1) is insufficient to drive the full activation of naïve T and B cells. A second, conditioning, signal is needed to promote and sustain the activation and cycling of lymphocytes. In the case of T cells, in addition to TCR recognition of Ag/MHC complexes expressed on an APCs, such as a virus-infected dendritic cell, costimulatory signaling occurs via interaction between the costimulatory molecule CD28 and B7.1 or B7.2 (CD80/CD86),[47,48] if the APC expresses them.[49] This leads to induction of both the high-affinity IL-2 receptor (IL-2Rα) and IL-2,[50] which provides sufficient signals for proliferation, and the development of effector (cytotoxic) functions such as the generation of cytolytic granules. Recognition of the Ag–MHC complex is sufficient to drive the T cell from G0 into the G1 phase of the cell cycle but not through S phase (DNA replication). As such, the production of IL-2 can almost be considered a go–no go signal for T cells. Because Lck can also phosphorylate CD28 (if it is in the SMAC),[51,52] it can lead to the recruitment of growth factor receptor-bound protein 2 (Grb2), ultimately leading to the generation of more PIP$_3$. This has the effect of supporting the signaling modules described previously: PLCγ and downstream transcription factors, AKT and Vav, and the stabilization of IL-2 mRNA. CD28 stimulation is considered as Signal 2 in T-cell activation.

In the absence of Signal 2, T cells enter a state of unresponsiveness termed *anergy*. Anergy is not passive but is sustained by the expression of ubiquitin ligases such as gene related to anergy in lymphocytes (GRAIL) and c-Casitas B-lineaage (c-CBL) that actively degrade components of the TCR signaling process, limiting T-cell activation.[53,54] As might be anticipated, high doses of IL-2 can overcome the induction of anergy, likely by binding to the low-affinity IL-2βγ chain receptor. Anergy is induced in T cells when APCs are insufficiently activated (because of limited inflammation) to upregulate CD80 and/or CD86 but do present MHC–peptide complexes. This can occur in situations of peripheral tolerance (when new antigens arise as a function of developmental stages such as puberty) or in the case of slow-growing tumors. Importantly, the expression of CTLA-4, which serves as a competitor to CD28 on T cells for binding with CD80/CD86,[55,56] mimics the effects of encountering antigen without strong costimulation. Approaches that impede CTLA-4 have had some beneficial effects in several cancer entities.[57] Other costimulatory molecules include IgSF members such as inducible costimulator (ICOS) and members of the tumor necrosis factor receptor superfamily (TNFRSF), such as CD27, OX40, and 41BB. Stimulation of TNF superfamily molecules promotes the expression and activity of c-Jun N-terminal kinase (JNK) via their regulation of tumor necrosis factor receptor-associated factor (TRAF) molecules and thus NF-κB.[58] TNFRSF stimulation is primarily associated with T-cell survival, although some aspects of metabolic activity and memory cell differentiation have been attributed to these costimulatory molecules. TNFRSF receptors are often expressed 2 to 3 days after initial activation of DCs, providing a sustaining signal to activated T cells.

For B cells, the source of costimulation differs between the two types of antigens. T cell–independent BCR signals require support from the CD91–CD21–CD81 complex, which engages complement-bound antigens. This results in SH2-mediated enhancement of BCR signaling and the engagement of scaffolding signaling complexes that promote and multiply initial BCR signals. Further T cell–independent costimulation is supported by sensing additional pathogen-associated molecular patterns (PAMPs) from invading pathogens.[59] These provide a MyD88-dependent activation of the NF-κB pathway that supports B-cell activation, analogous to the role of NF-κB in T cells.[60]

The BCR serves both as a signaling receptor, inducing the propagation of events that lead to functional changes within the B cell, and also as a mechanism for internalizing antigen for presentation on MHC class II molecules, both turning the B cell into a professional antigen-presenting cell (APC). This ability to process and present antigen on MHC class II molecules allows B cells to interact with antigen-specific CD4+ T cells (in this case, T follicular helper cells [Tfh] located in the lymph nodes), which in turn support B cells by providing cytokines and receptor ligands that support B-cell proliferation and differentiation into either antibody-secreting cells or memory B cells (T cell–dependent processes).[61] Tfh signals include CD40L, which provides survival advantages via the noncanonical NF-kB pathway (mediated by NF-kB-inducing kinase [NIK]) and the induction of the survival factor BCL2,[62] and IL-21, which signals via signal transducer and activator of transcription 3 (STAT3) to promote proliferation and differentiation into memory and plasma cells.[63] B cell–activating factor (BAFF; also known as B lymphocyte stimulator, BLyS), a member of the TNF superfamily, provides additional survival signals for maturing B cells.[64]

EXHAUSTION

T-cell responses to cancer will be limited by the lack of costimulation during antigen presentation, leading to anergy, as described previously. In addition to anergy, T-cell responses within the tumor microenvironment are often curtailed because of the effect of chronic antigen presentation.[65,66] In this context, the consistent presence of antigen prevents the programmed acquisition of memory T-cell characteristics and the loss of pluripotent stemness.[67] Aligned with this is a reduced expression of cytokines, reduced killing capacity, and limited proliferation. As with anergy, this altered state is driven by changes in transcriptional activity (e.g., the ratios of T-box expressed in T cells (Tbet): Eomesodermin (Eomes),[68] T cell factor 1 (TCF1): Thymocyte Selection Associated High Mobility Group Box (TOX),[69,70] and B-cell lymphoma 6 (Bcl6): B lymphocyte-induced maturation protein-1 (BLIMP-1)[71,72]) and the expression of a wide array of checkpoint inhibitor molecules, including Programmed Death-1 (PD-1), T cell immunoreceptor with Ig and ITIM domains (TIGIT), and T cell immunoglobulin and mucin domain-containing protein 3 (TIM-3)[73] (Table 7.2), whose ligands are commonly expressed in the tumor microenvironment (TME).[74] The need for such an extensive network of counterstimulatory molecules is unclear. Transcriptional changes in exhausted T cells are quite distinct from those found in anergic T cells. Mechanistically, many of these molecules work by recruiting phosphatases (e.g., SHP2 in the case of PD1) that disrupt signal transduction pathways, thus attenuating signals from the TCR. Exhaustion is accompanied by metabolic alterations and, with time, epigenetic repression of key effector cell activities.[75] Extensive studies in experimental models and in clinical trials have demonstrated

TABLE 7.2 ■ Examples of Checkpoint Inhibitors

Receptor	Potential Ligand	Possible Mechanisms of Action
CTLA-4	CD80/CD86	Competes against CD28 costimulation
PD1	PDL1; PDL2 receptors	Recruits SHP-2 phosphatase to SMAC via ITIM; limits TCR and CD28 signals
Unknown	B7H3 (CD276)	Unclear; T-cell proliferation reduced
LAG3	MHC class II; L-SECtin; Gal3; FGL-1; α-syn	Diminishes TCR signaling
TIM3 (CD366)	GAL9; phosphatidylserine; HMGB1	Impedes DC activation by DAMPs; induces apoptosis of Th1
TIGIT	CD112/CD155	Competes with CD226 costimulation
BTLA	HVEM	SHP-1 and SHP-2 recruitment
CD160	HVEM	Lower IL-2 mRNA; CD3ζ phosphorylation
PSGL-1; VSIG3	VISTA (B7-H5)	Induces FOXP3
2B4 (CD244; SLAMF4)	CD48 (SLAMF2)	ITSM-mediated SHIP, SHP-1, SHP-2 recruitment; CsK recruitment
Unknown	B7-H3	Limits IFN-γ production; indirect effects by modulating MDSC
Unknown	B7-H4	Arrests cell cycle

BTLA, B and T lymphocyte attenuator; CsK, C-terminal Src kinase; DAMP, damage-associated molecular pattern; FGL-1, fibrinogen-like protein 1; FOXP3, forkhead box P3; Gal-3, galectin-3; Gal-9, galectin-9; HMGB1, high mobility group box 1; HVEM, herpesvirus entry mediator; ITIM, immunoreceptor tyrosine-based inhibition motif; ITSM, immunoreceptor tyrosine based-switch motif; LAG-3, lymphocyte-activation gene 3; LSECtin, lymph node sinusoidal endothelial cell C-type lectin; MDSC, myeloid-derived suppressor cell; PDL-1/PDL-2, programmed death ligand -1/-2; PSGL-1, P-selectin glycoprotein ligand-1; SHIP, SH-2 containing inositol 5' polyphosphatase; SHP-1/-2, Src homology region 2 domain-containing phosphatase-1/-2; SLAMF2/-4, signaling lymphocyte activation molecule family-2/-4; SMAC, supramolecular activation cluster; Th1, T helper cell type 1; TIGIT, T cell immunoreceptor with Ig and ITIM domains; TIM-3, T cell immunoglobulin and mucin-domain containing-3; VISTA, V-domain Ig suppressor of T cell activation; VSIG3, V-set and Ig domain-containing protein 3; α-syn, alpha-synuclein the efficacy of targeting these checkpoint molecules for cancer immunotherapy. Correlates of responsiveness in patients include the presence of T cells within the patient's TME and tumor mutational burden (TMB), which reflects the array of putative tumor antigens available for T cells to target.[76,77] In some instances, high doses of IL-2[78] or IL-7[79] can revert exhausted phenotypes.

Evidence for a similar exhaustion phenotype in B cells is mostly derived from studies of chronic/latent pathogen infections. B-cell exhaustion is also characterized by the expression of ITIM-containing inhibitory receptors, such as Fc receptor-like 4 (FCRL4) and sialic acid–binding Ig-like lectin 6 (Siglec-6) and downregulation of proliferative activity and BCR signaling.[80] The presence and function of exhausted B cells in the tumor microenvironment has not been well documented.

SENESCENCE

As with exhaustion, cellular senescence is a state of limited responsiveness that arises because of chronic antigen engagement[81] and with aging[82] (see **T-cell subsets in cancer immunity**). Senescent T cells are characterized as having reduced telomere lengths and increased DNA damage, perhaps reflective of the combination of extensive replication and the age of the host. The DNA damage response found in senescent T cells can be induced both by tumor cells themselves as well as regulatory T cells found within the tumor microenvironment. Further characteristics that demark senescent T cells from exhausted include the absence of the costimulatory molecules CD27 and CD28, upregulation of molecules associated with terminal differentiation killer cell lectin like Rreceptor G1 (KLRG1; CD57), and the extensive production of proinflammatory and antiinflammatory cytokines. Some checkpoint molecules associated with exhaustion can also be expressed (e.g., TIM3, TIGIT) by senescent T cells.[83] Proliferation is compromised by lesions in the proteins that are normally activated by TCR signaling, limiting the accumulation of phosphorylated signal transduction complexes.

Metabolic Adaptations Used by Lymphocytes
T-CELL METABOLIC PROGRAMMING

Considering the rapid proliferation by lymphocytes and the engrailment of effector activities, significant modifications occur in their metabolic activity to support these changes.[84] At the simplest conceptual level, naïve and memory T cells are considered metabolically quiescent, or anabolic, whereas effector T cells use catabolic processes to convert glucose into the building blocks of protein, nucleotide, and lipid synthesis necessary for rapid proliferation (Fig. 7.4). Quiescent T cells uptake glucose at modest levels and use oxidative phosphorylation to generate adenosine 5'-triphosphate (ATP). Quiescent T cells rely on fatty acid oxidation to produce ATP and nicotinamide adenine dinucleotide (NAD) + hydrogen (H) (NADH) in the mitochondria via the electron transport chain. Importantly, inhibition of fatty acid oxidation impairs memory T-cell formation, persistence, and function.[85] With the engagement of the TCR, initial proliferation is dependent on oxidative phosphorylation, but then T cells rapidly increase their glycolytic activity.[86,87] In T cells, the induction of MYC results in the elevated expression of glucose transporters and the enzymes of the glycolytic pathway.[88] Because the production of ATP is substantially lower via glycolysis compared with oxidative phosphorylation, at first this seems counterintuitive. However, the amount of glucose uptake increases considerably, compensating for the potential shortfall. Additionally, the metabolic kinetics of boosting mitochondrial production to enhance oxidative phosphorylation, compared with augmenting glycolytic enzyme production, factor into this. Critically, in addition to ATP production, NAD^+ is reduced to NADH, the cofactor for a plethora of enzymes, during glycolysis. The intermediaries of

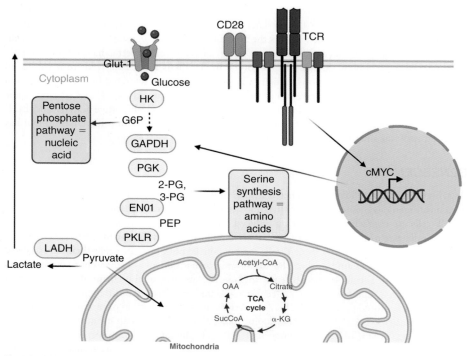

Fig. 7.4 Metabolic adaptations of lymphocytes. With receptor engagement, lymphocytes initiate metabolic alterations that arise with the induction of glycolysis. Activated lymphocytes induce the expression of transporters and enzymes that accumulate glucose and downstream intermediaries. Though ATP production is lower via glycolysis compared with oxidative phosphorylation, the increase in glucose uptake compensates for this and allows intermediaries to be shuttled into pathways that generate the building blocks of proliferating cells. (Created with BioRender.com.)

glycolysis are also used by the pentose phosphate pathway and other metabolic processes for the synthesis of nucleotides (e.g., glucose-6-phosphate), amino acids (e.g., 3-phosphoglycerate), and pyruvate/citrate and acetyl co-A, which are foundational for fatty acid and lipid synthesis. Importantly, impeding glycolysis shuts down both the latter stages of T-cell proliferation and effector function activity.[86,87] In the latter case, data suggest that enzymes involved in the glycolytic pathway can serve as translational inhibitors of cytokine production when not engaged in glycolysis. TCR engagement also activates amino acid uptake for incorporation into protein synthesis, glutamine metabolism, and fatty acid synthesis. It has been argued that competition between tumors (which commonly use glycolysis) and T cells for glucose is a major metabolic barrier for successful T-cell function in the tumor microenvironment.[89,90]

In contrast to effector T cell subsets, active regulatory T cells (Tregs) have been shown to use fatty acid oxidation as their primary metabolic activity.[91] Blocking fatty acid oxidation limits Treg suppressive activity and promotes tumor control, implicating fatty acid oxidation as an active repressor of effector activity. Further, engagement of PD-1 increases the expression of carnitine palmitoyltransferase 1A (CPT1A), which is responsible for fatty acid transport into mitochondria, and higher levels of fatty acid oxidation, linking checkpoint inhibition with T-cell metabolism.[92] It should also be noted that a variety of immunosuppressive mechanisms active in the tumor microenvironment involve the degradation, and thus availability, of nutrients necessary for

TABLE 7.3 ■ Metabolic Challenges in the Tumor Microenvironment

Metabolic Constraint	Example	Target
Fuel	Glucose	Glut receptors
	Glutamine	Glutaminase
Amino acid depletion	Tryptophan; arginine; cysteine	IDO; arginase
Immunosuppressive molecule production	Adenosine	CD39; CD73; A2AR
	Lactate	MCT1; MCT4
Hypoxia	Angiogenesis; PDL1 upregulation	VEGF

A2AR, Adenosine A2A receptor; *IDO,* indoleamine 2,3-dioxygenase; *MCT-1/-4,* monocarboxylate transporter -1/-4; *VEGF,* vascular endothelial growth factor

T-cell function. These include arginase which depletes arginine, and indoleamine-2-3-dioxygenase (IDO), which catabolizes tryptophan. Glucose availability is not the sole metabolic regulator of T-cell function in the tumor microenvironment; oxygen deprivation due to poor angiogenesis has also been implicated as a metabolic barrier for T-cell activity against tumors (Table 7.3).

B-CELL METABOLIC PROGRAMMING

Similar to T cells, naïve and memory B cells are maintained in a state of quiescence, primarily using oxidative phosphorylation to provide energy. Upon antigen receptor stimulation, B cells must undergo metabolic alterations to generate the secretory machinery that will be needed by plasma cells to produce copious quantities of antibodies.[93] BCR-stimulated B cells undergo metabolic adaptations that are highly similar to those of T cells, increasing glucose uptake, glycolytic activity, and the production of pyruvate for consumption in mitochondria via the TCA cycle. With B cells, the antigen receptor initiates glucose transporter protein type 1 (GLUT1) upregulation in a PI-3K-dependent manner and glycolysis via phospholipase C-γ2 (PLC-γ2)- mediated activation of protein kinase-C β (PKCβ).[94] Consistent with T cells, c-Myc promotes glycolysis, glutaminolysis, and amino acid uptake by B cells and is accompanied by the upregulation of a plethora of solute transporter proteins that enhance acquisition of metabolites from the extracellular environment. Indeed, the upregulation of CD98hc (Slc3a2) has been shown to be critical for B-cell proliferation. Hypoxia-inducible factor 1-alpha (HIF-1α) also contributes to the transcription of genes involved in solute transport and glycolysis. In contrast to T cells, nutrient sensing by B cells (and thus metabolic regulation) is apparently independent of AMP-activated protein kinase (AMPK) and the increase in glycolysis that occurs with antigen receptor stimulation is more coordinated with glucose oxidation. Notably, plasma cells also engage de novo lipogenesis to augment sufficient phospholipids to promote antibody secretion, and the hexosamine pathway repurposes glucose to allow antibody glycosylation.

Tumor Antigen Presentation: Dendritic Cells

ROLE IN THE LYMPH NODE

In order for T-cell responses to be initiated, naive T cells bearing cognate TCRs, as described above, must encounter an MHC–peptide complex that has sufficient affinity to trigger signal transduction in the surveilling T cell. In addition to this first signal (Signal 1), the context in which antigen presentation occurs is critical to generate a productive T-cell response (the subsequent proliferation and differentiation of the stimulated T cell). The qualitative nature of antigen presentation is referred to as *costimulation*, or Signal 2. To successfully stimulate a primary T-cell response, Signal 1 and Signal 2 must be achieved simultaneously, meaning that the antigen-presenting cell responsible for initiating this response must be appropriately supplied with antigen and also educated, or activated, to become a professional APC. Dendritic cells are the predominant cell with these capabilities[95] and thus play a critical role in eliciting immunity to tumors, whether, for example, as part of a cancer vaccine therapy or cells that participate in responses after initial tumor destruction elicited by standard of care therapies or targeted therapies. Each of these stages will be explained later.

ANTIGEN PRESENTATION

The fundamental basis for activation of T cells is the presence of cognate MHC–peptide complexes on the cell surface. For CD4$^+$ T helper cells, which will be explored in more detail later, this requires MHC class II molecules. In contrast, antigen presentation to cytotoxic CD8$^+$ T cells requires MHC class I molecules. These two molecules are used because they generally acquire antigen from different cellular compartments. In most instances, MHC class I molecules acquire the peptides they present at the cell surface from proteins that have been expressed in the host cell (e.g., normal host proteins, proteins that contain alterations as a function of the transformed nature of the cell, or proteins that result from pathogenic infection). To access MHC class I molecules, protein products of translation are degraded in the cytoplasm by the proteosome and transported into the endoplasmic reticulum (ER) by the transporter associated with antigen processing (TAP) molecules where they can meet empty, recently translated MHC I molecules (Fig. 7.5). Various editing proteins trim and enhance

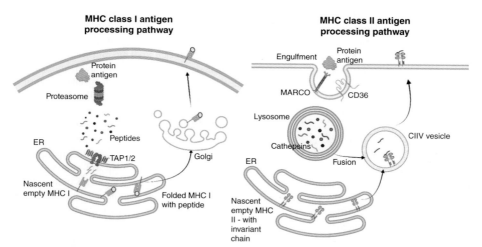

Fig. 7.5   MHC class I and MHC class II antigen processing pathways. MHC molecules presented fragments of proteins derived from different sources. Peptides for MHC class I–restricted presentation are generated by the action of the proteasome on ubiquitinated substrate proteins. Peptide fragments are shuttled into the ER by TAP1/2 molecules where they encounter nascent, empty MHC class I molecules. If the MHC molecule and peptide match with respect to the MHC binding site (determinant selection), the MHC class I molecule alters its conformation and leaves the ER to the cell surface. cDC1 dendritic cells can shuttle antigen from external sources into this pathway, a process referred to as cross-presentation. Peptides that are destined to be presented on MHC class II, which engage CD4$^+$ T cells, are generally derived from extracellular sources. After engulfment, antigen is proteolytically degraded in lysosomes by cathepsin. Lysosomes fuse with vesicles containing nascent MHC class II molecules that are kept empty by having the invariant chain bound to them. Chaperoning by HLA-DO and HLA-DM allows peptides to bind to MHC class II and transit to the cell surface. (Created with BioRender.com.)

the binding of peptides to the MHC. Most peptides bound to MHC class I molecules are 8 to 10 amino acids in length. Subsequently, folding with β2-microglobulin induces the release of the complete MHC–peptide complex to the cell surface. In contrast, nascent MHC class II molecules move from the ER to endosomal vesicles containing antigen that has been acquired, by either endocytosis or phagocytosis, from the extracellular environment. As antigen-containing endosomes move inward, proteolytic enzymes such as cathepsins are responsible for digesting the antigen cargo, resulting in polypeptides that can, with the help of chaperone molecules such as human leukocyte antigen (HLA)-DM and HLA-DO, bind in the MHC class II binding cleft (Fig. 7.5). Peptides derived from endogenous proteins are less commonly found on MHC class II molecules because the coexpressed invariant chain blocks peptide access until late endosomes, where it is also cleaved, allowing peptide binding to the MHC class II molecule. The different antigenic requirements for MHC molecules play a considerable role in the design of subunit cancer vaccines. Short, precise peptides are used for MHC class I binding and CD8[+] T-cell responses, and longer peptides can be used to elicit MHC class II binding and CD4[+] T-cell responses.

CROSS-PRESENTATION

An implication of discrete antigen sources for MHC class I and class II molecules with respect to CD8[+] T-cell responses is that either DCs express tumor antigens themselves or somehow tumor antigen must gain access to the cytoplasm and MHC class I antigen-processing and presentation machinery. Indeed, some subsets of DCs have the unique ability to extract phagocytosed material from endosomes into the cytoplasm, allowing interaction with proteasomes and entrance to the ER to engage with nascent MHC class I molecules.[96] Two pathways are thought to be responsible for this: (1) the active export or partially degraded proteins from specialized endosomes and (2) fusion and regurgitation of degraded cargo with the ER itself, again allowing initial engagement with nascently translated empty MHC class I molecules. Conventional type 1 DC (cDC1) have the greatest capacity to perform this function.

DC ONTOGENY AND ROLES

It is now clear that various DC subpopulations are derived from common myeloid precursors. Two major subsets of conventional DC (cDC) exist. The first subset, cDC1, which express the X-C Motif Chemokine Receptor 1 (XCR1) in mice, were identified in 2020 as the major cross-presenting cDC subset for tumor cell antigens.[97] The second major subset, cDC2, which express CD11b and Signal regulatory protein α (SIRPα), primarily presents exogenously derived antigen to CD4[+] T cells in a manner analogous to macrophages.[98,99] Though the mechanistic basis that differentiates the ability of cDC1 and cDC2 to cross-present cellular antigen remains to be determined, it should be noted that both cDC subsets can cross-present cell-free antigen.[98] Human equivalents to these subsets have been identified and express CD141 and CD1a/c (Table 7.4), respectively, though their relative importance in cross-presentation in vivo in humans has not been demonstrated for practical reasons. Given that the presence of cDC within tumors is a strong prognostic indicator for response to cancer immunotherapy, approaches are being taken to increase the presence of cDCs within tumors or to directly target antigen to cDCs to increase the chances that cDCs will acquire antigen and process for presentation to T cells. On the one hand, fms-like tyrosinse kinase 3 ligand (FLT3L) has been shown to drive the expansion of cDC1. On the other, granulocytic myeloid cell–stimulating factor (GM-CSF) promotes cDC2 expansion.[100] cDCs have two main sites of residency. In the periphery they exist in tissues and are constantly surveying for the presence of cells that express "eat me" signals that will initiate phagocytosis. In the lymph node, cDC have either migrated from the periphery or are residential subsets that are responsible for surveying the efferent lymph for extracellular material that drains via lymphatics,

TABLE 7.4 ■ DC Subsets and Markers

Subset	Mouse Markers	Human Markers	Function
Conventional cDC1	XCR1; CD8αα; CD103 (migratory)	Clec9A; CADM1; CD141; XCR1	Cross-presentation to CD8 T cells; CD4 T-cell activation
Conventional cDC2	CD11b; SIRPα; CX3CR1	CD1c; CD32b (cDC2-A); CD36, CD163 (cDC2-B)	CD4⁺ T-cell activation
Plasmacytoid pDC	B220+	CD123, BDCA-2	IFN-1 production; NK activation by IL-12/IL-18
Langerhans	CD207 (langerin); F4/80	CD1a; CD207; Birbeck granules	
CD16+DC (cDC4)		CD11c+; CD1c−CD141− CD16+	Cytokine production and costimulation Low MHC class II Maybe monocytes
Inflammatory/ monocyte DC	Ly6C	CD1a; CD1c; CD14; SIRPα	

BDCA-1, Blood dendritic cell antigen-1; CADM1, cell adhesion molecule 1); CLEC9A, C-type lectin domain containing 9A; IFN-1, interferon, type 1; SIRPα, signal regulatory protein alpha; XCR-1, X-C motif chemokine receptor 1

or acquire antigen from other DCs that have migrated to the lymph node. Peripheral cDC1 expresses CD103 in mice, and lymph node–resident cDC1 expresses CD8α. Peripheral cDC2 and lymph node–resident cDC2 are harder to separate based on phenotypic markers.

Two additional major subsets of DCs have been well documented. First are plasmacytoid DCs (pDCs), which reside primarily within lymph nodes. These cells are poor at priming naïve T cells because of limited antigen-presenting ability but, in contrast, can produce copious quantities of type 1 interferon (IFN-1). Second, Langerhans cells (LCs) which were in fact the first DC subset identified that are more aligned with macrophages and are derived from embryonic precursors rather than common myeloid precursors (CMP) (and thus are radio-resistant) and are self-renewing. The contribution of these two subsets to innate and adaptive immune control of tumors is less well characterized.

ANTIGEN ACQUISITION BY cDCS

In order for cDCs to perform their role as antigen-presenting cells with MHC molecules loaded with pathogen- or tumor-derived peptides, they must either be directly infected by an invading pathogen or acquire the antigenic material from infected or transformed cells. Given the importance of this step, an extensive series of studies has shown that cDC use a variety of mechanisms to take up antigen from dead or dying cells.[101] cDCs have a large capacity for pinocytosis, the nonspecific uptake of extracellular soluble material, and a non-clathrin-dependent endocytic pathway that is linked to rapid membrane ruffling activity. Macropinosomes shrink and then target their material to MHC class II–containing compartments where they are degraded and become available for presentation on MHC II molecules. Clathrin-coated pits are also well represented on cDCs, making them permissive for receptor-mediated endocytosis. A variety of surface receptors, particularly C-type lectin receptors, formyl peptide receptors, and Fc receptors, authorize cDCs to engulf particulate material based on the ligands displayed by that material. For example, mannose receptors complex efficiently with exposed carbohydrates; DEC-205 (CD205) and DC-specific ICAM-grabbing non-integrin (DC-SIGN; CD209) receptors recognize glycosylation through their carbohydrate recognition domains. Fc receptors engage opsonized target cells decorated with antibodies and facilitate the endocytosis of this material. Scavenger receptors such as macrophage receptor with collagenous structure (MARCO) bind and ingest unopsonized particles. As with pinocytosis, the cargo of receptor-mediated endocytosis is targeted to late endosomes that undergo acidification, activating the lysosomal enzymes responsible for degrading the cargo for MHC class II binding. Important from the perspective of tumor immunology, a variety of receptors, such as T-cell immunoglobulin and mucin domain containing 4 (TIM-4) and MER proto-oncogene tyrosine kinase (MERTK), recognize phosphatidyl-serine (PS) exposed on the flipped membranes of cells undergoing apoptosis, leading to the phagocytosis of these dying bodies.[102] Notably, cDCs are in competition with other myeloid cells for these dying cells as scavenger receptors and PS receptors are expressed on macrophages and granulocytes in addition to cDCs. In the mid-2000s, studies indicated that chemotherapy-induced cell death results in the mobilization of calreticulin to the surface of dying cells, and the release of cDC-activating DAMPs.[103] Cell surface calreticulin serves as a potent "eat me" signal to phagocytes via binding the low-density lipoprotein–related protein (LRP), leading to their engulfment. In the face of all of these molecules that drive the targeted acquisition of tumor-derived material by cDCs, there also exist inhibitor molecules such as SIRPα, which negate phagocytosis after engagement of CD47. Tumor cells commonly upregulate CD47 to prevent engulfment. Given this deep insight into the molecules that regulate antigen acquisition, clinical opportunities exist to promote antigen delivery to cDCs and also to disarm inhibitory molecules that limit phagocytosis.

MATURATION AND MIGRATION OF cDCS

An essential element in the ability of DCs to promote adaptive immune responses is that not only do they present antigen to surveilling T cells but they do so in a manner that is considered "productive." This is achieved by presenting antigen while simultaneously expressing the costimulatory molecules, CD80 and CD86 (also known as B7.1 and B7.2), that engage CD28 on T cells. Many inflammatory pathways can promote the expression of CD80 and/or CD86 on the surface of cDCs. The most well described are the engagement of pathogen recognition receptors (PRRs) such as Toll-like receptors (TLRs) and NOD-like receptors (NLRs) by invariant elements of invading pathogens (e.g., lipopolysaccharide [LPS]; double-stranded RNA) that are collectively termed *pathogen-associated molecular patterns* (PAMPs).[104] Importantly, studies have revealed that these receptors can also respond to endogenously derived ligands, referred to as *damage-associated molecular patterns* (or DAMPs).[105] DAMPs are molecules that are generally released from cells that are not undergoing normal programmed cell death (and thus hidden from innate receptors) and include molecules such as ATP and high-mobility group box 1 (HMGB1) that are normally sequestered in healthy cells and degraded before release during the process of programmed cell death.[106] The engagement of PRRs not only results in the initial upregulation of costimulatory molecules but promotes the migration of cDCs to draining lymph nodes via the efferent lymphatics, where they can encounter naïve T cells and initiate primary T-cell responses. This is achieved by the upregulation of the CCR7 chemokine receptor, which in turn detects a gradient of CCL19 and CCL21 on the lymphatic endothelial cells.[107] These, in combination with sphingosine-1-phosphate gradients, direct trafficking of cDCs to the lymph nodes (Fig. 7.6).

Once in draining lymph nodes, cDCs secrete chemokines that recruit naïve T cells to their vicinity, providing them the opportunity to detect the presence of their cognate antigen.[108] Interestingly, the degree of cDC maturation achieved by PRR stimulation is seldom sufficient to drive durable CD8[+] T-cell responses. Many studies have shown that CD4[+] T cell–mediated help is needed to elevate cDCs to a level of activation needed to fully license CD8[+] T-cell responses.

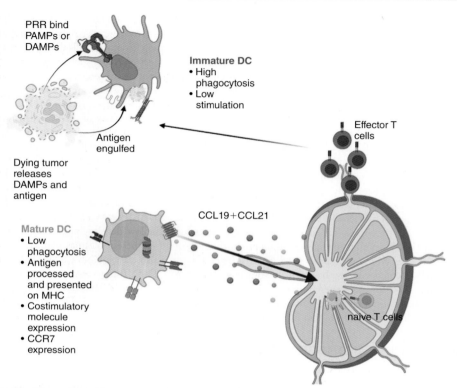

Fig. 7.6 Maturation and migration of DC. Dendritic cells acquire antigen and activation signals from dying or infected cells, using pattern recognition receptors (PRRs) to sense damage-associated molecular patterns (DAMPs), and lectins and phosphatidylserine receptors to engulf antigen. With activation, DCs upregulate antigen processing, MHC molecules, and costimulatory molecules. Upregulation of CCR7 allows DCs to follow a CCL19 and CCL21 gradient through the lymphatics to the lymph node, where they can engage naïve T cells and provide antigen to B cells. Activated naïve T cells then exit the lymph node and traffic back to the site of inflammation. (Created with BioRender.com.)

Landmark studies demonstrated that the expression of CD40-ligand (CD40L) by activated CD4$^+$ T cells engages CD40 on cDCs, and this stimulation pathway is critical to fully activate cDCs.[109] There is some evidence that natural killer (NK) or NKT cells may also be able to raise the activation level of cDCs.[110] Targeting CD40-mediated activation of cDCs is a continuing area of translational and clinical research, and many cancer vaccines include MHC class II–restricted epitopes to recruit CD4$^+$ T cells into the response. Alternatively, agonists of CD40, including antibodies and recombinant ligands, are being explored in clinical trials.

T cells that initiate signaling via the TCR in the absence of CD28 costimulation signal undergo an alternative activation pathway that results in unresponsiveness or anergy. Thus immunotherapeutic regimens that are intended to promote antigen release and availability must also concurrently induce the availability of DAMPs (as seen in the case of certain chemotherapies, irradiation, and oncolytic viruses[111]) or have PRR-activating molecules delivered at the same time to ensure that costimulatory molecules are induced on cDCs that have acquired tumor antigen. Beyond PRR ligands, proinflammatory cytokines such as type 1 interferons (IFN-1) and tumor necrosis factor alpha (TNF-α) can also support the expression of CD80 and CD86 and some cytokine production.

Beyond Signal 2, additional molecules are expressed by activated cDCs that can be highly influential in the quality of the ensuing T-cell response. Appropriately activated cDCs can express proinflammatory cytokines such as IFN-1 and IL-12. Both of these stimulatory pathways have been shown to influence effector T-cell differentiation, as described later. Further, fully activated cDCs can express members of the TNF superfamily, such as 4-1BB (CD137), OX40 (CD134), GITR (CD357), and CD70. Each of these molecules can support antiapoptotic programs in T cells and further development into both effector and, importantly, memory T-cell populations.

Thus, it is important to know whether targeted therapies or other antitumor interventions result in the release of DAMPs in sufficient quantity and activity to promote the activation of cDCs to full antigen-presenting cells.

ROLE OF DC IN THE TUMOR

There is some debate as to whether tumor-resident cDCs play a role beyond serving as precursors for the migratory cDCs that are responsible for the initial priming of T cells in lymph nodes. Pertaining to this, studies have shown that fewer effector-activated T cells (bypassing the role of cDCs in T-cell priming) accumulate and persist in tumors devoid of cDCs compared with those replete with cDCs.[112] Further, elegant studies have shown that cDCs in the parenchyma can provide IL-2 in support of tissue-resident effector T cells.[86] Additionally, the formation of tertiary lymphoid structures, comprising cDCs, B cells, and fibroblasts, in tissue adjacent to or associated with tumors has significant prognostic utility in many cancer types. Together, these data suggest that tissue-resident cDCs provide a supporting role in sustaining effector T cells once they extravasate into the target tissue and boost the rationale for studies that intend to recruit cDCs to the tumor microenvironment.

Integrating Innate and Adaptive Immunity to Cancer

STAGES OF T-CELL RESPONSE

Adaptive T-cell immune responses are divided into several stages. The initial encounter with antigen-bearing APCs by naïve cells is termed *priming*, and the subsequent massive expansion and dissemination of the effector daughter clones is referred to as the *primary response* (Fig. 7.7). The vast majority (~95%) of these effector cells, referred to as *short-lived effector cells* (SLECs), will undergo cell death shortly after the peak of the response in what is termed the *contraction phase*.[114,115] Embedded within the primary response are clones that have not undergone terminal differentiation (possibly owing to less engagement of TCR, exposure to proinflammatory cytokines) and have the capacity for further self-renewal. These cells are referred to as *memory precursor effector cells* (MPECs).[116] Residual memory cells can populate several different regions of the body. Those that patrol the circulation are called *effector memory T cells* (T_{EM}). Those that reside in secondary lymphoid organs are called *central memory* T cells (T_{CM}).[117] Those that persist in the tissue, in isolation from circulating memory cells, are called *tissue-resident memory cells* (T_{RM}).[118,119] Each of these populations has different longevity and speed of reactivation and can play significant and varied roles in the protective response to tumors. Hallmarks of T-cell memory include a decreased dependence upon costimulation for activation, a higher sensitivity to antigen, the capacity to self-renew, and larger precursor frequencies for specific antigen than found in the naïve population.[120]

LYMPHOCYTE TRAFFICKING

A critical element that supports the efficiency of adaptive immune responses is the coordinated movement of naïve and effector lymphocytes and antigen-presenting cells, so that they are

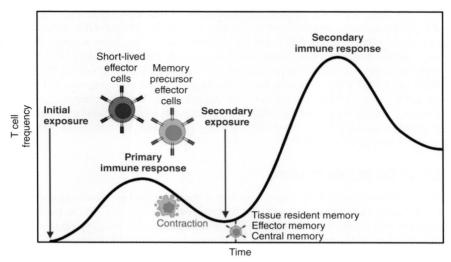

Fig. 7.7   Stages of CD8⁺ T-cell response. Activated CD8⁺ T cells expand rapidly after TCR engagement with costimulation. Depending on the cytokines produced by DCs and in the lymph node during expansion, primary T cells become either terminally differentiated short-lived effector cells (SLECs) or memory precursor effector cells (MPECs). Within the MPEC population are long-lived memory cells that can either reside in lymph nodes (central memory), circulate in blood (effector memory), or remain in the tissue (tissue-resident memory). The vast majority of SLECs die by apoptosis during the contraction phase. Upon reexposure to antigen, memory T cells expand rapidly to generate the secondary response, which is larger and more potent than the primary response. (Created with BioRender.com.)

positioned in lymph nodes to increase the likelihood of encountering their cognate antigen at either the priming or the effector stage.

Naïve T cells survey the secondary lymphoid organs by constantly circulating through the vasculature. They move from the blood into the organ by interacting with cell adhesion molecules expressed by naïve T cells and their ligands expressed on the surface of high endothelial venules (HEVs). The process of extravasation is initiated by rolling of lymphocytes that is mediated by L-selectin binding to vascular addressins, followed by CCL21 chemokine–mediated structural rearrangement of lymphocyte function-associated antigen 1 (LFA-1) that increases its binding affinity, resulting in firm adhesion.[121,122] Finally, transmigration occurs across the endothelial cells in response to CCL21 and CXCL12.[123,124] Once in the lymph node cortex, further chemokines attract T cells to the T-cell zone, positioning them to survey incoming and resident DCs.[125] Activated DCs express CCL3 and CCL4, recruiting naïve T cells and further reducing the randomness of a rare T cell encountering its cognate ligand in the lymph node.[126]

After T cells encounter their cognate antigen in the draining lymph node, the signals derived from the TCR and costimulatory molecules drive a program of proliferation and differentiation that imbue these cells with their different qualities, defined further in below. Follicular T helper cells stay resident in the lymph node but traffic to the B-cell zones to support B-cell differentiation, and many activated T cells exit the lymph node to traffic to the site where the antigen originated. During the earlier proliferation steps, now-activated T cells downregulate the sphingosine-1-phosphate receptor (S1PR) that senses gradients of S1P and is used by naïve T cells to exit lymph nodes back into the circulation. After several rounds of proliferation, exiting from the lymph node and finding the site of origin require a coordinated series of changes in the homing receptors expressed on activated T cells. This process aligns them with the address posted on the endothelial cells of the site of origin. Exiting from the lymph node requires the downregulation of the homing receptors that support naïve T-cell transit into lymph nodes, namely, the chemokine receptor CCR7 and the integrin CD62L (L-selectin). Additionally, the reexpression of S1PR, which is transiently downregulated after initial TCR engagement, allows activated T cells to follow a S1P gradient into the circulation. Stimulating SIP1R with agonists such as FTY-720 to prevent egress of effector T cells from lymph nodes not only is a novel therapy to enhance transplant engraftment but is a useful experimental tool for understanding the site of origin of T cells invoked by immunotherapeutic interventions. L-selectin expression is replaced by the expression of P-selectin glycoprotein ligand-1 (PSGL-1), which permits tethering and rolling of T cells on the activated endothelial cells that express P- and E-selectin at the site of inflammation. Expression of PSGL-1 is accompanied by the upregulation of other integrins that contribute to the process of T-cell extravasation, including very late antigen-4 (VLA-4) (binding vascular cell adhesion protein 1 [VCAM1] on the endothelial cells) (Fig. 7.8). Importantly, the site of origin of the cDC that primes the T cell influences the expression of other specialized homing receptors expressed by the activated T cell. For example, DCs from the intestines will imprint the expression of the mucosal addressin cell adhesion molecule 1 (MAdCAM-1), which is expressed on the endothelial cells of the gut mucosa. Similar observations have been made for skin-homing T cells, which express cutaneous lymphocyte antigen (CLA). An additional layer of regulation of T-cell trafficking is coordinated by the expression of chemokines. Chemokines can be expressed constitutively to help naïve T cells traffic to lymph nodes (CCL19 and CCL21, which bind to CCR7) and as a permanent part of tissue homing (such as CCL17 and CCL27, which bind to CCR4 and CCR10, respectively, and are expressed on cutaneous endothelial cells). Varied chemokines can also be induced by cytokines that are activated in response to infection and other inflammatory events. These chemokines decorate the endothelial surface. For example, CXCL9, -10, and -11 are induced by IFN-γ and promote the recruitment of effector cells, particularly CD8[+] T cells, T helper (Th) 1 CD4[+] T cells, and NK cells that express the cognate receptor CXCR3. Engagement of chemokine receptors on homing T cells leads to structural alterations of the integrins involved in tethering and rolling, increasing the likelihood that a T cell will egress from the vasculature at the appropriate sites. Notably, different subsets of T cells can express different chemokine

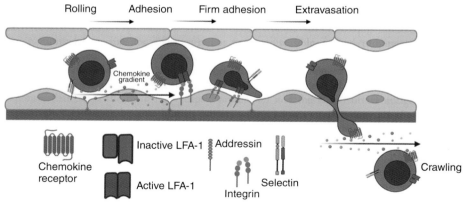

Fig. 7.8 Lymphocyte trafficking and extravasation. Lymphocytes use addressins and selectins to initiate rolling on activated endothelial cells. Engagement of chemokine receptors results in confirmational changes in LFA-1, allowing firm adhesion to ICAM-1. Once adhered, lymphocytes undergo diapedesis to extravasate across the endothelial cell barrier, where they can follow other chemotactic gradients. A similar process is used for the entrance of naïve T cells into the lymph node and effector T cells into the periphery. (Created with Biorender.com.)

receptors, allowing them to be recruited in a semiselective manner according to the chemokines that are expressed by different subsets of innate immune cells at the site of inflammation. As a coordinated exercise, this process allows a more efficient targeting of T cells to the relevant parts of the body, enhancing the rapidity of recruitment and limiting off-target immunopathology. Notably, the vasculature of tumors presents several different challenges for effective recruitment and is illustrated by the relatively poor infiltration of solid tumors by CAR-T and other cellular therapies. There is emerging evidence that the chaotic nature of tumor vasculature limits its ability to induce the expression of appropriate homing receptor ligands for T cells, and strategies that enhance the normalization of tumor vasculature promote T-cell entrance.

Naïve B cells enter lymph nodes from the vasculature in a similar manner to naïve T cells via HEV and using CCR7 to respond to CCL19 and CCL21 produced by lymph node stromal cells and follicular DCs. Recruitment to the follicles is mediated by an attraction to CXCL13 that is sensed by CXCR5.[127] Once B cells are activated by opsonized antigen presented by follicular dendritic cells or subcapsular sinus macrophages, B cells upregulate CCR7 and another chemokine receptor, EBI2; migrate to the outer follicle regions to further sample antigen; and then follow CCL21 to the interface of the T- and B-cell zones where they can encounter follicular T helper cells, increasing the chance that T and B cells that are specific for the same antigen can interact.[128] Upon receiving T-cell support, B cells proliferate and differentiate at the follicle border and then decrease CCR7 expression and increase EBI2. On the one hand, this allows B cells to move back to the interfollicular region to seed the primary focus, a cluster of differentiating B cells. Plasmablasts are derived from these primary foci. Plasma cells can originate from plasmablasts but can also arise separately and ultimately seed the bone marrow to generate long-lived antibody-secreting cells. This requires the downregulation of CXCR5 and increased expression of CXCR4 and $\alpha4\beta1$ integrin to populate the periphery. On the other hand, B cells and Tfh can migrate to a germinal center if they downregulate EBI2 expression and begin somatic hypermutation and affinity maturation and class switching of their antibodies (in response to cytokines produced by Tfh). Movement within the germinal center is regulated by CXCR4 and CXCR5 and the chemokine CXCL12. Downregulation of CXCR4 then permits cells to migrate to the light zone, which contains follicular DCs that express CXCL13.

It has been appreciated that lymph node–like structures, containing dendritic cells, B cells, and T cells, can form in association with tumors. These clusters, termed *tertiary lymphoid structures* (TLS) are commonly associated with better prognosis for patients, in the context of both standard of care therapies and immunotherapies.[129] The generation of TLS has been scrutinized, and a coordinated expression of T cell– and B cell–recruiting chemokines including CCL19, CCL21, CXCL13, and peripheral node addressin (PNAd) by cancer-associated fibroblasts and on tumor endothelium is needed,[130] demonstrating how the identification of chemokines and integrins that are associated with both B- and T-cell recruitment could be exploited to improve the immunologic landscape of cancer.

T-Cell Subsets in Cancer Immunity

CYTOTOXIC CD8$^+$ T CELLS

Cytotoxic T cells primarily express the CD8 coreceptor, which enhances the interaction between the TCR with intermediate affinity for the MHC class I molecule, promoting their survival. MHC class I molecules are thereafter the selecting molecule for CD8$^+$ T cells. CD8 expression becomes engrained, as is the restriction for antigen presented on MHC class I molecules.

Cytotoxic CD8$^+$ T cells are a particular focus of cancer immunotherapy due to the variety of studies that have shown that in their absence tumors form more commonly in murine models. Further, their presence in human tumors correlates with better prognosis in a variety of tumor types[3,131] and response to checkpoint immunotherapy.[132,133] Thus considerable attention is paid to interventions and therapies that enhance their presence within the tumor microenvironment. The importance of this cell type within the TME is likely a manifestation of their varied activities, referred to as *effector functions*, that cause death of their target cells.

Cytolysis

After recognition of their MHC–peptide ligand in the draining lymph node, naïve CD8$^+$ T cells transcribe and epigenetically impress the expression of the components needed for cytolysis. Cytolysis describes the extrusion of cytolytic enzymes, such as granzymes, through a pore, formed by perforins, in the target cell wall. These cytolytic proteins (granzymes, perforins, and granulysins) are stored in an active form in modified lysosome *granules*.[134] These enzymes initiate caspase-dependent cell death both by directly activating cytosolic caspases and by damaging the target cell mitochondria via degrading members of the B-cell lymphoma 2 (Bcl2) family and disrupting mitochondrial membrane integrity. Critically, to limit immunopathology, bystander cells that do not express the appropriate MHC–peptide complex are not killed by activated CD8$^+$ T cells, because the release of cytotoxic granules is directed through a highly polarized tight point of contact between the effector cell and the target cell. TCR engagement in the periphery results in further transcription and translation of cytolytic molecules in CD8$^+$ T cells. Thus cytotoxic T cells can "serially" kill multiple target cells.

Fas Ligand–Mediated Lysis

Activation of T cells via their receptor results in the upregulation of the expression of Fas ligand (CD178). Subsequent encounter with cells that express the Fas (CD95) initiates a cell death pathway that uses the death domain in the tail of Fas to induce apoptosis.[135] This mechanism of cell death also plays a role in the programmed elimination of T cells at the end of the primary immune response.

Cytokine Secretion

In addition to direct and indirect lysis of target cells, CD8$^+$ T cells secrete cytokines that also directly and indirectly inhibit the survival of their target cells. The cytokines produced by CD8$^+$ T cells that are most relevant to tumor control are tumor necrosis factor alpha (TNF-α) and interferon gamma (IFN-γ).[136-138] The production of TNF-α results in death of the target cell via the Fas Associated via Death Domain (FADD)-containing TNF receptors. The expression of IFN-γ has pleiotropic effects on target and allied cells. IFN-γ promotes the expression of MHC class I molecules and the proteins involved in antigen processing and presentation.[139] Further, it enhances the activation of myeloid cells within the vicinity, enhancing their expression of tumoricidal molecules such as reactive oxygen species (ROS) and inducible nitric oxide synthase (iNOS). IFN-γ also induces the expression of chemokines that can support the recruitment of additional effector immune cells to the tumor microenvironment.[140] Finally, IFN-γ has potent antiangiogenic functions that limit the development of tumor vasculature. Not surprising, early immunotherapies tested whether the infusion of patients with these cytokines would eliminate tumors. However, it was quickly recognized that systemic cytokine therapies had significant toxicities associated with them, limiting their utility. Current studies are investigating the effectiveness of intralesional delivery of these and other cytokines.

Helper CD4$^+$ T Cells

CD4$^+$ T cells are selected by MHC class II peptide complexes. The expression of MHC class II is much more restricted than MHC class I. In general, only professional antigen-presenting cells such as macrophages, activated B cells, and dendritic cells express MHC class II, though it can

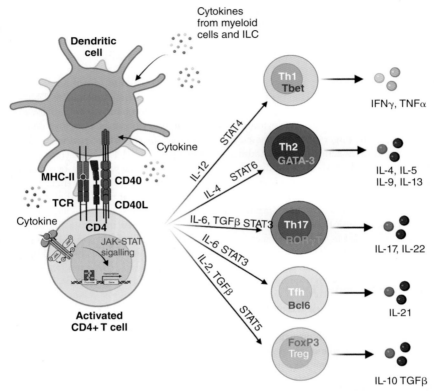

Fig. 7.9   CD4⁺ T-cell differentiation is driven by cytokines and transcription factors. During priming by dendritic cells, CD4⁺ T cells are exposed to cytokines either from DCs, myeloid cells, or innate-like lymphocytes (ILCs). Cytokine receptors drive JAKs to activate STATs, which mobilize to the nucleus and orchestrate differing transcriptional programs. Different cytokines work with different STATs, resulting in the induction of transcription factors that drive cytokines production from the different lineages of CD4⁺ T cells.

be induced on tumor cells under certain circumstances. Upon activation, helper CD4⁺ T cells (Th) differentiate into subsets defined by the transcription factors and cytokines that they can express. Th1, Th2, Th17, and TfH are the major effector CD4⁺ T cell subsets, and regulatory T cells (Treg) represent an immunosuppressive subset of CD4⁺ T cells (Fig. 7.9). Different T helper cell subsets evolved to deal with different pathogen challenges: intracellular (Th1), extracellular bacteria (Th17), and helminths (Th2). TfH supports B cell maturation and class switching. Each subset has been described to have differing contributions to antitumor immunity, depending on the time and context of their encounter with a cancer cell, because their prominent interaction with cells of the innate immune system, such as innate lymphoid cells (ILC) and macrophages.[141] These interactions are driven by both the surface molecules and the cytokines secreted by T helper cells.

Th1

Traditionally characterized by their expression of both IFN-γ and TNF-α, these cells are considered to have the most value in controlling tumor growth. Th1 signatures are driven by the expression of the transcription factor Tbet (*tbox22*)[142] and are induced by the secretion of IL-12 by dendritic cells during priming. IL-12 drives STAT4 phosphorylation and access to the nucleus, which is reenforced by exposure to IFN-γ, which uses STAT1 phosphorylation to influence transcriptional profiles. Some studies have suggested that IL-1 also has the capacity to support Th1 differentiation.

Th2

Polarization toward Th2 characteristics, which include the production of IL-4, IL-5, and IL-13, is driven by exposure to IL-4 and signaling via STAT6. This in turn induces the expression of the transcription factor GATA binding protein 3 (GATA3). IL-10 is a major immunosuppressive cytokine, via STAT3 induction, that diminishes both DC-mediated T-cell activation and can directly suppress T-cell function.[143] In contrast, IL-10 can promote resistance to T-cell exhaustion in the TME.[144] Th2 signatures within tumors have been associated with worse prognosis and commonly with the recruitment and differentiation of M2 macrophages, which possess a repertoire of immunosuppressive activities.

Th17

Th17 cells are characterized by the production of IL-17, IL-21, and IL-22. Notably, polarization to the Th17 subset has similarities to Treg differentiation, using transforming growth factor beta (TGF-β) and IL-6 and being reinforced by IL-21 and IL-23. The driving transcription factor for Th17 cells is RAR-related orphan receptor gamma T (RORγT). On the one hand, Th17 cells have been associated with inflammation-induced tumorigenesis; on the other, many of the cytokines that Th17 cells produce have effector activity against tumors, and infusion of tumor-specific Th17 cells can suppress tumor growth.[145] Th17 cells can exhibit a degree of plasticity and convert to Th1 cells in vivo.

Follicular T Helper Cells

Follicular T helper cells are a specific subset that has the responsibility of assisting B cells in germinal centers, and their ensuing antibody responses, by providing cofactors that support B-cell proliferation and antibody class switching. TfH are characterized by the expression of Bcl6, which is induced by STAT3 signaling in response to IL-6 and IL-21. They also commonly express PD-1 and CXCR5, a chemokine receptor that helps position them in the B-cell zone of the lymph node. Although their role in normal conditions is primarily to support B cells, the presence of TfH in varied solid tumors has been associated with enhanced survival.[146,147] This may reflect their contribution to the development of tertiary lymphoid structures that can assist in sustaining immune responses in the hostile environment of the tumor. Also, it should be noted that TfH has the capacity to secrete varied cytokines, including IFN-γ and IL-4, that direct class switching, and this capacity may also influence immune responses in the tumor.

Regulatory T Cells

Tregs arise in the thymus after surviving negative selection against self-antigens and play a critical role in peripheral tolerance and preventing autoimmunity. In mouse models and genetic diseases, the absence of the prototypical Treg transcription factor forkhead box P3 (FOXP3) results in overwhelming autoimmune pathology. In contrast, high levels of Tregs within tumors are associated with poor outcomes and resistance to immunotherapy.[148] The CD8:Treg ratio is commonly used as a surrogate marker of the "immunologic fitness" of the tumor. Tregs are considered natural (produced in the thymus) or induced. In the latter case, the cytokine milieu present at their activation (predominantly TGF-β and IL-23) promotes the induction of FOXP3 expression.[149] Tregs are dependent on and scavenge IL-2 from effector T cells. Tregs possess an armamentarium of mechanisms for limiting effector T-cell responses. They produce cytokines including IL-10, IL-35, and TGF-β that have been shown to impede varied effector activities.[150] They express CTLA-4, which competes with CD28 on primary T cells for CD80/CD86-mediated costimulation. They express enzymes that produce extracellular adenosine, inducing metabolic deficiency in effector T cells.

Biologic Variables in Adaptive Immunity

EFFECT OF AGING ON IMMUNE COMPETENCE

Multiple facets of adaptive immunity are influenced by the process of aging.[151] Lymphocyte production and persistence are reduced, leading to potential gaps in the immune repertoire capable of either responding directly to developing cancers, responding to cancer vaccines, or serving as tools to be manipulated for immunotherapeutic interventions such as CAR-T.[152] Collectively, these alterations are described as *immunosenescence*.

Lymphocyte Development

In the aging process, the accretion of an inflammatory state, termed *inflammaging* can result in the chronic presence of inflammatory cytokines. Studies suggest that, as a consequence, common hematopoietic precursor cells more commonly differentiate to the myeloid pathway. This limits the production of novel T and B cells that are destined to repopulate the peripheral immune system. Precursor B-cell production in bone marrow is limited with age, perhaps because of a reduction in IL-7, a lymphocyte survival factor. Additional limitations in the naïve T-cell repertoire, particularly in CD8[+] T cell populations, arise because of the process of thymic involution. Involution substantially limits thymic output, reducing the pool of potential naïve T cells available to respond to de novo exposures to antigen.

Lymphocyte Priming

In addition to limitations in the T-cell repertoire, several physiologic alterations that are present in the geriatric hematopoietic cell populations have the potential to compromise both de novo primary and memory lymphocyte populations. Chronic inflammation and cytokine exposure can desensitize myeloid cells, including dendritic cells, limiting their ability to respond to both cytokines and pattern recognition molecules and thus reach full activation. Evidence also exists that geriatric dendritic cells have deficiencies in antigen processing, constraining the presentation of MHC–peptide complexes at the cell surface.[153] Finally, global alterations in host metabolism can lead to biochemical insufficiencies in lymphocytes. For example, limitations in cholesterol can compromise the presence of cholesterol in lymphocyte membranes. This in turn leads to a reduction in the efficiency of formation of the lipid rafts needed for efficient receptor signaling, disrupting the coordinated steps necessary for lymphocyte activation.

Lymphocyte Persistence

A hallmark of adaptive immunity is the capacity for self-renewal resulting in memory lymphocyte populations that are poised to proliferate in response to reexposure to antigen. Though the vaccine formulation/composition can play a substantial role in the qualities and durability of memory lymphocyte populations (e.g., the durability of protective memory to smallpox after vaccinia immunization is decades long compared with studies that suggest that mRNA vaccines against coronavirus disease 2019 [COVID-19] induce relatively ephemeral antibody production),[154] the persistence of memory lymphocytes to common antigens is different in young vs aged vaccinated populations. Normally, each lymphocyte division reduces telomere length, ultimately leading to the induction of cell death. Lymphocytes can induce the expression of telomerase after antigen stimulation, which initially compensates for telomere loss by adding back nucleotides. However, this only occurs for a few rounds of antigen stimulation. Thus with repetitive antigen stimulation, there is attritional reduction in telomere length that leads to constricted replication, as evidenced by effector memory T cells. During the natural aging process, naïve T cells and memory lymphocytes generated by either inoculation or vaccination have reduced telomerase activity and show signs of premature senescence and reduced ability to proliferate.[155]

SEX DIFFERENCES IN IMMUNITY

Many disease states with immunologic associations exhibit a sex dimorphism, and sex has been shown to influence the strength of immune responses to vaccinations and infections.[156] Many aspects of sex differentiation could contribute to dimorphism, but although recent studies have begun to demonstrate some intrinsic differences between male and female adaptive immune responses, it remains a profoundly understudied area.[157–159] Plasmacytoid dendritic cells (pDCs) from women produce more IFN-α on a per cell basis than do those from men when stimulated with TLR agonists.[160] In the example discussed, TLR-7 is X-linked and female pDCs express higher levels of TLR7.[161] FoxP3, the master transcription factor of regulatory T cells, is also expressed on the X chromosome, and mutations in FOXP3 lead to immune dysregulation, polyendocrinopathy, enteropathy, and X-linked syndrome (IPEX) in humans. Indeed, mosaicism and escape from X-chromosome silencing may perturb the expected balancing effect of chromosome silencing on expression of immune-related genes in females and males. Newer studies have suggested that differences in microRNA, which are encoded at a much higher density on the X chromosome compared with the Y chromosome,[155] can influence the quality and quantity of adaptive immune responses. Further examples of sex-based immune influences include sex hormones and the wide expression of estrogen receptors on T cell subsets. A direct effect of estrogen receptor stimulation on T-cell differentiation, according to dose and receptor subtype, has been demonstrated.[162,163] Thus, both the natural reduction of estrogen production with age and the potential that patients are taking estrogen supplements may influence the differentiation state of T cells responding to cancer antigens.

Key References

1. Dunn GP, Old LJ, Schreiber RD. The three Es of cancer immunoediting. *Annu Rev Immunol.* 2004;22:329-360.
4. Pagès F, Berger A, Camus M, et al. Effector memory T cells, early metastasis, and survival in colorectal cancer. *N Engl J Med.* 2005;353:2654-2666.
14. Cox AL, Skipper J, Chen Y, et al. Identification of a peptide recognized by five melanoma-specific human cytotoxic T cell lines. *Science.* 1994;264:716-719.
17. Lu LL, Suscovich TJ, Fortune SM, Alter G. Beyond binding: antibody effector functions in infectious diseases. *Nat Rev Immunol.* 2018;18:46-61.
23. Wu W, Zhou Q, Masubuchi T, et al. Multiple signaling roles of CD3ε and its application in CAR-T cell therapy. *Cell.* 2020;182:855-871.e23.
26. Love PE, Hayes SM. ITAM-mediated signaling by the T-cell antigen receptor. *Cold Spring Harb Perspect Biol.* 2010;2:a002485.
34. Iwashima M, Irving BA, Van Oers NSC, Chan AC, Weiss A. Sequential interactions of the TCR with two distinct cytoplasmic tyrosine kinases. *Science.* 1994;193:4279-4282.
40. Macian F. NFAT proteins: key regulators of T-cell development and function. *Nat Rev Immunol.* 2005;5:472-484.
44. Chi H. Regulation and function of mTOR signalling in T cell fate decision. *Nat Rev Immunol.* 2012;12:325.
57. Leach DR, Krummel MF, Allison JP. Enhancement of antitumor immunity by CTLA-4 blockade. *Science.* 1996;271:1734-1736.
61. Crotty S. T follicular helper cell biology: a decade of discovery and diseases. *Immunity.* 2019;50: 1132-1148.

65. Blackburn SD, Shin H, Haining WN, et al. Coregulation of CD8+ T cell exhaustion by multiple inhibitory receptors during chronic viral infection. *Nat Immunol.* 2009;10:29-37.

73. Anderson AC, Joller N, Kuchroo VK. Lag-3, Tim-3, and TIGIT: co-inhibitory receptors with specialized functions in immune regulation. *Immunity.* 2016;44:989-1004.

81. Crespo J, Sun H, Welling TH, Tian Z, Zou W. T cell anergy, exhaustion, senescence, and stemness in the tumor microenvironment. *Curr Opin Immunol.* 2013;25:214-221.

84. O'Neill LAJ, Kishton RJ, Rathmell J. A guide to immunometabolism for immunologists. *Nat Rev Immunol.* 2016;16:553.

97. Ferris ST, Durai V, Wu R, et al. cDC1 prime and are licensed by CD4+ T cells to induce anti-tumour immunity. *Nature.* 2020;584:624-629.

103. Obeid M, Tesniere A, Ghiringhelli F, et al. Calreticulin exposure dictates the immunogenicity of cancer cell death. *Nat Med.* 2007;13:54-61.

112. Spranger S, Dai D, Horton B, Gajewski TF. Tumor-residing Batf3 dendritic cells are required for effector T cell trafficking and adoptive T cell therapy. *Cancer Cell.* 2017;31:711-723.e4.

126. Castellino F, Huang AY, Altan-Bonnet G, Stoll S, Scheinecker C, Germain RN. Chemokines enhance immunity by guiding naive CD8+ T cells to sites of CD4+ T cell–dendritic cell interaction. *Nature.* 2006;440:890-895.

136. Grasso CS, Tsoi J, Onyshchenko M, et al. Conserved Interferon-γ signaling drives clinical response to immune checkpoint blockade therapy in melanoma. *Cancer Cell.* 2020;38:500-515.e3.

Visit Elsevier eBooks+ (eBooks.Health.Elsevier.com) for complete set of references.

CHAPTER 8

Cancer—Avoiding Immune Detection

John E. Niederhuber

SUMMARY OF KEY FACTS

- The natural history of a human malignancy and its relationship to the host immune system has been described as comprising the "three Es": elimination, equilibrium, and escape.

- In order to progress, the tumor needs to escape immune control by the cell destructive capacities of the CD8$^+$ T cells of the adaptive immune system and of the NK cells of the innate immune system.

- While attempting to eradicate the tumor, the immune system undergoes what has been described as a process of immunoediting to alter the immune system's recognition of the tumor as nonself, resulting in the tumor escaping immune destruction.

- Despite initial immune recognition of the tumor, as the tumor progresses, clones of tumor cells with lower capacity for antigen recognition and/or greater resistance to immune cell destruction are preferentially selected for tumor progression (immunoediting).

- The many diseases called cancer are characterized by their genetic instability and, as such, are prone to mutations and structural genetic variants occurring in the genes coding for proteins responsible for performing the many normal processes of the cell, including the complex mechanisms of transcription and translation. A tumor cell may have more than 1000 genetic variants, confirming the complexity of cancer as a disease.

- Tumor cells can avoid immune recognition and destruction in multiple ways:
  - a silencing of intrinsic tumor cell processes to generate and to select for MHC presentation of strong antigenic peptides (TSAs and TAAs).
  - a silencing of or mutations in the HLA genes of MHC class I and MHC class II molecules.
  - by co-opting immune checkpoint processes to enable immune suppression.
  - by recruiting inflammatory cells to the tumor and TME with immunosuppressive capacity.
  - by molecular alterations to intrinsic T-cell signaling pathways.

- Genetic alterations in the control mechanisms for mRNA translation can be a cause of tumor antigen loss despite normal MHC antigen-presenting molecules.

- MHC class II antigen presentation requires the classic antigen-presenting cells, especially dendritic cells, to first take up tumor antigenic peptides released from tumor cells and internally process these for loading on the MHC class II molecule. The multiple steps required in this process provide ample opportunity for a failure to generate the stimulatory pMHC class II molecule for TCR presentation.

- Tumor-derived antigenic peptides can undergo self-tolerance within the thymus. This process appears to be selective for tumor antigenic peptides that survive tapasin editing for MHC class I presentation and DM editing for MHC class II presentation.

Continued on following page

Introduction

We have come to understand the many diseases we call cancer by their genetic and epigenetic instability and the relationship the growing tumor has with its surrounding cellular microenvironment and with the host's extensive immune system. Genetic instability in the tumor leads to the development of tumor-specific neoantigenic peptides and, on occasion, ectopic overexpression of genes not normally expressed in the tissue in which the tumor has developed. These non-self-antigenic peptides have an opportunity for presentation by major histocompatibility (MHC) class I molecules expressed on the tumor cells and for cross-presentation by MHC class II molecules expressed by classic antigen-presenting cells. The peptide-loaded MHC molecules present the antigenic epitopes to the T-cell population of the adaptive immune system and to natural killer (NK) cells of the innate immune system. The level of antitumor response by both innate and adaptive compartments of the immune system depends on numerous interactions between the tumor cells and various immune cells and with inflammatory cells of the tumor microenvironment (TME). Antitumor immunity occurs at multiple levels within the host, both locally at the tumor site and peripherally in the immune system. The patient's antitumor response must react to a changing tumor burden and to therapeutic interventions requiring constant efforts of response renewal.

The intimate relationship between the tumor and the immune system occurs over the entire course of disease, from initiation through the progressive stages of growth, local invasion, and metastasis to distant sites. For tumors to survive and progress along this path requires that the tumor develop mechanisms that actively inhibit antitumor cell immune responses.[1,2] Much like the complexities of the antitumor immune response, there are multiple, equally complex mechanisms that function to enable the tumor cells to resist immune destruction.[3,4] Though much has been learned regarding the development of immune resistance to avoid immune tumor cell destruction, developing effective immune therapies that overcome this resistance remains a tremendous challenge. This chapter will address the intimate relationship between the tumor as it progresses and interacts with the patient's immune system with a focus on the mechanisms that enable the tumor to evade immune destruction.

The Presence of Tumor Immune Suppression

The concept of the three "Es" of cancer—elimination, equilibrium, and escape—was first introduced in 2004 as a way of describing the relationship between the initiation and development of cancer and the host's immune system.[3] In the elimination phase, potentially malignant cells arising during the early initiation stage of cancer development are detected as nonself and eliminated as a result of their MHC class I presentation of neoantigens. They are recognized as foreign by the NK cells of the host's innate immune system and by cytotoxic T lymphocytes (CTLs) of the adaptive

> **BOX 8.1 ■ Mechanisms for Tumor Immune T-cell Escape**
>
> Genetic downregulation or loss of MHC class I and II molecule expression.
> Downregulation or genetic alterations in mechanisms controlling immunogenic antigenic peptide creation and MHC antigenic peptide loading.
> Upregulation of immune checkpoint ligands inhibitory to CTLA-4 and PD-1 receptors expressed on NK cells, CD8$^+$ CTLs, and CD4$^+$ T cells.
> Antigen loss: silencing of or mutations altering tumor antigenic epitope translation.
> Tumor-derived immune suppression: membrane bound and secreted.
> TME chronic inflammation suppression of antitumor immune response.

immune response. This stage has been equated with the historic concept of immune surveillance. If the tumor cells escape elimination, they may enter the second stage, termed the *equilibrium phase*. In the equilibrium phase, surviving tumor cells, not eliminated by the immune system, are instead held in check by the immune system without being destroyed but without progression.

Most cancer clinicians recognize a second clinical component of this equilibrium phase. For example, it is not uncommon for aggressively treated newly diagnosed cancer to enter a period of complete response (CR) only to recur many years later. Clearly, these CR patients have undetected micrometastases after treatment and remain in a state of equilibrium or at least controlled slow progression. Clinically, we refer to this phase of cancer as *disease-free survival* (DFS) or in some cases *stable disease* (SD). During this phase of DFS or SD, the relationship between the tumor and the host's immune system is one of controlled equilibrium.[1-5] Finally, should the tumor progress to the third escape stage, its capacity to be immunogenic has been significantly altered and on balance it is no longer completely susceptible to immune cell destruction by the host.

As the tumor progresses through these three stages, it is said to undergo immunoediting.[4] Immunoediting has been described as the complex process(s) by which the host immune system can either inhibit tumor growth or be suppressed/edited in ways that promote tumor progression. There are multiple targets and intracellular pathways that provide mechanisms by which tumor cells can escape both the innate and adaptive immune systems. These escape mechanisms will be described individually but almost certainly occur in a combinatory fashion for successful tumor escape (Box 8.1).

Downregulation of or Actual Loss of MHC Class I and II Expression

As presented in Chapter 5, the MHC class I molecules are the mechanism by which nonself tumor neoantigenic peptides are presented on the surface of tumor cells to the CD8$^+$ T cells of the adaptive immune system. Though MHC class I molecules are essential for the presentation of foreign antigens such as infectious viral peptides or cancer antigens, conditions in which the expression of the MHC molecules is structurally defective or even absent are not uncommon in the genetically altered cancer cell. Importantly, defective or absent tumor cell MHC molecules does not interfere with tumor cell survival. It is recognized that tumor cell surface MHC class I neoantigen presentation is generally not a very efficient method of tumor antigen T-cell stimulation. In fact, cross-antigen presentation by MHC class II molecules expressed on antigen-presenting cells (APCs) is generally the more effective mechanism for stimulating the CD8$^+$ T cells and other T cells of the immune system. Tumor antigen cross-presentation requires the antigenic peptides produced in the tumor cell to be released and taken up by APCs such as the dendritic cells (DCs) and presented to T cells via the MHC class II molecules rather than MHC class I.

Nevertheless, any impairment in tumor cells to the normal expression of genes involved in the processing of potential tumor antigenic proteins and in their presentation to the T-cell receptor (TCR) of the CD8$^+$ T cells will have a significant negative effect on the host's antitumor response. For example, let us begin with the dysregulation of the MHC chromosome 6p region's human leukocyte antigen (HLA) genes. The class I region of the polymorphic HLA locus includes, among others, the highly polymorphic *HLA-A*, *HLA-B*, and *HLA-C* genes (Fig. 8.1). These genes generate the 45 kDa classic α-chain (362–366 amino acids) of the class I molecule. The MHC class I β$_2$ microglobulin chain of 12 kDa is coded for by a gene on chromosome 15, a site different from the HLA region located on chromosome 6p21.3. Two of the three class I α domains, α$_1$ and α$_2$, create the MHC domain containing the neoantigen peptide-binding cleft. The class II MHC molecule has a similar overall physical structure but is the product of two HLA genes containing one α$_1$ and one β$_1$ domain that fold to generate the groove that holds the antigenic peptide[6] (for an in-depth review, see Monos and Winchester[6]).

It is easy to understand that within the genomically unstable tumor cell there is ample opportunity for somatic mutations to occur in the HLA genes, resulting in aberrant expression or actual silencing of HLA class I and II molecules. An example of HLA-I gene dysregulation and dysregulation of genes involved in antigen processing and presentation can be found in studies at the University of Cologne reported by Thelen and colleagues.[7] They determined the expression level of 24 genes known to be involved in antigen presentation. The genes were selected based on their known downregulation in at least a portion of patients for one or more of the tumor types selected.[7,8] They found that the mean expression levels for 7 of 24 genes were increased greater than twofold in the tumor microenvironment (TME) of tumor samples compared with normal tissues. They selected a twofold change as a cutoff in order to determine evidence for impaired gene expression. They found TME downregulation to occur in at least one patient of the following genes β*2M*, *HLA-A*, *HLA-B*, *HLA-C*, *ERAP1*, *ERAP2*, *PDIA2*, *NLRC5*, *UBB*, *UBC*, and *LMP10*. This downregulation was reported in >10% of analyzed tumor samples and occurred in more than 3 (>12.5%) of the included genes in 45 of 142 patients (32%). No alterations in expression level were found in 23% of patients. They noted that expression patterns of the 24 genes across tumor types were quite heterogeneous. Though this represents an early effort to show HLA-I gene dysregulation as an important aspect of immunoediting during cancer progression, it clearly emphasizes both the complexity and the critical relationship of HLA expression to immunotherapy.[7]

Human HLA genes
(chromosome 6p21)

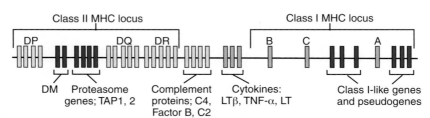

Fig. 8.1   A schematic map of the human leukocyte (HLA) genes on chromosome 6p coding for human MHC class I and II molecules. The HLA genes HLA-A, HLA-B, and HLA-C were initially serologically defined. This was followed by the use of mixed leukocyte reactions between allogeneic cells to define the HLA-D region (HLA-DR). C4, factor B, and C2 are complement proteins coded for by genes located as depicted on the map close to the HLA genes. Also coded in this region are proteasome genes coding for proteins DM, TAP1, and TAP2 that are involved in antigenic peptide processing within the cell.

The loss of both copies of MHC class I heavy chain genes or of β2M will, of course, eliminate the expression of a major component of the antigen presentation molecule and has been observed in cancers such as melanoma with the loss of HLA-A2 expression.[8-14] Many cancers have also been found to have a loss of only one copy of the heavy chain or of only β2M (heterozygous).[15,16] MHC class I heavy chains are codominantly expressed but the genetic alteration at the level of the heavy chain gene may be heterozygous. Montesion and colleagues surveyed 59 different cancer types and observed that in 17% there was a significant loss of MHC I expression secondary to a loss of heterozygosity[17,18] (for an in-depth review, see Dhatchinamoorthy et al.[18]).

There are a few facts to keep in mind regarding the function of MHC class I molecules. First, as part of their normal functions, all cells generate essential proteins and, as a result, present short peptides derived from those proteins on their cell surface as part of the peptide–MHC (pMHC) complex. When the peptide is nonself as in cancer, it is recognized as such by the immune system—innate or adaptive—for the cell to be destroyed. In all cells, the expression of the MHC complex on the cell surface is governed by interferons, especially interferon gamma (INF-γ) and the IFN signaling pathway. Stimulation with INF-γ increases the expression of MHC class I and therefore of detectable MHC class I molecules on the surface of tumor cells. The loss of MHC in cancer or the suppression of MHC expression correlates significantly with the progression of the cancer, indicating the significance of this mechanism in tumor resistance and poor prognosis (Fig. 8.2).

MHC low expression metastases are also known to respond poorly to immunotherapy. Many genes coding for proteins intimately involved as factors in the ubiquitin–proteasome production of the neoantigenic peptides can also be subject to genetic alteration in the tumor cell. Such genetic alterations in the proteins comprising the processing machinery of the proteasome can

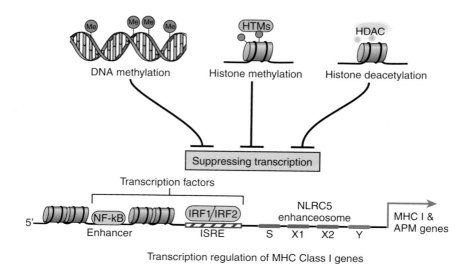

Transcription regulation of MHC Class I genes

Fig. 8.2 **The process of transcription of MHC class I genes is illustrated in this schematic.** As shown, successful transcription is at risk should genetic variants occur in any of the required transcription factors NF-κB, IRF1, IRF2, and the NLRC5 of the enhanceosome. Transcription is also subject to further impairment by the occurrence of DNA methylation, by methylation of histone H3K27me3, by histone methyltransferases (HTMs), and by histone deacetylases (HDACs) that can remove histone acetylation sites. Any of these alterations have the potential to suppress or silence transcription, eliminating the production of MHC molecules for antigen presentation.

alter the neoantigenic peptide, causing a loss of its antigenic epitope or simply a loss of the peptide altogether. Such alteration can also occur as the potential antigenic peptides leave the proteasome and enter the endoplasmic reticulum where they are loaded on the MHC class I molecules (see also Chapter 5, Fig. 5.2).

Many of the genes involved in the preparation of immunogenic peptides have similar transcription and translation governance, and many of the genes for these processing factors are actually chromosomally located in association with the HLA heavy chain genes on chromosome 6p. Thus genetic alterations affecting these genes may manifest in low expression of MHC molecules. Studies show that within the tumor itself there exists significant tumor cell heterogeneity in terms of MHC expression and therefore the robustness of T-cell antigen presentation.[18] This heterogeneity in levels of pMHC cell expression is also found in relationship to the various metastases of a given tumor both as to the metastatic site (lung, liver, brain, etc.) and within the actual individual metastases. Low or absence of detectable MHC class I has been reported to varying degrees in patients for many of the most common human malignancies including breast, prostate, colorectal, melanoma, head and neck, and non-small cell lung cancer (NSCLC), for example. It also appears that the level of expression may vary over the course of disease and in association with therapy. Finally, a loss of MHC class I has been reported to be associated with resistance to anti-programmed cell death protein-1 (PD-1) immunotherapy.[19,20]

It is easy to understand how in a genomically unstable tumor cell there exists ample opportunity (see Chapter 5) for genetic variants to cause defects that prevent optimal MHC molecule formation and optimal tumor antigen generation suitable for pMHC class I presentation. For example, any loss of the key molecules such as transporter for antigen processing (TAP), tapasin, or endoplasmic reticulum aminopeptidases (ERAP1 and ERAP2) will cause a loss of pMHC expression and presentation on the cell surface. Tumor cells that sustain homozygous deletion or frameshift variants of the HLA region of chromosome 6p will result in low expression or complete loss of MHC class I antigenic peptide presentation. Some alterations are unique to a specific cancer, whereas others may be found in numerous patients and in a variety of cancer types (Box 8.2).

A number of clinical correlations with low or absent MHC class I are important to note. For example, the presence of low MHC class I expression in breast cancer is associated with tumors that contain fewer tumor-infiltrating lymphocytes (TILs) than the tumors demonstrating a high degree of MHC class I expression.[21-24] Second, though the low expression of pMHC molecules or even a total absence prevents activation of the T cells and triggering of adaptive immune response against the tumor, it does not have a negative effect on cancer cell viability or tumor cell proliferation. The low expression or loss of MHC, as expected, does strongly indicate a worse cancer prognosis. Third, and perhaps even more important, is the association of low or absent MHC class I expression with development of resistance to anti-PD-1 and anti-PD-L1 immunotherapy.[25-27] A similar negative correlation is associated with MHC class I loss in other epithelial tumors such as melanoma, cancers of the colon and rectum, and head and neck cancer[18,25] (for an in-depth review, see Gettinger et al.[25]).

BOX 8.2 ■ Loss of pMHC Class I Expression in Cancer

Mutations or deletions of HLA structural genes.
Variants in genes or loss of genes involved in the tumor antigen MHC presentation pathway.
Variants affecting the transcription of genes critical to the pathway.
Epigenetic silencing of pathway gene regulatory elements.
Variants affecting mRNA fidelity and/or stability in generating pathway elements, pre and posttranscription.

MHC class I molecules are more densely presented on the cells of the hematologic lineage. MHC class II molecules, in contrast, are predominantly found on the surface of antigen-presenting cells such as dendritic cells (DCs), B cells, and classic macrophages. Their major role is the presentation of antigenic peptides such as from viral infections and cancer cells produced in other cells from which these peptides are released. The released antigenic peptides are internalized by the APCs for further processing and for loading onto the MHC class II molecules for surface presentation. The antigenic peptide–MHC class II molecule is primarily interactive with the CD4$^+$ T cells. CD4$^+$ T cells function to support and enhance the CD8$^+$ CTL of the adaptive immune response and to generate effective memory T cells.

In addition to a direct interaction of the antigenic peptide bearing tumor-specific MHC class II molecule (tsMHC class II) with the TCR of CD4$^+$ T cells, tsMHC class II molecules have been implicated in the stimulation directly or indirectly of other T-cell subsets. Secretion of several known activating cytokines, such as IFN-γ, can be triggered by tsMHC II interaction with CD4$^+$ T helper (Th) cells. On the other hand, the stimulation of CD4$^+$ T cells may result in activation of the subclass of regulatory T cells (Tregs), which function to suppress the immune response favoring cancer progression.

Some tumor cells during the cancer's progression have been shown by immunofluorescence to actually present both MHC class II and MHC class I molecules. Tumor-specific MHC class II expression may increase the immune response to the tumor.[28] In fact, this finding has been associated with improved prognosis in response to immunotherapy. The binding groove of the MHC class II molecules can bind longer peptide chains than can be held in the groove of the MHC class I molecule and also accept peptide chains having more branched side chains that are more immunostimulatory when interacting with the TCR.[29]

The MHC class II molecule is heterodimeric in contrast to MHC class I, and studies have demonstrated that expression of the class I and class II molecules is independently regulated in cancer. This independent regulation may in part account for observed variations in immunotherapy responses. For example, MHC class I molecular assembly and expression are not normally controlled except in T cells. Its expression, however, can be induced and enhanced by IFN-γ and by activation of the NF-κB signaling pathway. The expression of MHC class II, in contrast, is tightly controlled by the "master transcription control factor," a protein (class II major histocompatibility complex transactivator) encoded by the *CIITA* gene located on 6p.

There are a number of intracellular alterations in signaling pathways that can contribute to the suppression of MHC class II expression. For example, JAK/STAT cell signaling is necessary for upregulation of MHC class II molecule expression and, as such, mutations occurring in JAK result in suppressed IFN signaling and suppressed expression of MHC class II molecules. Also, with activation of RAS/MAPK signaling in breast cancer, there is suppression of MHC class II expression. Clearly, from clinical studies the extent to which MHC class II expression is suppressed is a strong biomarker for a poor response to immunotherapy.[29,30]

In summary, increasing evidence from clinical studies of solid tumors suggests the following: (1) the presence of a significant increase in tsMHC class II expression is associated with an improved disease-free survival (DFS) and overall survival (OS) perhaps as a result of increased antigenic recognition by the adaptive immune system, (2) significant surface expression of tsMHC class II is required for CD4$^+$ T-cell (including T-cell subsets Th1 and Treg) activation, and (3) the increased presence of tsMHC class II correlates with improved response to anti-PD-1 and anti-PD-L1 immunotherapy. The apparent significant role that the neoantigen-loaded MHC class II molecule plays in the immune control of the tumor's progression highlights why it is extremely important when anticipating the use of immunotherapy to determine whether the tumor is showing a low or possible absence of tsMHC class II expression or an intermediate or high level of expression, as well as upon which cell types the expression is occurring. This information is increasingly predictive of likely response.

Immune Checkpoints and Checkpoint Ligands

Tumors, as noted, not only escape recognition and destruction by the host's immune system but can actively block normal T cell–directed antitumor activity. One such method is by modulating immune inhibitory signals termed *immune checkpoints*. The immune checkpoints and their biologic pathways represent one of the most exciting anticancer therapeutic opportunities since their introduction in 2011 and, as such, one of the most intensely studied. In normal health, these immune checkpoints operate to prevent immunity to self (autoimmune diseases) and to self-proteins when the host is responding to infectious pathogens.

Cytotoxic T lymphocyte–associated antigen 4 (CTLA-4) was the first immune checkpoint receptor to be studied clinically. CTLA-4 functions primarily to depress the early T-cell response to tumor neoantigens by countering the TCR costimulatory receptor CD28.[31,32] Antigen recognition by the TCRs of T cells and the subsequent activation of CD8+ CTLs increases the expression of the CTLA-4 receptor on the T cells. TCR activation also suppresses the numbers of CD4+ T helper cells and their activity, along with an increase in numbers of CD4+ Tregs, which have an immunosuppressive effect. Taken together, these multiple actions have a suppressive effect on the antitumor immune response and favor tumor progression.

Another important checkpoint inhibitor is the programmed cell death protein 1 (PD-1). PD-1 receptor protein is expressed on T cells with the function of limiting T-cell activity in peripheral tissues at the time of pathogenic inflammation and of cancer initiation and development. In cancer, the ligand to PD-1 (PD-L1) is expressed in tumor cells and other cells of the TME. A high or enhanced expression of the ligand PD-L1 by the tumor causes increased stimulation of the T-cell PD-1 receptor, resulting in suppression of these T cells and their functions; in doing so, it promotes tumor growth. PD-1 activation generates suppression of two important antitumor activities. It triggers the induction of apoptosis to antigen-specific T cells and blocks the apoptosis of Tregs. PD-1 is a member of the immunoglobulin gene superfamily and is expressed as a transmembrane protein with a C-end cytoplasmic tail and an N terminus IgV-like domain.[33] PD-1 is found to be highly expressed on TCR-activated tumor-specific T lymphocytes and is also found expressed to some extent on NK cells, B cells, dendritic cells, macrophages, and monocytes.[34]

PD-1, in conditions where the immune T cells are challenged with a pathogen and inflammation, functions in the antigen-reactive T cell to prevent ineffective or harmful immune responses to self-tissues, helping to maintain a condition of immune self-tolerance. When expressed on immune cells that are being activated by cancer antigens, PD-1 has a very different role. When faced with cancer, PD-1 acts to interfere with the antitumor response by downregulating the T-cell responses, causing a decrease in T-cell proliferation and clonal expansion, a decrease in secretion of cytokines, and an increase in T-cell demise (Fig. 8.3).[35] Other described checkpoints include YIM-3, LAG-3, and VISTA. Targeting the immune checkpoints with blocking humanized monoclonal antibodies has emerged as a strategy to generate beneficial antitumor immune responses[36] (for an in-depth review, see Han et al.[36]).

The ligand that binds to the PD-1 receptor, PD-L1, is expressed by cancer cells and, as such, plays the role of enabling the tumor cells to escape immune attack. PD-L1 is a small (33 kDa) B7 transmembrane glycoprotein with extracellular domains of Ig- and IgC.[33] PD-L1 is also found to be expressed by DCs, macrophages, and B cells, as well as some epithelial cells, during inflammation. IFN-γ is known to increase the expression of PD-L1 in most cancers, and the pathway involved in PD-L1 expression also appears involved in several additional protumor stimulatory actions such as tumor cell proliferation, epithelial-to-mesenchymal transition, and expansion of the tumor stem cell population in some tumors.[36-38] A presentation of all of the intrinsic cell signaling pathways involved in interacting to provide influence/control over the PD-L1/PD-1 axis in cancer is beyond the scope of this chapter but it has been well reviewed by others.[30-38] Of increasing interest is how the genetic variants that define and alter the tumor

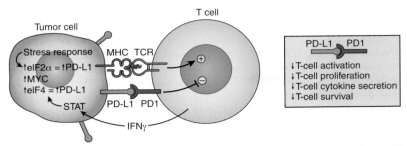

Fig. 8.3 This schematic depicts an MHC class I molecule presenting a tumor antigenic peptide to the CD8$^+$ T cell along with the engagement of the immune checkpoint ligand PD-L1 with the PD-1 receptor on the T cell. PD-L1/PD-1 interaction acts to interfere with the antitumor immune T-cell response. Mechanisms for upregulating the tumor cell expression of PD-L1 include interferon gamma (IFN-γ) activation of the intracellular STAT signaling pathway, tumor hypoxia stress response signaling pathway through eIF5B-mediated translation, and increased activation of *MYC* oncogene signaling.

microenvironment (TME) over time also manifest themselves in the up- and downregulation of various microRNAs that directly affect these signaling pathways. Undoubtedly, this will be a critical map to develop to optimally guide the integration of future immunotherapies.

Antigen Loss Variants—Loss of mRNA Translation

In Chapter 5 of this text, a good deal of effort was devoted to providing a detailed overview of the intracellular mechanisms involved in the generation and characterization of tumor-specific antigens (TSAs) and tumor-associated antigens (TAAs). As repeatedly noted in Chapter 5 and in this chapter, the genetically unstable cancer cell provides ample opportunity for the development of non-self-peptides containing antigenic epitopes of varying degrees of antigenicity when presented to CD8$^+$ T cells. As presented, there is a complex multistep process involving many cytoplasmic proteins and enzymes required to fashion an appropriately sized antigenic peptide within the immunoproteasome and transporter molecules required to shuttle the peptide to and through the endoplasmic reticulum and to chaperone its loading into the MHC class I molecule's groove for transport to the cell surface.

Mutations and structural variants, aspects of immunoediting, have the potential of affecting any of these factors directly or indirectly via variants that disrupt other critical signaling pathways. Any of these genetic alterations may affect this process, resulting in (1) selection of a short peptide with a weakly immunogenic epitope and (2) the generation or selection of an antigenic peptide that is not well sized or structured for optimal stable positioning in the MHC groove, interfering with optimal TCR recognition and T-cell immune activation. All throughout the process of tumor-specific neoantigen creation there are opportunities for mutations and structural variants to occur, resulting in a loss of optimal antigen presentation and a weakening of the tumor's immunogenicity that facilitates the escape of the growing tumor from immune control.[39,40] Tumor antigen loss includes any of the possible alterations described that lead to a decrease or absence of the expression of any of the components required (1) to create and select an optimally antigenic short TSA peptide in the immunoproteasome, (2) for the formation of a competent MHC class I molecule for antigen presentation, and/or (3) for a loss of costimulatory molecules involved in T-cell activation as well as ligands for NK cell–activating receptors.

Studies have uncovered yet an additional cause of tumor-specific antigen loss. In these experiments, it has been demonstrated that tumor antigen loss may result from a unique posttranscriptional process by which tumor cells lose antigen expression by suppressing the translation of the tumor antigen's mRNAs. There is increasing indication that RNA-binding proteins and microRNAs are involved in the active suppression of the translation of tumor cell TSAs.[41-44] Evidence to support this mechanism of antigen loss can be found in a series of experiments reported recently (2019) by Han and colleagues using a CT26/HER2 murine protective tumor model to induce CTL and HER2 immunity. These experiments demonstrated that CT26/HER2 tumor cells could develop resistance to primed antitumor CTL through the loss of antigen expression while continuing to express MHC class I molecules. The authors concluded from their experiments that the CT26/HER2-A2 tumor cells lost antigen expression and tsMHC class I presentation secondary to a defect occurring at the posttranscriptional level. They demonstrated that the CT26/HER-A2 tumor cells expressed HER2 mRNAs but not HER2 antigenic proteins.[45]

This observation of a tumor cell defect in translation should not be surprising, but certainly it requires a careful examination of the mechanisms involved and the extent of specificity involved in targeting tumor-generated neoantigens. The most critical and highly regulated step in mRNA translation is the initiation of translation by the eukaryotic initiation factors (eIFs). These initiation factors have a critical role to play in controlling both the specificity of mRNA translation and the rate of translation of a given mRNA. Thus, the initial step in translation involves the assembly of the appropriate protein factors into the eIF4F complex. It has also been shown that oncogenes such as *MYC* can upregulate the transcription of ribosomal proteins, including the initiation factor protein components of eIF4F, enhancing translational output in the tumor cell.[46,47]

A number of studies, both in animal models and in humans, provide increasing evidence that tumor cells can use the tightly controlled mechanisms regulating mRNA translation as a protective measure to force immune suppression and enable tumor progression. Another example of tumor cells controlling translation is the use of the integrated stress response, which, when activated appears to promote the priority selection of mRNAs with upstream open reading frames (uORFs) in their 5′ UTRs for translation.[47,48] It is also important to note that evidence suggests that alterations in the control of translation of mRNAs can occur in cells of the immune system as well as in the dividing tumor cells. Altered translation control occurring in cells of the immune system and in cells of the TME, for example, could cause degradation of neoantigenic peptides in dendritic cells, reduce CTL activity in CD8⁺ T cells, and, by phosphorylation of eIF4F factors in neutrophils, promote the trafficking of neutrophils to the TME, facilitating tumor metastasis.[47,49,50]

The Development of Actual Tumor Cell Tolerance

From past and current studies using both animal models of cancer and the application of whole genome sequencing (WGC) and RNAseq technologies to dissect the intricacies of the human immune response to cancer, CD8⁺ T cells have evolved as central to a successful and sustained antitumor response.[32] The development of the T cells critical to this response requires the generation of the large diversity of T-cell receptors (TCRs) required to generate the antigen recognition repertoire through extensive random recombination events. TCRs that could be harmful to the host by recognition of self-peptides under normal conditions enter into a process of self-tolerance to maintain the health of the individual. This, as we know, is a process dependent on thymic development. As a result, there are a number of mechanisms that serve to regulate and limit T-cell activation in the periphery of the immune system to maintain health and nonrecognition of self-antigens. In cancer, much like the immune response to inflammation and infectious disease, the blocking of self-reacting peripheral T cells serves to restrict activation of TCRs and to downregulate T-cell effector functions including clonal expansion and tissue infiltration.[51]

Evidence has shown that the progressing tumor itself can acquire a variety of additional ways to enhance its ability to evade immune control and to even exclude CD8⁺ T cells from invading the tumor and the TME. Studies suggests that even outside the confines of the tumor and its TME, as, for example, in the tumor's draining lymph nodes of the peripheral immune system, tumor cells are being protected from immune destruction, a form of tumor cell tolerance. This peripheral immune protection or tumor cell tolerance has been observed when antibody therapies directed against CTLA-4, PD-1, and PD-L1 have shown increased CTL tumor cell destruction, effectively breaking this tolerance in a percentage of patients, resulting in a significant period of therapeutic benefit.[52]

In another example of what might be considered tumor cell tolerance, immunologists have for years marveled at the relationship of the developing fetus to the mother's immune system and frequently noted similarities between the immune tolerance of the fetus during pregnancy and the ability of the tumor to develop tolerance to the anticancer immune attack in a patient with cancer. It has been noted by cancer biologists that during pregnancy a number of immune-active placental proteins can be identified including the numerous isoforms of pregnancy-specific β-1-glycoproteins (PSGs).[52,53] PSGs are produced by the placenta's syncytiotrophoblast cells and consist of a gene family (PGS-1 to PGS-9 plus PGS-11) located on chromosomes 19.1–19.3. More than 30 PSG isoforms have been identified and PSG proteins are readily measured in the maternal peripheral blood, especially during the third trimester.[54]

In a recent very interesting and innovative study published in 2021, investigators set out to determine whether cancers took advantage of similar preprogrammed immunosuppressive mechanisms that provided a similar form of tolerance for cancer.[55] To ask this question, they determined the level of PSG gene family member expression cancers using The Cancer Genome Atlas (TCGA) of over 10,000 tumors and consisting of 33 cancer types. In normal tissues the expression of PGS genes is rare. The authors found that PGS genes were in fact significantly upregulated in the majority of the tumors they studied; for example, kidney chromophobe carcinoma, 85%; thyroid carcinoma, 74%; adrenocortical carcinoma, 73%; head and neck squamous cell carcinoma, 68%; and cholangiocarcinoma, 67%. They found elevated PGS mRNA expression in at least 10% of all tumors and that PSG-9 was the most commonly upregulated of the PSG gene family in ~25% of tumors. Perhaps most important, they found that patients with breast cancer, lung mesothelioma, and ovarian tumors identified with higher PGS expression levels had a significantly worse disease outcome. These results highlight the possibility that PGS proteins may play an added important role in generating tumor tolerance.[55] As such, they may prove to be interesting targets to block.

Tumor Cell–Derived Immune Suppression

Tumors have been shown to express a variety of immune suppressive membrane-bound determinants and soluble factors released into the TME that can suppress antitumor immunity. Tumor membrane–bound vesicles contain molecules such as FasL, which is recognized by Fas receptors on CD8[+] CTL, suppressing CTL function and stimulating the expression and secretion of a number of inhibitory inflammatory cytokines such as interleukin (IL)-10, IL-35, and transforming growth factor beta (TGF-β).[56] This dynamic between antitumor immunity and protumor progression takes place to a large extent within the cellular microenvironment surrounding the tumor and in association with tumor metastases—the collective microenvironment (TME). The tumor and surrounding tissues that comprise the TME include cancer cells, cancer stem cells, cancer-associated fibroblasts, antigen-activated T cells, NK cells, B cells, dendritic cells, endothelial cells, and bone marrow–derived proinflammatory myeloid cells that further differentiate into macrophages, neutrophils, and monocytes.[57] Evidence has been accumulating to place the inflammatory TME in the key position of being an important determinant, if not the determinant, of the effectiveness of both standard anticancer therapies and the newer immunotherapies. For example, conventional therapies (chemotherapy, radiotherapy, and surgery) targeted directly at tumor cell destruction may enhance dendritic cell maturation, antigen presentation, and CD8[+] T-cell recruitment, enhancing the antitumor adaptive immune response. In contrast, genomic variants occurring within the cancer cells as well as those variants induced by the cancer in noncancer cells of the TME can cause recruitment and activation of inflammatory cells in the TME, resulting in immunosuppression and tumor progression.[57]

Characteristic of carcinogenesis, the immune system and the chronic inflammation associated with the developing tumor cogenerate a conflicted environment of antitumor suppression and protumor progression. The interaction of these forces is edited in multiple ways during the progression of the disease by the introduction of externally derived cell destructive therapies (chemotherapy, radiation therapy, and surgery); what is even more confounding to this environment of combined pro and con activities is the use of immunotherapies. From the efforts to introduce immune therapeutics into the mainstream of cancer treatment, it is more apparent than ever that there is much work to do to understand how the immune system and the inflammatory response can be effectively joined to treat cancer.

The Tumor Microenvironment, Inflammation, and Immune Escape

Though much of the discussion in this chapter has centered on the tumor cell itself and its direct interaction with the cells of the immune system, it is critical in any review of the ways in which tumors avoid host immune destruction to recognize that the growing epithelial tumor exists within a desmoplastic complex stroma, the tumor microenvironment (TME). This multicellular supporting environment is a network of stromal cells including cancer-associated fibroblasts (CAFs), vascular endothelial cells, pericytes, various cells of the immune system, and a variety of bone marrow–derived inflammatory cells including mesenchymal cells.[58] As the tumor progresses, it is readily apparent that the TME becomes increasingly supportive of the tumor and increasingly suppressive of antitumor immunity. The cellular heterogeneity of the TME is well recognized, but even more important is the dynamic nature of the environment reflected in the shifting nature of its different cellular composition. This creates changes in cell-to-cell interactions and differential transcriptomics regulating the secretion of specific cytokines and chemokines. This qualitative and quantitative difference in cytokines and chemokines determines differences in inflammatory cell recruitment to the TME. In addition to recruitment of immune cells such as immunosuppressive Tregs, other tumor-promoting cells such as macrophages, monocytes, neutrophils, or innate lymphoid cells are attracted to the TME and to infiltrate the tumor itself. Expansion of specific cell populations within the TME may occur by clonal expansion or by recruitment from the bone marrow (Fig. 8.4).

It is also relevant that the therapeutic interventions of chemotherapy, radiotherapy, and surgery are injurious to tissues, generating additional inflammatory responses secondary to tumor cell and tissue cell injury and cell death. These inflammatory responses are further contributed to by innate mechanisms of tissue repair. As the tumor continues to expand, hypoxia and areas of tumor necrosis occur within the tumor and further contribute to the inflammation in the TME. Collectively, these events result in release of proteins from damaged tissues, neoantigenic peptides, and immunostimulatory cytokines with the potential for generating a period of actual enhanced antitumor response. On the other hand, the collective release of a number of factors such as IL-10, transforming growth factor β (TGF-β), Fas ligand, tumor necrosis factor (TNF), a loss of cell adhesion molecules, an increase in PD-1 expression, and an increase in antiapoptosis occurring in the tumor and the TME may collaborate to enhance immunosuppression and therefore tumor progression[59-62] (for an in-depth review, see Greten and Grivennikov[62]).

Extensive reviews describe in great detail the repertoire of TME cells and their capabilities to either support the antitumor immune response of the host or enhance the growth and spread of the tumor. Many of the TME cellular phenotypes actually have the capacity to play both roles depending on the stimulating signals they receive and the state of their maturation, a set of circumstances that can be confusing to anyone attempting to gain a full understanding of the

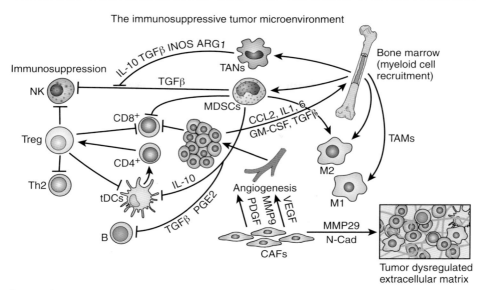

Fig. 8.4 The developing tumor leads to the formation of the tumor microenvironment (TME). The tumor and the TME involve the recruitment of a variety of different cells, some of which are recruited from the bone marrow. Immunocytes are recruited from the peripheral immune system. Many of the cells in the TME have been shown to have undergone tumor-specific alterations to their genetic expression profile. Angiogenesis occurs in the TME to support tumor growth. Cancer-associated fibroblasts secrete factors to alter the extracellular matrix and express both upregulated and downregulated microRNAs that demonstrate changes to intracellular signaling pathways of the tumor. The tumor cells in collaboration with the chronic inflammatory response occurring in the TME act to suppress the antitumor immune response. Myeloid-derived suppressor cells (MDSCs), tumor-associated macrophages 1 and 2 (TAMs, M1, M2), tumor-associated neutrophils (TANs), natural killer cells (NKs), and matrix metalloproteinase (MMP) collectively suppress the immune response against the tumor.

growth controlling nature of the TME. It is worth, however, focusing on a few of what one might term "major players" (not an exhaustive review) with an emphasis appropriate for this chapter on the support of tumor progression[63,64] (for an in-depth review, see Farc and Cristea[63]).

Dendritic Cells and Inflammation

Certainly, the DCs deserve considerable attention. The immature DCs attracted to the TME encounter, engulf, and normally are stimulated by tumor generated non-self-peptide antigenic fragments. As a result, the antigen-activated DCs go through a process of maturation and acquire the capability to present internally processed tumor antigens complexed to MHC class II molecules to the TCR of CD4[+] T cells. Mature DCs also secrete IFN-γ1, which triggers T helper (Th) cell activation and differentiation, actions that enhance the antitumor immune response of CTL and NK cells.[65] However, it has been shown that when this process of attracting immature DCs to the TME fails to properly cause appropriate DC maturation, the immature DCs actually present tumor antigens in a tolerogenic manner to T cells. Tolerogenic DCs have a high expression of PD-1 and CTLA-4 as well as other immunosuppressive molecules and, as such, also enhance the generation of Tregs.[66-69] The tumor has a great deal of influence over the cellular makeup of the TME because of the ability of tumor cells and the cells of the tumor stroma to release chemokines that influence the quality and quantity of the tumor-infiltrating lymphocytes.

A greater extent of this infiltration is an indicator of favorable outcomes. During the growth of the tumor, however, this antitumor chemokine environment can be reversed and an increase in M2 macrophages and other cells with an immunosuppressive action can become dominant, enhancing tumor progression.[70]

Myeloid-Derived Tumor Suppressor Cells

Classically, the myeloid cells, granulocytic neutrophils, and mononuclear myeloid cells such as monocytes, macrophages, and dendritic cells are activated and mobilized from the bone marrow in a response to pathogens and to tissue damage. In the setting of tumor initiation and progressive tumor growth, there is a steady presence of growth factors and a recognition by the innate and adaptive immune systems of non-self-neoantigens. The activation of T cells by tumor TSAs triggers inflammatory signaling pathways and the production of cytokines such as granulocyte–macrophage colony-stimulating factor (GM-CSF) and macrophage colony-stimulating factor (M-CSF). In this context, both granulocytic and monocytic myeloid-derived suppressor cells (MDSCs) are key components of the tumor microenvironment that favor cancer progression.

The most recognized function of MDSCs is one of suppressing antitumor immune responses. They are among the most important cells facilitating cancer dissemination and metastatic growth. MDSCs can produce nitric oxide, which is inhibitory to the JAK/STATS signaling pathway, decreasing T-cell proliferation and induces T-cell apoptosis. MDSCs also have the ability to produce reactive oxygen species also known to suppress T-cell function. Other actions of MDSCs include interfering with T-cell trafficking to tumor-draining lymph nodes and to the TME. MDSCs are a major producer of the cytokine IL-10, and this secretion is enhanced in the presence of tissue hypoxia. IL-10 is a suppressor of antigen presentation and of certain T-cell functions and an apparent enhancer of Tregs. MDSCs are also a significant source of TGF-β, which in certain circumstances is immunosuppressive (Fig. 8.5).

As a major cellular component of the TME, MDSCs have multiple functions, including dispersing the various actions of different MDSC subsets within the TME, making the MDSC a versatile participant in the suppression of the immune response. It has been shown that MDSCs' suppressive activities extend beyond the antigen activated T cells to include natural killer (NK) cells, antigen-presenting dendritic cells, and B cells. Functions of the various subsets of MDSC cells include facilitating epithelial–mesenchymal transition, cancer stem cell formation, tumor angiogenesis, the complex process of establishing the premetastatic niche, the physiologic and metabolic support of cancer cell survival, and the growth of tumor in metastatic sites. As noted, the complexity of the potential actions of MDSCs and the multiple levels of TME influence or control of a diverse group of activities make therapeutic targeting of MDSCs problematic. MDSCs are short-lived once they have entered the TME, but they are continuously recruited to maintain their presence and actions. Clinical studies confirm that the presence in the TME of a high level of MDSCs correlates with a poor response to current immune therapy[71] (for an in-depth review, see Yang et al.[71]).

MDSCs also play an essential role in the process of developing metastasis, with much of it taking place initially in the TME. The TME must be prepared to facilitate the entry of tumor cells into the circulation (lymphatic and vascular) for these cells to reach distant organs and form metastatic tumors. Studies have demonstrated that the sites for development of future metastatic lesions (liver, lung, bone, etc.) undergo preparation for engraftment of the tumor cells. Polymorphic neutrophil MDSCs (PMN-MDSCs) are recruited from the TME to the premetastatic "niche" by chemokines. It is postulated that in the niche they are immunosuppressive to both NK cells and T cells, induce matrix remodeling, and promote angiogenesis[72,73] (for an in-depth review, see Veglia et al.[73]).

This process of developing metastases, as complex and varied as it is, also depends on the entry of viable cancer cells into the circulation and their survival. This stage in cancer progression

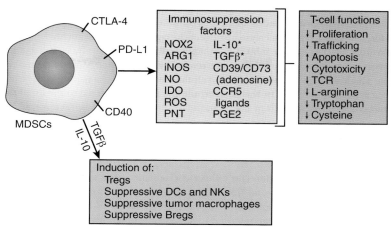

Fig. 8.5 **Myeloid-derived suppressor cells (MDSCs) are mobilized from the bone marrow in response to progressive tumor growth.** MDSCs, both monocytic and granulocytic, are central components of the TME and function to support progression of the malignant process. The main function of MDSCs as depicted in this figure is the suppression of the antitumor immune response through the release of a series of immunosuppressive factors that act on T lymphocytes. A description of these factors includes nicotinamide adenine dinucleotide phosphate (NADPH) oxidases that give rise to NO, NOX2 nitric oxidase; arginase 1 (ARG1); inducible nitric oxide synthase (INOS); indoleamine 2,3-dioxygenase (IDO); reactive oxygen species (ROS); peroxynitrite (PNT); interleukin-10 (IL-10) cytokine; transforming growth factor-beta (TGF-β). CD39 and CD73 are ectonucleotidases, adenosine triphosphate is first hydrolyzed by CD39 (the rate limiting step) into adenosine monophosphate and then dephosphorylated by CD73 into immunomodulatory adenosine; C-C chemokine receptor type 5 (CCR5) is a G protein–coupled receptor that regulates trafficking and effector functions of T cells, macrophages, and immature dendritic cells; prostaglandin E2 (PGE2) regulates the activation, maturation, migration, and cytokine secretion of immune cells including T cells, neutrophils, macrophages, and dendritic cells.

also requires escape from immune detection and is essential for the development of lethal metastases. These circulating tumor cells (CTCs) are frequently found in clusters with neutrophils (neutrophil extracellular traps or NETS), and patients with a high percentage of such clusters have been shown to have a worse prognosis.[74,75]

CD4⁺ T Cells and Tregs in Cancer Inflammation

Certainly, another important cell phenotype to review is CD4⁺ T cells. CD4⁺ T cells recognize tumor antigenic peptides presented primarily on antigen-presenting cells to the T-cell receptor by MHC class II molecules. CD4⁺ T cells play a critical role because of the number of different regulatory cellular phenotypes that antigen triggering can stimulate. CD4⁺ T cells generate both immune help (Th) and immune suppressive regulation (Treg). The functionally different subsets of T helper cells include Th1, Th2, Th9, Th17, and Th22. Th1 cells are recognized for secretion of IL-2 and IFN-γ, which together act to enhance the presence of CD8⁺ CTLs and their activation. In addition to the Th cell subsets, CD4⁺ T cells are responsible for differentiation into the Treg subline. Tregs produce several chemokines and their respective receptors and in the TME suppress antitumor immunity, support tumor growth, and facilitate the metastatic process. Tregs suppress the antitumor immune response by releasing IL-10, TGF-β, and IL-35.

As noted, there are a number of Th phenotypes. It should be understood that these subsets have the capability of both supporting and suppressing the physical (vascular) and metabolic growth needs of the tumor and also under specific circumstances suppressing antitumor immune responses. Th2, for example, can increase angiogenesis to support tumor growth.[76,77] The role that each of the Th and Treg cellular subsets play individually and collectively, as well as the research defining their individual phenotypes, is well reviewed in the immunology literature and is certainly an evolving science. A detailed presentation of all the identified mechanisms used by each specific cell subtype is beyond the scope of this chapter, and the reader is referred to the listed reviews.

Cancer-Associated Fibroblasts

The TME represents the interface between the expanding tumor (primary or secondary) and the host's normal surrounding tissues. In normal tissues, connective tissue fibroblasts, derived from mesenchymal cells, form the main cellular component of the tissue's extracellular matrix. They produce collagens, elastin, and fibronectin, all of which are important to defining tissue morphology. As in normal tissues, cancer-associated fibroblasts (CAFs) are the most common cells comprising the TME and are involved in supporting tumor growth. Several observations regarding CAFs are important to recognize. First, CAFs in the TME are responsible for synthesizing growth factors that regulate tumor cell proliferation, tumor cell survival, proteins involved in remodeling of the extracellular matrix, and proteins involved in the process of tumor cell egress for metastasis development.[78-80] Interestingly, though studies of CAF derived from a number of human epithelial carcinomas have confirmed that they do not undergo malignant transformation while a functioning part of the TME, they do undergo significant changes in their gene expression patterns and consequently in their TME functions.[81]

Some years ago (2006-2011), in a series of experiments in my lab, we obtained fresh tissues from patients undergoing hysterectomy for localized endometrial cancer. Samples of normal-appearing peritumoral tissue were paired with a tissue sample of normal endometrium as anatomically removed as possible from the tumor and served as a source of cultured fibroblasts. These experiments using paired cultured fibroblasts demonstrated that in 9 of 20 pairs the human endometrial cancer–associated fibroblasts showed significantly lower levels of detectable miR31 compared with their normal paired endothelial fibroblasts. miR31 is just one example of a number of microRNAs in CAFs that were found to be either upregulated or significantly downregulated in terms of their expression. The low expression of miR31, for example, was shown to have a relationship with the SATB2 pathway in tumor cells. These and similar experiments have supported the conclusion that the various cellular components of the TME depend on alterations in their transcriptional regulation, on epigenomic modifications, on alterations in chromatin structure, and in other variations to their genome organization to be transformed and as a result perform their highly specific TME functions.[82,83]

Studies by Donnarumma and colleagues first published in 2017, also demonstrated the presence of CAF-generated extracellular vesicle exosomes expressing miRNA-21, miRNA-143, and miRNA-378e, which were not found in exosomes from normal fibroblasts. Very clearly, CAFs function to collaborate in tumor-specific immune suppression as well as function to support tumor growth, tumor cell invasion, and tumor metastasis[57,84] (for an in-depth review, see Labani-Motlagh et al.[57]).

Overall, the ability of the progressing tumor to avoid immune destruction requires a number of information-carrying cells of different phenotypes and genetic backgrounds. The ability of these different cells, whether located within the tumor, the TME, or the peripheral immune system, requires the generation of many unique chemokines and cytokines, as has been noted throughout this chapter. These soluble factors are the communication system, and there is increasing awareness of the role that extracellular microvesicles and exosomes released by TME cells play in transferring intracellular factors between cells and the role they play in the cell–cell communication and cell trafficking in the TME, producing a more aggressive tumor. Immuno-cytes, similar to CAFs and the various inflammatory cells of the TME, also release exosomes and, again, these exosomes may contain enhancing factors supporting increased CTL activity or they can be immunosuppressive and can facilitate tumor growth directly.

The ability to identify and functionally characterize cancer-associated fibroblast (CAF) heterogeneity, as well as the heterogeneity that exists within other inflammatory cells in the TME, has previously depended primarily on immunohistochemistry and cell sorting approaches. The iden-tification and functional characterization defining subclasses within cell populations has been revolu-tionized by the development of single-cell RNA sequencing technology. This approach has already identified several functionally distinct fibroblast subpopulations such as inflammatory CAFs, myofibroblast CAFs, and antigen-presenting CAFs expressing MHC class II antigen presentation complexes, as well as subpopulations within other cell phenotypes comprising the TME.[85-89]

Tumor-Associated Macrophages

Tumor-associated macrophages (TAMs) are another prominent cellular component infiltrating the tumor and are early residents of the developing TME. TAMs are generally divided into the M1 class and M2 class primarily related to the roles they play in inflammation. M1 TAMS are classically functioning macrophages found early as resident tissue macrophages in tumor development and demonstrate antitumor activities similar to activities observed in viral infections such as direct cell killing and antibody-dependent cell-mediated cytotoxicity. M2 TAMS, in contrast, inhibit T-cell tumor destruction, produce cytokines maintaining a state of immunosuppression, and function pri-marily to support tumor growth, angiogenesis, tumor invasion, and tumor spread. They also appear to play a role in the tumor's resistance to chemotherapy[56,90] (for an in-depth review, see Zhao et al.[56]).

The cellular origin of TAMs has variously been proposed to be from one of two sources. M1 TAMs have generally been assigned as coming from tissue-specific embryonic-derived resident macrophages that infiltrate the tumor and the associated TME. Alternatively, M2 TAMs are thought to be derived from the monocyte-like myeloid-derived suppressor cells (M-MDSCs) attracted to the tumor from the bone marrow.[91,92] Thus, M2 TAMs are considered to be almost exclusively of the monocyte origin recruited from stem cells in the bone marrow. TAMs, like so many of the cell types that populate the tumor and the TME, demonstrate significant plasticity influenced by the changing biochemical environment of the TME or as a result of the adminis-tration of anticancer therapies. This plasticity of function appears to be triggered by cytokines and chemokines produced by tumor cells and by lymphocytes residing in the TME.

Nonclassic HLA Molecules—HLA-G

Previously in this chapter, the similarities of immune evasion that exist during pregnancy and those that develop in cancer were noted. Nonclassic HLA molecules, specifically HLA-G, originally identified as expressed on placental trophoblasts cells, have become of interest when focusing on mechanisms of tumor immune escape.[93] HLA-G expression has been detected on the cell surface of a number of solid tumors and hematologic malignancies and is generally more prominent in late-stage malignancies. It is rarely found on the cells of normal, healthy tissues.[94,95] HLA-G has four membrane-expressed isoforms and is structurally formed as a classic MHC class I molecule although without significant polymorphism. As a result, HLA-G is not a source of TSA presentation but rather functions as an immune checkpoint. The degree of its expression is often associated with tumor hypoxia. HLA-G also has three immunosup-pressive soluble isoforms secreted by tumor cells. It is still quite early in the application of clinical research studies designed to further determine the true significance of HLA-G tumor expression. An important question is whether, as an immune checkpoint, it offers therapeutic targeting opportunities. Nevertheless, it is clearly evolving to be a serious mechanism for tumor immune escape.

Some Concluding Thoughts

The future development of immunotherapies that target the patient's tumor directly while enhancing the patient's own adaptive immune system to reject the tumor will require a comprehensive knowledge of all of the many ways that tumor(s) have at their command to avoid immune destruction. Though some of the escape pathways are common across tumors, there does exist considerable tumor site specificity to the immune avoidance process, as well as individual patient differences. The complexity of cell phenotypes and cellular functions supporting tumor progression is positioned in juxtaposition to the active pro and con processes that exists within the host's own immune system. Experimental efforts to better understand the mechanisms supporting tumor progression and suppression of antitumor responses must be carefully designed to account for the metabolic stress of tumor growth and for the effect on the immune system generated by administered therapies.

Because T lymphocytes and especially CD8$^+$ CTLs are central to carrying out the antitumor immune response, the tumor's ability to avoid immune destruction must be considered first in the context of the tumor-infiltrating T cells and T cells in the TME. The family of T lymphocytes differentiates into several phenotypes with different functional roles. Across the T-cell compartment, T lymphocytes comprise memory cells, a phenotypic series of cell subtypes termed T helper cells, and a suppressive or regulatory T-cell population (Tregs). Studies have also identified CD8$^+$ CTL cells as existing in a state termed *T-cell exhausted* (Tex). Tex, it is surmised, results from chronic tumor antigen exposure. Though Tex, as its name suggests, is considered to be mainly a terminal state for the CD8$^+$ CTL, it now appears that the Tex cells with appropriate TME support can be rescued and reactivated as effective CTLs.

To consider the varied opportunities for the tumor to avoid immune destruction (downregulation or loss of MHC molecules, loss of effective tumor neoantigens, upregulation of immune checkpoint ligands, loss of tumor antigen translation) a considerable effort is required to place the immune system in the context of the TME and the tumor-induced inflammatory reaction. Much like the complex altered genetics that characterizes cancer as a disease, the cancer paths to avoid immune system control are equally focused on genetic mutations and structural variants. The very real promise of immuno-oncology in cancer therapeutics resides in the realization that the dissection of the complexity of the TME is continuing to evolve at an increasingly rapid pace. Success has been realized in efforts to better define specific cell subtypes and to describe intricate cell–cell communication pathways that are critical to both enhancing the antitumor response and suppressing the response. The introduction of microfluidics and single-cell mRNA sequencing to the challenge of cell identification and to defining cell function is already promising tremendous benefit, providing a clear roadmap of all of the mechanisms involved at the level of a single cell. This is the type of knowledge required to optimally guide future immunotherapy clinical trials.

Key References

3. Dunn GP, Old LJ, Schreiber RD. The three Es of cancer immunoediting. *Ann Rev Immunol.* 2004;22:329-360.
4. Schreiber RD, Old LJ, Smyth MJ. Cancer immunoediting: integrating immunity's roles in cancer suppression and promotion. *Science.* 2011;331(6024):1565-1570.
5. Quail DF, Joyce JA. Microenvironmental regulation of tumor progression and metastasis. *Nat Med.* 2013;19(11):1423-1457.
6. Monos DS, Winchester RJ. Chapter 5. The major histocompatibility complex. In: Rich RR, Shearer WT, Frew AJ, et al., eds. *Clinical Immunology.* Elsevier; 2019:79-92.
7. Thelen M, Wennhold K, Lehman J, et al. Cancer-specific immune system evasion and substantial heterogeneity within cancer types provide evidence for personalized immunotherapy. *NPJ Precis Oncol.* 2021;5:52. doi:10.1038/s41698-021-00196-x.

8. McGranahan N, Rosenthal R, Hiley CT, et al. Allele-specific HLA loss and immune escape in lung cancer evolution. *Cell*. 2017;171(6):1259-1271.e11. doi:10.1016/jcell.2017.10.001.
9. Maleno I, Aptsiauri N, Cabrera T, et al. Frequent loss of heterozygosity in the beta2-microglobulin region of chromosome 15 in primary human tumors. *Immunogenetics*. 2011;63(2):65-71. doi:10.1007/s00251-010-0494-4.
10. Maeurer MJ, Gollin SM, Storkus WJ, et al. Tumor escape from immune recognition: Loss of HLA-A2 melanoma cell surface expression is associated with a complex rearrangement of the short arm of chromosome 6. *Clin Cancer Res*. 1996;2:641-652.
17. Montesion M, Murugesan K, Jin DX, et al. Somatic HLA class I loss is a widespread mechanism of immune evasion which refines the use of tumor mutational burden as a biomarker of checkpoint inhibitor response. *Cancer Discov*. 2020;11:282-292. doi:10.1158/2159-8290.CD-20-0672.
18. Dhatchinamoorthy K, Colbert JD, Rock KL. Cancer immune evasion through loss of MHC class I antigen presentation. *Front Immunol*. 2021;12:636568. doi:10.3389/fimmu,2021.636568.
20. Sade-Feldman M, Jiao Yi, Chen JH, et al. Resistance to checkpoint blockade therapy through inactivation of antigen presentation. *Nat Commun*. 2017;8:1136.
25. Gettinger S, Choi J, Hastings K, et al. Impaired HLA class I antigen processing and presentation as a mechanism of acquired resistance to immune checkpoint inhibitors in lung cancer. *Cancer Discov*. 2017;7:1420-1435. doi:10.1158/2159-8290.CD-17-0593.
28. Kambayashi T, Laufer TM. Atypical MHC class II-expressing antigen presenting cells: can anything replace a dendritic cell? *Nat Rev Immunol*. 2014;14:719-730.
30. Johnson DB, Estrada MV, Salgado R, et al. Melanoma-specific MHC-II expression represents a tumour-autonomous phenotype and predicts response to anti-PD-1/PD-L1 therapy. *Nat Commun*. 2016;7:10582.
36. Han Y, Liu D, Li L. PD-1/PD-L1 pathway: current researches in cancer. *Am J Cancer Res*. 2020; 10(3):727-742.
39. Dunn GP, Bruce AT, Ikeda H, Old LJ, Schreiber RD. Cancer immunoediting: from immunosurveillance to tumor escape. *Nat Immunol*. 2002;3(11):991-998. doi:10.1038/ni1102-991.
41. Vyas M, Müller R, von Strandmann EP. Antigen loss variants: catching hold of escaping foes. *Front Immunol*. 2017;8:175-182. doi:10.3389/fimmu.2017.00175.
51. Nüssing S, Trapani JA, Parish IA. Revisiting T cell tolerance as a checkpoint target for cancer immunotherapy. *Front Immunol*. 2020;11:589641. doi:10.3389/fimmu.2020.589641.
55. Zhao J, Rabadan R, Levine AJ. Pregnancy-specific glycoproteins: a possible mediator of immune tolerance of cancers. *J Cell Immunol*. 2021;3(2):109-117.
56. Zhao H, Wu L, Yan G, et al. Inflammation and tumor progression: signaling pathways and targeted intervention. *Signal Transduct Target Ther*. 2021;6:263. doi:10.1038/s41392-021-00658-5.
57. Labani-Motlagh A, Ashja-Mahdavi M, Loskog A. The tumor microenvironment: a milieu hindering and obstructing antitumor immune responses. *Front Immunol*. 2020;11:940. doi:10.3389/fimmu.2020.00940.
62. Greten FR, Grivennikov SI. Inflammation and cancer: triggers, mechanisms, and consequences. *Immunity (Cell Press)*. 2019;51:2738. doi:10.1016/j.immuni.2019.06.025.
63. Farc O, Cristea V. An overview of the tumor microenvironment, from cells to complex networks (Review). *Exp Ther Med*. 2021;21:96-115. doi:10.3892/etm.2020.9528.
67. Kushwah R, Wu J, Oliver JR, et al. Uptake of apoptotic DC converts immature DC into tolerogenic DC that induce differentiation of Foxp3+ Treg. *Eur J Immunol*. 2010;40:1022-1035. doi:10.1002/eji.200939782.
71. Yang Y, Li C, Liu T, Dai X, Bazhin AV. Myeloid-derived suppressor cells in tumors: from mechanisms to antigen specificity and microenvironmental regulation. *Front Immunol*. 2020;11:1371. doi:10.3389/fimmu.2020.01371.
73. Veglia F, Sanseviero E, Gabbrilovich DI. Myeloid-derived suppressor cells in the era of increasing myeloid cell diversity. *Nat Rev Immunol*. 2021;21:485498.
75. Rayes RF, Moubanza JG, Nicolau I, et al. Primary tumors induce neutrophil extracellular traps with targetable metastasis promoting effects. *JCI Insight*. 2019;5:e128008. doi:10.1172/jciinsight.128008.
80. Lorusso G, Ruegg C. The tumor microenvironment and its contribution to tumor evolution toward metastasis. *Histochem Cell Biol*. 2008;130:1091-1103.
85. Zheng GXY, Terry JM, Belgrader P, et al. Massively parallel digital transcriptional profiling of single cells. *Nat Commun*. 2017;8:14049.
92. Pan Y, Yu Y, Wang X, Zhang T. Tumor-associated macrophages in tumor immunity. *Front Immunol*. 2020;11:583084. doi:10.3389/fimmu.2020.583084.

Visit Elsevier eBooks+ (eBooks.Health.Elsevier.com) for complete set of references.

CHAPTER 9

Vaccines and Active Immunization Against Cancer

Luis A. Rojas ▪ Vinod P. Balachandran

SUMMARY OF KEY FACTS

- Cancer vaccines represent a promising strategy to activate immunity in cold tumors.
- The complexity and heterogeneity of human tumors remains a challenge to developing cancer vaccines.
- Sipuleucel-T is the first therapeutic vaccine approved for cancer.
- Cancer vaccines targeting unmutated tumor-associated antigens (TAAs) have had poor results in the clinic.
- Neoantigens that arise from tumor-specific mutations are immunogenic, drive antitumor immune responses, and are promising new are targets for cancer vaccines.
- Early results with neoantigen vaccines have shown the most promise in the clinic.

Introduction

Immunotherapy has now emerged as one of the most promising therapeutic approaches to treat cancer. Evidence that the immune system can recognize human cancer and that this recognition can be therapeutically leveraged to control, and even eradicate, widespread cancer has highlighted the power and promise of the immunotherapeutic approach. Antibodies that inhibit immune checkpoint pathway proteins (Programmed Cell Death Protein 1 (PD-1), Cytotoxic T-Lymphocyte Associated Protein 4 (CTLA-4), Lymphocyte Activation Gene 3 (LAG3)) have now demonstrated antitumor efficacy and are U.S. Food and Drug Administration (FDA)-approved for use in melanoma, renal cell carcinoma (RCC), colorectal cancer (CRC), non-small cell lung carcinoma (NSCLC), and Hodgkin lymphoma (HL), among other cancers. Engineered T cells equipped with chimeric antigen receptors (CARs) are FDA-approved for hematologic malignancies including acute lymphoblastic leukemia (ALL), B-cell lymphoma, follicular lymphoma (FL), mantle cell lymphoma, and multiple myeloma. Yet because these approaches undoubtedly represent merely a fraction of the myriad ways through which the immune system controls cancer and could potentially be future therapeutic cudgels, immuno-oncology appears to be in its infancy, with a bright future.

The success of immune checkpoint inhibitors (ICIs) and CAR T cells notwithstanding, what has emerged is that these immunotherapy strategies appear to be successful in only certain tumor types. The impressive results obtained with CAR T cells have appeared restricted to hematologic cancers, and these successes have not so far extended beyond liquid cancers to solid tumors. Similarly, though ICIs have shown broader efficacy across multiple solid and some liquid tumors, their success appears to be mostly restricted to the so-called hot tumors—tumors with greater inherent antigenicity (for instance, due to a higher mutational burden or viral transformation)—which

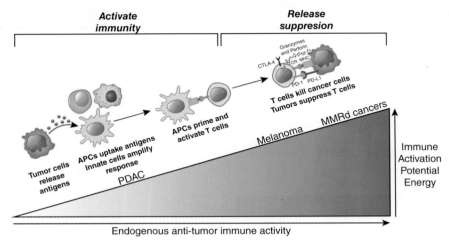

Fig. 9.1   The cancer immune incline. Cold tumors such as pancreatic ductal adenocarcinoma (PDAC) appear to arrest earlier on a "cancer immune incline" than immune checkpoint inhibitor (ICI)-responsive tumors such as melanoma or mismatch repair–deficient (MMRd) tumors. Cold tumors thus have lower immune activation potential energy, and blockade of suppression alone with ICIs is insufficient to generate a clinical response. *APC,* Antigen-presenting cell; *TCR,* T-cell receptor. © 2021 Memorial Sloan Kettering Cancer Center. All rights reserved.

provoke baseline antitumor immune responses that are subsequently disinhibited by ICIs. In fact, ~80% of cancers appear to be "cold" given lower inherent antigenicity; because they thus provoke weaker baseline antitumor immune responses, they remain insensitive to ICIs.

Thus it is likely that cold tumors, which comprise the majority of current cancers, fail to mount sufficient endogenous antitumor immune responses to render them sensitive to ICIs.[1,2] Such cold tumors hence appear halted at an early stage of an immunologic incline (Fig. 9.1) and therefore may require therapies that activate immunity rather than release immune suppression. Cancer vaccines represent one promising strategy to activate immunity.[3]

Cancer Vaccines

Vaccination is arguably the most important breakthrough in the history of medicine. Vaccines have proven highly effective in preventing infectious diseases caused by viruses or bacteria and have saved hundreds of millions of lives by protecting from, and even eradicating, several deadly infectious diseases such as smallpox, polio, and diphtheria. The success of vaccination stems from its ability to therapeutically harness the inbuilt circuitry of immunologic memory against foreign antigens, namely, that when the human immune system encounters a foreign antigen, it not only rapidly activates immune cells to expand and clear the threat but empowers a subset of these cells to persist long term in the absence of the antigen to reexpand with subsequent exposures. Thus prophylactic exposure to the antigen (i.e., vaccination) activates this circuitry to protect against a future foreign encounter. It remains simple, elegant, and highly effective.

Despite the proof that the immune system protects not only against foreign infectious agents but also oncogenically transformed host cells, unlike vaccination against pathogens, vaccination against host cancer cells has proven significantly more challenging. Though several factors contribute to this challenge, the central hurdle with cancer vaccination has remained the difficulty of choosing optimal tumor antigens for vaccines. Unlike pathogens, tumor cells are intrinsically host cells; thus the majority of proteins in tumors are "self" and hence restricted by central tolerance with their cognate T cells thymically deleted during development. Thus an optimal tumor antigen for a vaccine must be both tumor specific and sufficiently "nonself" to escape central tolerance and allow antigen-specific T cells to escape thymic deletion, enter the peripheral repertoire, and expand upon antigen delivery. Furthermore, given that cancers are genetically heterogeneous collections of transformed cells (more akin to a clade of viruses), further raises the possibility that different on-cogenic clones may possess different antigens. These characteristics impose two requirements to identify optimal cancer vaccines: specificity, namely, to discover cancer-specific antigens that are absent from the host proteome during T-cell development, and heterogeneity, namely, to identify cancer antigens that are both sufficiently abundant and antigenic across cancer cell clones and subclones. This necessitates individualized comparisons of tumor and normal host cell genomes and proteomes to identify optimal targets, which has for decades remained technically challenging.

However, breakthroughs in next-generation sequencing technology have made significant advances in this regard—now, comparison of entire genomes of tumor and normal cells is possible. Such analyses have unveiled that most cancers accumulate mutations as they grow, and a fraction of these mutations can generate novel protein sequences completely absent from the human proteome. These "neoantigens" are absent in normal tissues, escape central tolerance to T cells in the thymus, and become T cell targets in cancers.[4] Next-generation sequencing advances have also revealed that T cells recognize neoantigens in cancer[5] (for an in-depth review, see Schumacher et al.[5]) and induce the success of clinical immunotherapies. Tumors with more immunogenic or "high-quality" neoantigens correlate with greater patient survival[6,7] and response with immune checkpoint inhibitors in multiple cancers.[8-10] Neoantigen-specific T cells induce these clinical responses[11] as well as responses with transfer of autologous tumor-infiltrating T cells.[12] Thus neoantigens have emerged as specific and fundamental immunogenic by-products of cancer pathophysiology, and thus are highly attractive targets for cancer vaccines. Nevertheless, generating effective long-lasting immune responses through vaccination against a tumor has proven much more challenging compared with viruses or other infectious agents because of different factors that will be discussed in subsequent sections.

Antigen Choice

A central requirement to develop an effective cancer vaccine is to choose an appropriate antigen. An ideal cancer vaccine antigen would have following ideal characteristics:

1. High immunogenicity (less/not restricted by central tolerance)
2. Tumor specificity
3. Homogeneity across
   (a) cancer clones
   (b) patients with cancer.

In this regard, tumor antigens can be categorized under two groups: (1) tumor-associated antigens (TAAs) and (2) tumor-specific antigens (TSAs) (Table 9.1).

TUMOR-ASSOCIATED ANTIGENS

Tumor-associated antigens (TAAs) are nonmutated self-proteins with preferential or abnormal expression in tumor cells but also some level of expression in normal cells. TAAs can be classified into three main groups:

Overexpressed antigens: This category includes proteins expressed at higher levels in tumors compared with normal tissues. These could be products of genetic amplification or increased transcription, resulting in elevated protein levels. Examples of overexpressed TAAs include human epidermal growth factor receptor 2 (HER-2/neu), human telomerase reverse transcriptase (hTERT), mesothelin, and mucin 1 (MUC-1).[13]

TABLE 9.1 ■ **Characteristics of Antigens Employed in Cancer Vaccines**

Antigen Type		Tumor Specificity	Central Tolerance	Shared Among Patients
Tumor-associated antigens (TAA)	Overexpressed antigens	Low	High	Yes
	Differentiation antigens	Low	High	Yes
	Cancer/testis antigens	Intermediate	Low	Yes
Tumor-specific antigens (TSAs)	Oncogenic viral antigens	High	Absent	Yes
	Public neoantigens	High	Absent	Yes
	Private neoantigens	High	Absent	No

Differentiation antigens: This category includes proteins selectively expressed in differentiated cell types and their derived tumors. Differentiation antigens studied as immunotherapy targets include several in melanomas, including tyrosinase, glycoprotein 100 (gp100), and melanoma antigen recognized by T cells 1 (MART-1), and in prostate cancer, including prostate-specific antigen (PSA) and prostatic acid phosphatase (PAP).[14]

Cancer/testis antigens: This category includes proteins with restricted expression in male germ cells, fetal ovaries, and trophoblasts. Thus these types of antigens are absent in healthy somatic cells but are expressed in a wide variety of tumors. Examples of cancer/testis antigens include the large melanoma-associated antigen (MAGE) family (MAGE-A, MAGE-B, MAGE-C) and New York esophageal squamous cell carcinoma-1 (NY-ESO-1).[15]

Several obstacles limit inclusion of TAAs in cancer vaccines. One of the main disadvantages of TAAs is their low immunogenicity. As outlined previously, TAAs are self-antigens and thus TAA-specific T cells are subject to central tolerance and TAA-specific high-affinity lymphocytes are typically deleted by central or peripheral tolerance. Furthermore, TAA expression is not restricted to tumor cells. These obstacles hamper efforts to use TAAs to induce an immunogenic, tumor-specific immune response.

For overexpressed antigens and differentiation antigens, high levels of protein expression can presumably break tolerance and activate lower affinity lymphocytes.[16] However, they primarily target low-affinity lymphocytes, thus contributing to overall low immunogenicity. The use of highly immunogenic adjuvants and effective costimulators has been proposed to increase the immunogenicity of TAAs. Yet an additional disadvantage remains their lack of tumor specificity and thus the possibility to induce reactivity against corresponding normal tissues and lead to autoimmunity. In support of this, such phenomenon has been observed after adoptive transfer of tumor-reactive T cells directed against overexpressed self-derived differentiation antigens in melanoma.[17] In terms of tumor specificity, cancer/testis antigens theoretically represent a more attractive option because they are not expressed in normal adult tissues but only in germline and embryonic cells. Conversely, one logistic advantage of the use of TAAs for cancer vaccines is that because they are self-proteins and do not arise from patient-specific mutations, they are shared by many patients' tumors and thus permit universal tumor-specific vaccines rather than personalized vaccines.

Initial clinical trials of cancer vaccines preferentially targeted TAAs because of their easier identification compared with mutation-derived tumor antigens. Preclinical studies have shown that TAAs can be immunogenic in vitro and in murine models in vivo,[18] leading to tumor-protecting immunity. Despite promising results in preclinical studies, results from clinical trials using cancer vaccines targeting TAAs have been in general disappointing.[19-22] Evidence of TAA-specific CD8$^+$ T-cell responses in vaccinated patients was found, yet clinical efficacy has been rarely reported. The main exception to this would be sipuleucel-T (Provenge, Dendreon Corporation), the first and only therapeutic cancer vaccine approved by the FDA for the treatment of metastatic castration-resistant prostate cancer (mCRPC).[23] Sipuleucel-T is an autologous dendritic cell vaccine prepared by culturing peripheral blood mononuclear cells (PBMCs) from the patient with a recombinant fusion protein of the prostate differentiation antigen PAP and granulocyte-macrophage colony-stimulating factor (GM-CSF), which are then reinfused to the patients. Antigen-presenting cells (APCs) activated by GM-CSF further activate and induce replication of PAP-specific T cells with the capacity to recognize and kill PAP-positive prostate cancer cells. Sipuleucel-T was approved in 2010 based on the results of a phase III trial that showed improved overall survival compared with placebo.[23] Despite their theoretical low immunogenicity, TAAs are still being evaluated as antigens for therapeutic cancer vaccines, and new clinical trials that combine them with other immune checkpoint inhibitors show more promising clinical results and possible correlations with increased survival.[24]

TUMOR-SPECIFIC ANTIGENS

Tumor-specific antigens (TSAs) are proteins that are completely absent from normal tissues but only expressed in cancer cells. Thus two obvious advantages over TAAs are that: (1) TSAs are more immunogenic than TAAs because they are not subject to central or peripheral tolerance and thus high-affinity TSA-specific lymphocytes are not eliminated, and (2) TSAs are tumor specific and thus targeting TSAs should less likely induce immune reactivity against healthy tissues and autoimmunity. TSAs can be classified in two groups: (1) oncogenic viral antigens and (2) neoantigens.

Oncogenic Viral Antigens

Oncogenic viral antigens are viral proteins expressed in cells infected with oncogenic viruses that have subsequently undergone cellular transformation. Viruses can induce cancers,[25] and vaccinating with antigens derived from cancer-inducing viruses is an effective vaccination strategy against such tumors. Because expression of these antigens will be shared among different patients' tumors, universal vaccines for different tumor types are feasible. Indeed, prophylactic vaccines have been approved to prevent cancers of the cervix, anus, penis, and head and neck induced by human papilloma virus (HPV) and hepatocellular carcinoma induced by the hepatitis B virus (HBV). Both vaccines consist of recombinant virus–like particles (VLPs) that induce immune responses that target the main HPV capsid protein L1 and the HBV surface antigen HBsAg, respectively.[26] However, because human cancers with a known viral etiology are the exception, neoantigens represent the only TSAs targetable for the majority of human tumors.

Neoantigens

Mutations cause cancer and accumulate in cancers as they grow. These mutations can generate novel protein sequences completely absent from the human proteome called *neoantigens*. These abnormal proteins are degraded in the cytosol by the proteosome to generate short peptides termed *neopeptides* or *neoepitopes*. Neoepitopes are then transported to the endoplasmic reticulum, loaded onto major histocompatibility complex (MHC) class I molecules and transported to cell membranes for peptide presentation. Because neopeptides are absent in normal tissues, they escape central tolerance to T cells in the thymus to become T-cell targets in cancers. CD8$^+$ T cells can then recognize the presented neoepitope and acquire cytolytic potential to directly kill tumor cells.[5] Additionally, it is now evident that CD4[+] T cells can recognize neoepitopes presented by MHC class II molecules, and their role is also clinically important in controlling tumors in both mice and humans.[27-29]

Neoantigens are thus both highly immunogenic and tumor specific, which makes them ideal candidates for cancer vaccines. Mounting clinical evidence also indicates that neoantigens are critical antigens targeted by host T cells in human cancers. Advances in next-generation sequencing that now enable neoantigen discovery have revealed that T cells recognize neoantigens in cancer[5] and induce the success of clinical immunotherapies.

Neoantigens are classified based on the type of somatic mutation that alters the protein sequence. The most common somatic mutations that generate neoantigens are as follows:

Single-nucleotide variants (SNVs): Neoantigens are generated by the substitution of an individual nucleotide within an exonic sequence of a gene. Such alterations result in neoantigens with a single amino acid substitution and represent the most common source of neoantigens.[30]

Mutational frameshifts (indels): Single-nucleotide insertions or deletions generate novel amino acid sequence strings because of the shift in the gene reading frame, which may also result in premature stop codons. Such premature stop codons can induce nonsense-mediated decay (NMD) of the translated RNA and prevent protein translation. Nonetheless, indel-derived neoantigens have been correlated with higher immunogenicity and increased clinical response to ICIs.[31]

Fusion genes: Novel amino acid sequences are generated owing to genetic rearrangements that fuse two unrelated genes. Evidence shows that these types of neoantigens can be immunogenic.[32] However, because the frequency of these gene fusions is relatively low, their efficacy as cancer vaccine targets remains unexplored.

Splicing alterations: Mutations can both disrupt and generate de novo splicing sites. Such events can lead to retained introns and alternative exon junctions ("neojunctions") that generate novel amino acid sequences absent in normal cells that can be presented by MHC molecules. Pharmacologic modulation of RNA splicing has been shown to induce neoantigen generation and to enhance antitumor immunity in mouse models.[33] The use of these types of neoantigens for personalized cancer vaccines has also been proposed, but their efficacy as vaccine targets remains unknown.

The main disadvantage of neoantigens as cancer vaccine antigens is that, because they most frequently arise from stochastic somatic passenger mutations, each tumor has its own profile of neoantigens that is rarely shared among patients. Thus application of neoantigens as a source for vaccine antigens is most common in the context of individualized vaccines, where every patient receives their own private set of mutated epitopes. This is in contrast to TAAs or oncoviral antigens where universal vaccines are feasible. However, advances in next-generation sequencing technologies and bioinformatics now allow for rapid identification of candidate neoantigens on a per patient basis.

Although the vast majority of neoantigens arise in passenger genes and are thus private, public neoantigens arising from driver genes are also possible therapeutic targets. Theoretically, targeting public neoantigens for therapy offers advantages over targeting private neoantigens. First, it avoids many of the challenges of developing personalized vaccines. Manufacturing a therapeutic vaccine de novo for each patient requires complex logistics and higher costs, which have in general raised doubts about the widespread accessibility and feasibility of the personalized approach. Additionally, the extended timeline of design and manufacture increases the risk of disease progression before treatment can be initiated. Second, because driver gene mutations drive tumorigenesis and are indispensable for tumor growth, they should be present in most cells within the tumor. Furthermore, because losing the mutation would result in a loss of tumor fitness, tumor cells are less likely to acquire therapy resistance by means of neoantigen loss.[34] This is in contrast to passenger neoantigens, which are subclonal, do not usually provide an advantage in tumor fitness, and thus are more likely to be lost during clonal evolution and induce therapy resistance.[35] Despite these theoretical advantages, public neoantigens also present some important limitations that hinder their applicability as off-the-shelf therapeutic cancer vaccines. One potential problem is that most patients have just one or very few public neoantigens in their tumors, in contrast to private neoantigens, which are present at a much higher multiplicity. Multiepitope vaccines are thus less feasible when targeting neoantigens in driver genes, which increases the risk of therapy resistance. Another important barrier of public neoantigen therapy is that most driver mutations appear to not be immunogenic, with immunogenic driver mutations requiring the presence of rare human leukocyte antigen (HLA) alleles. Thus for a public neoantigen-targeted therapy to be applicable to different patients, it needs to share not only the specific driver mutations but also the specific HLA alleles that can allow the neopeptide to be presented as immunogenic. Considering frequencies of the most common HLA alleles and most common driver mutations, it was calculated that patients with pancreatic cancer that could potentially benefit from anti-KRAS G12D therapy is around 10%.[36] If a collection of public neoantigen-targeted therapies is developed, they could potentially treat millions of patients with cancer. Yet personalized approaches will still be necessary for the vast majority of cases.

Neoantigens are currently conceived as the most promising antigens in cancer to induce antitumor immune responses. Several studies have shown that higher neoantigen burden is associated with increased baseline immune cell tumor infiltration and T-cell activation[37] and improved clinical outcome in patients with different types of cancer.[38,39] Clinical response to ICIs has also been associated with mutations and thus neoantigen load in patients with different tumors including melanoma,[9] NSCLC,[10] and CRC with mismatch repair deficiency.[40] Furthermore, expansion of neoantigen-specific T cells was found in patients showing clinical responses to anti-CTLA4[9,11] and anti-PD-1 treatment.[10] However, tumor mutational burden and neoantigen load do not always predicts immunotherapy response,[5] suggesting that there might be other immunologic factors that predict neoantigen immunogenicity. For example, in patients with pancreatic cancer[6] or glioblastoma,[7] survival was not correlated with neoantigen quantity but with neoantigen quality (see **Nonselfness of microbial vs tumor antigens**). In any case, this suggests that even in cancer with low mutational burden and baseline T-cell activation (cold cancers), tumor neoantigens might drive antitumor immune responses and play a key role in patient survival.[6,7] Overall, it has now been demonstrated through mouse models and human studies that neoantigens elicit cytolytic responses that contribute to tumor regression and that neoantigens are key targets of the most successful immunotherapies[4] including immune checkpoint blockade and adoptive cell transfer.

Cancer vs Pathogen Vaccines

PROPHYLACTIC VS THERAPEUTIC APPROACH

Infectious diseases are caused by specific microbes. Developing a vaccine against such diseases requires previous knowledge of the etiologic agent, its genome, proteome, and therefore the potential immunogenic antigens. Hence, barring putative mutations that could lead to antigenically distinct variants, the antigens that could elicit a protective immune response will be common among the pathogen and thus shared among all infected individuals. Thus a universal vaccine that contains such antigens can be prophylactically administered to healthy individuals who are yet to contract the disease. This can lead to immunologic memory that can prevent future infection and therefore pathogen spread. In the case of a new disease like the coronavirus disease 2019 (COVID-19) pandemic, modern technologies have allowed for an exceptionally rapid identification of the virus, its genome, and the lightspeed development of several effective vaccines. Since the first cases were reported in China, the first severe acute respiratory syndrome coronavirus 2 (SARS-CoV-2) genome sequence was released approximately 1 month after, the first phase I clinical trials started 3 months after, and the FDA approved the first two vaccines 1 year after. This unprecedented speed of vaccine development supports vaccination as the most effective approach to fight infectious diseases.

This is in contrast to tumors, which rarely have universal antigens. Genome instability and accumulation of mutations are a hallmark of cancer, and during tumor evolution most genetic mutations are acquired stochastically. As a result, each person's cancer has a unique combination of genetic alterations, and even different cells within the same tumor harbor different mutations. This high antigenic variability adds significant complexity to developing universal cancer vaccines and thus hinders the feasibility to treat cancer prophylactically.

An exception to this is infection-associated cancers. In 2018, approximately 13% of all cancers diagnosed worldwide were associated with infection.[41] Although the bacteria *Helicobacter pylori* is responsible for most cases, viruses represent the most common etiologic agent overall. At least eight viruses have been identified to cause cancer, HPV, HBV, hepatitis C virus (HCV), Epstein-Barr virus (EBV), Kaposi sarcoma–associated herpesvirus (KSHV or HHV-8), Merkel cell polyomavirus (MCV), human T-lymphotropic virus type-1 (HTLV-1), and human immunodeficiency virus (HIV).[25] These viruses can induce oncogenesis either directly through expression of viral oncoproteins (HPV, HTLV-1), or indirectly by inducing chronic inflammation (HBV or HCV) or compromising the immune system and the immunosurveillance of malignant cells (HIV). The theoretical advantage of virus-induced tumors is that vaccines can be developed to target the viral antigens and therefore can be used prophylactically. Indeed, prophylactic vaccines against two virus-inducing tumors have been approved by the FDA, including vaccines against HPV (associated with cancers of the cervix, anus, penis, and head and neck) and HBV (associated with hepatocellular carcinoma [HCC]). The HBV vaccine can be considered the first FDA-approved vaccine to prevent cancer. The first version approved in 1981 was a blood-derived product that was replaced in 1986 by a safer recombinant virus–like particle (VLP) vaccine.[26] Twenty years later, in 2006, the FDA approved the first HPV vaccine, also a VLP-based vaccine. Overall, three vaccines have been approved conferring protection against different HPV subtypes: Gardasil (Merck) against subtypes 6, 11, 16, 18; Cervarix (GlaxoSmithKline) against subtypes 16 and 18; and Gardasil 9 (Merck) against subtypes 6, 11, 16, 18, 31, 33, 45, 52, and 58.[26]

Because preventing virus infection is an effective mechanism to prevent virally induced cancers, the efficacy of these vaccines is mostly attributed to the induction of virus-neutralizing antibodies. Hence, although these vaccines work prophylactically, they have limited therapeutic efficacy for patients with already established virus-induced tumors,[25] where T-cell responses are more desirable. In the case of HPV, tumor progression is often associated with the lack of virus-specific T-cell immunity or the presence of dysfunctional and suppressive HPV-specific T cells.

Looking more broadly, despite these advances, human cancers with a known viral etiology are a minority. Vaccination approaches for the remaining 87% of human cancers will require the use of tumor antigens arising from the patient's own genome, impeding the prophylactic approach.

NONSELFNESS OF MICROBIAL VS TUMOR ANTIGENS

Arguably, one primary function of the immune system is to protect the host from pathogens. For that purpose, the peripheral T-cell repertoire is pruned to recognize non-self-antigens and, to avoid autoimmunity, thymic selection deletes T cells with high affinity to antigens derived from the human proteome. Therefore our peripheral lymphocyte repertoire has been shaped to avoid recognition of self-antigens. In theory, this poses a great challenge to vaccination against cancer because unlike microbial pathogens, tumor cells are in principle self. This lack of immunogenicity against self-proteins is likely one of the key factors why cancer vaccines using unmutated tumor-associated antigens (TAAs) have in general been ineffective.[22]

Nevertheless, it is now widely accepted that another key function of the immune system is to surveil for aberrant cells that could potentially lead to cancer. Although this "cancer immunosurveillance" theory was proposed in 1957, newer studies from 2002 have strengthened this concept, demonstrating that the immune system not only eliminates nascent transformed cells but also sculpts developing tumors.[42] Multiple studies have demonstrated that the relevant targets of the immune system in such transformed cells do not seem to be unmutated TAAs but rather neoantigens that arise as a result of somatic mutations in the cancer cell genome.[5] Theoretically, because neoantigens are absent in normal cells, putative T cells recognizing them are not deleted during thymic selection and populate the peripheral repertoire.[4] As in the case of microbial antigens, this bypass of central tolerance would render them as non-self-antigens. Indeed, neoantigens have been shown to induce protective responses against cancers and are targets of adoptive T-cell transfers or immune checkpoint therapies.[10,11,29] But are neoantigens as nonself as microbial antigens? In reality, a large fraction of computationally predicted neoantigens fail to induce detectable immune responses. This could be attributable to different factors, such as inaccurate in silico predictions, immunodominance, or the suppressive microenvironment of a tumor. However, another possibility is that many neoantigens might still fall within the self-peptide space. Although neoantigens can arise from different types of mutations (see **Neoantigens**), efforts have been especially focused on nonsynonymous SNVs, mainly because they are the most common type in most cancers.[30] SNV neoantigens differ only by one amino acid from the wild-type self-peptide. However, some of these amino acid changes might generate neopeptides that are too antigenically similar to self and thus not sufficiently immunogenic to trigger an immune response.[43]

Mechanisms underlying neoantigen immunogenicity are still not fully understood, which creates difficulty in rational design of neoantigen vaccines. Dissimilarity to the self-proteome has been proposed as a predictor of peptide immunogenicity.[44] If an amino acid substitution results in a presented neopeptide with a high degree of similarity to the self-antigen, namely, three-dimensional shape or T-cell receptor (TCR) contacts, one would think that putative self-antigen-specific T cells that could cross-react against the neoantigen would have been deleted by thymic selection.

Interestingly, another possible theory postulates that neoantigens with high similarity to non-self-peptides, namely microbial antigens, may possess higher immunogenic potential.[6,9,45] The most accepted mechanism for this theory is molecular mimicry, where lymphocyte receptors with specificity to microbial epitopes could potentially cross-react against highly homologous neoantigens. This phenomenon of cross-reactivity has been widely documented in the context of autoimmune diseases and has gained more strength in the last few years in the context of cancer. Snyder et al. showed that tumors from patients who exhibited long-term clinical benefit from CTLA-4 inhibition contained immunogenic neoantigens that shared sequences that were homologous to many viral and bacterial antigens from the Immune Epitope Database (IEDB).[9] Such a sequence signature was absent in patients with minimal or no benefit from the immune checkpoint treatment. Furthermore, this neoantigen signature showed stronger correlation with survival than did mutational load. Additional support for the clinical relevance of the mimicry theory was shown with the development of a neoantigen quality fitness model. This model, which confers a higher immunogenicity score to neoantigens with differential MHC presentation and homology to infectious disease–derived peptides, predicted survival in two independent cohorts of immunotherapy-naïve patients with pancreatic cancer based on neoantigen quality.[6] Moreover, T-cell clones with specificity to both high-quality neoantigens and predicted cross-reactive microbial peptides were found to infiltrate the tumors of long-term survivors of pancreatic cancer. The same model also predicted survival in anti-CTLA-4-treated patients with melanoma and anti-PD-1-treated patients with lung cancer.[8] Subsequent studies further confirmed the predictive power of the quality model in glioblastoma.[7] In the aforementioned cohorts, neoantigen quality was a better predictor for survival than neoantigen burden. Subsequent improvements to this model to rationally select immunogenic neoantigens based on immunogenic features of "high quality" have identified immunogenic neoantigens naturally targeted by the endogenous repertoire in cancers and longitudinally edited.[43]

In addition to pathogenic microbes, the commensal microbiota has been described to play an important role in molecular mimicry. Theoretically, the gastrointestinal tract is considered a tolerogenic environment to avoid immune rejection of commensal gut microbiota. Thus it would be logical to posit that neoantigen homology to epitopes of commensal microbiota would be tolerated and lowly immunogenic. However, evidence seems to point otherwise. Indeed, it has been proven in different mouse models that having a specific bacterial strain in their gut microbiota confers better tumor protection and that such protection was mediated by cross-reactive microbiota-specific T cells.[46,47] Similarly, the gut microbiome also seems to play an important role in responsiveness to immune checkpoint blockade. *Bifidobacterium* was found to be associated with the antitumor effects of anti-PD-L1 therapy,[48] whereas *Bacteroides thetaiotaomicron* or *Bacteroides fragilis* was associated with response to CTLA-4 blockade.[49] The latter association was also found in patients with cancer in whom T-cell responses specific for such bacterial strains correlated with improved efficacy of CTLA-4 blockade.[49]

The likely explanation for this phenomenon remains skewing of the peripheral T-cell repertoire toward recognizing common immunogenic features in antigenic peptides, which is then reflected as cross-reactivity of T cells between peptides that harbor such features (e.g., microbial peptide and neopeptide). One interesting therapeutic potential of this cross-reactivity is that heteroclytic vaccination with microbial peptides could elicit potential cross-reactive protection against homologous tumor antigens.[50] These concepts remain areas of active investigation and will be critical to elucidate the features that distinguish immunogenic and nonimmunogenic neoantigens.

Antigen Delivery Systems

Human tumors are complex, with varying antigens and levels of expression. For this reason, efficient cancer vaccination platforms should ideally capture the breadth of the tumor antigenic space and theoretically include vaccines with multiple tumor antigens to prevent outgrowth of antigen-negative tumor cells. To achieve this, different vaccination platforms have been tested in the clinic. Among those, cell-based vaccines, peptide vaccines, and mRNA vaccines are the most advanced. These strategies can either be antigen agnostic, where whole tumor cells or tumor cell lysates are used as an antigen source without selection, or antigen specific, where prior antigen identification and selection is performed. The characteristics of these vaccine platforms and their application in the clinic are discussed later (Table 9.2).

CELL-BASED VACCINES

Whole-Cell Cancer Vaccines

Whole–tumor cell vaccines can be generated from irradiated tumor cells, tumor cell lysates of autologous tumor cells, or heterologous tumor cell lines.[58] The main advantage of this approach is that because the tumor cells provide a source of all potential antigens, it avoids the need to identify the most immunogenic antigens for each patient. To further stimulate immune responses, these vaccines are typically genetically modified to express cytokines, chemokines, or costimulatory molecules. Among those, expression of GM-CSF was found to be superior to

TABLE 9.2 ■ Selected Clinical Trials of Neoantigen Cancer Vaccines

Delivery	Reference	Tumor Type	Phase	Antigens/Patient	Formulation	Route of Administration	Vaccine Responses
DC	Carreno et al. 2015[51]	Melanoma	I	7 HLA-A*02:01-restricted private neoantigens + gp100	DCs pulsed ex vivo with antigen peptides	Intravenous	NA-specific responses in 3/3 patients. 43% of neoantigens were immunogenic (67% vaccine-induced).
Peptide	Ott et al. 2017[52]	Melanoma	I	13–20 private neoantigens restricted to HLA-A and -B	15- to 30-mer SLPs + poly-ICLC	Subcutaneous	NA-specific responses in 6/6 patients. 60% of NAs elicited CD4 responses, 16% of NAs elicited CD8 responses.
	Keskin et al. 2019[53]	Glioblastoma	Ib	7–20 private neoantigens	15- to 30-mer SLPs + poly-ICLC	Subcutaneous	Patients not treated with dexamethasone (2/5) developed NA-specific CD4 and CD8 responses.
	Hilf et al. 2019[54]	Glioblastoma	I	9 TAAs (APVAC1) + 2 private neoantigens (APVAC2) restricted to HLA-A*02:01 and HLA-A*24:02	19-mer SLPs + poly-ICLC + GM-CSF	Intradermal	TAA-specific responses in 12/13 patients. NA-specific responses in 8/10 patients. 84.7% of NAs were immunogenic.
	Ott et al. 2020[55]	Melanoma NSCLC Bladder	Ib	Up to 20 private neoantigens restricted to HLA-A and -B	14- to 35-mer SLP + poly-ICLC	Subcutaneous	NA-specific responses in 34/34 patients in all cohorts. 52% of NAs were immunogenic in patients with melanoma, 47% in patients with NSCLC, and 52% in patients with bladder cancer.
mRNA	Sahin et al. 2017[56]	Melanoma	I	10 private neoantigens	Naked mRNA 2 pentatopes encoding 27-mers	Intranodal	NA-specific responses in 13/13 patients. 60% of NAs were immunogenic. 60% CD4 responses, 20% CD8 responses, 20% both.
	Cafri et al. 2020[57]	Gastric Colorectal	I/II	Up to 20 private neoantigens in driver genes	LNP-RNA Single molecule encoding 25-mers	Intramuscular	NA-specific responses in 3/4 patients. 15.7% of NAs were immunogenic. 54% CD4 responses, 41% CD8 responses.

DC, Dendritic cell; NSCLC, non-small cell lung carcinoma; SLP, synthetic long peptide; GM-CSF, granulocyte-macrophage colony-stimulating factor; LNP, lipid nanoparticle; NA, neoantigen; TAA, tumor-associated antigen.

other cytokines such as interleukin (IL)-2, IL-4, IL-6, tumor necrosis factor alpha (TNF-α), or interferon gamma (IFN-γ), inducing accumulation of dendritic cells (DCs), macrophages, eosinophils, and T cells at the vaccination site.[58] GM-CSF-expressing whole–tumor cell vaccines have now been tested in the clinic for two decades. These group of vaccines, collectively known as GVAX, showed promising signs of immunologic responses[59,60] and have induced tumor-reactive CD8$^+$ T cells in early clinical trials in multiple solid and hematologic cancers. However, clinical responses of GVAX used as a single therapy have been overall disappointing. A phase II trial was reported where GVAX vaccination showed no survival improvement after hematopoietic stem cell transplantation (HSCT) in patients with myelodysplastic syndrome (MDS) or acute myeloid leukemia (AML).[61] In pancreatic ductal adenocarcinoma (PDAC), a heterologous prime-boost vaccination strategy with allogeneic GVAX and a *Listeria monocytogenes* vaccine expressing mesothelin (a TAA overexpressed in PDAC) resulted in extended patient survival,[62] suggesting that combinatorial approaches might be required to improve clinical outcomes. Combination of GVAX with ICIs has shown strong antitumor responses in mice and is being tested in the clinic (NCT03190265, NCT02451982).

One main disadvantage of this vaccination approach that might compromise its efficacy is the dilution of the most immunogenic and relevant tumor antigens with the remaining antigenic pool in the tumor cell, the majority of which are nonimmunogenic self-antigens[63] (for an in-depth review, see Hu et al.[63]). With technologies that allow identification of individual tumor-specific antigens in an efficient and increasingly rapid manner, most vaccination strategies have evolved to an antigen-specific approach.

Dendritic Cell–Based Vaccines

Dendritic cells (DCs) are the most potent professional APCs and are critical to generating effective adaptive immune responses. DCs surveil peripheral tissues where they uptake antigens to present them to naive T cells at tissue-draining lymph nodes. DCs can present exogenous antigens by MHC class II molecules to stimulate CD4$^+$ T cells but also by MHC class I molecules to stimulate CD8$^+$ T cells via cross-presentation, a process crucial to rejection of tumors. Thus autologous DCs generated ex vivo represent attractive vaccination platforms and have been widely studied for this purpose. Autologous DCs can be directly isolated from patient PBMC samples, derived from monocytes, or derived from CD34$^+$ hematopoietic stem cells.[64] DCs are then expanded and matured in vitro with cytokine cocktails. Mature DCs have enhanced antigen processing and presentation potential, improved migration to lymphoid tissues, and increased capacity to stimulate T cells.[64] Cancer antigens are then loaded onto DCs, which act as delivery vehicles, and are administered back into the patients to induce antitumor immunity. This approach can be antigen-specific by loading DCs with tumor-specific antigens using peptides, proteins, DNA, RNA, or recombinant viruses. Alternatively, an antigen-agnostic approach can be employed by loading DCs with lysates of autologous or allogeneic tumor cells or by fusing DCs to autologous tumor cells. In the clinic, only mature DCs have had the capacity to induce antigen-specific T-cell responses in patients with cancer. Overall, the process of generating DCs ex vivo is complex and shows low reproducibility because of patient variability. Additionally, generating the numbers required for patient vaccination is costly and time-consuming.

The first clinical trials with DC-based cancer vaccines were conducted in the late 1990s and mainly used DCs pulsed with tumor lysates or peptides encoding TAAs. Many of these trials were tested in melanoma targeting different TAAs including Mage-3A1, MART-1, tyrosinase, or gp100.[14] Additionally, DC vaccines have been tested in prostate cancer, renal cell carcinoma, and glioma. Overall, DC vaccines have been shown to be safe and able to induce and expand tumor antigen–specific T cells in patients with cancer. In some cases, preliminary clinical responses were reported, and regression of metastases have been observed.[65,66] In general, the leukapheresis process to isolate PBMCs and cell culture processing to obtain DCs is laborious and has been shown to limit the number of vaccinations.

The most successful example of such a vaccine is sipuleucel-T (Provenge), which was approved by the FDA in 2010 for the treatment of metastatic castration-resistant prostate cancer (mCRPC). This vaccine consists of autologous antigen-presenting cells (APCs) isolated from leukapheresis-collected PBMCs and incubated with recombinant protein PA2024, a fusion protein of the TAA prostatic acid phosphatase (PAP) with GM-CSF. The vaccine is then reinfused back into the patients within 48 hours of the leukapheresis. Phase I and II trials have demonstrated that sipuleucel-T is safe and immunogenic and induces reactivity against the fusion protein. The randomized phase III IMPACT clinical trial showed that vaccination improved the median overall survival (OS) by 4.1 months compared with the placebo group (25.8 months versus 21.7 months, respectively).[23] Additional studies further demonstrated that sipuleucel-T induces infiltration of CD4[+] and CD8[+] T cells in the tumor microenvironment and facilitates antigen spreading to other prostate cancer TAAs like PSA or galectin-3. Combination of sipuleucel-T with immune checkpoint blockade is currently being investigated in the clinic to improve its efficacy (NCT01420965, NCT01832870), although initial reports with anti-CTLA-4 have shown modest clinical activity.

Advances in technologies that allow rapid identification of patient-specific mutations have allowed the incorporation of neoantigens into DC vaccines. The first cancer neoantigen DC vaccine was published by Carreno et al. in 2015. They performed whole-exome sequencing on tumors from three patients with melanoma to identify somatic mutations, loaded monocyte-derived DCs (MoDCs) with HLA-A*02:01–restricted neoantigen peptides, and reinfused them back into the patients.[51] The results showed that the vaccine augmented preexisting as well as induced de novo expansion of polyclonal CD8[+] T cells with specificity to multiple tumor neoantigens. This clinical trial provided a proof of concept that personalized neoantigen vaccines based on patient-specific neoantigens were feasible and immunogenic in the clinical setting. Given their promising results of neoantigen immunogenicity, they extended their studies to treat a larger cohort of patients with melanoma (NCT00683670). The safety and immunogenicity of neoantigen DC vaccines have been further confirmed in subsequent trials, and encouraging duration of response was observed in some patients.[67] Additionally, clinical trials of neoantigen DC vaccines in breast cancer (NCT04105582), HCC (NCT03674073), and lung cancer (NCT04078269) are underway and should shed light into the clinical efficacy of these vaccines.

PEPTIDE-BASED VACCINES

Peptide vaccines comprise amino acid (AA) sequences containing the immunogenic epitopes and thus offer the most direct way to vaccinate against tumor antigens. Historically, they have also been the most commonly used form of cancer vaccine.[22] Peptide-based vaccines are more time-efficient and cost-effective than autologous vaccines that require isolation and culture of patients' cells. Conceptually, two types of peptides have been used in therapeutic vaccines: minimal peptide epitopes (~8–11 AA) or synthetic long peptides (SLPs, ~25–30 AA). Minimal peptide epitopes have the appropriate length so they can directly bind to HLA-I molecules without the necessity of being internalized or processed. However, one must consider that HLA-I molecules are expressed by most nucleated cells, and thus most peptide molecules will bind to nonprofessional HLA-I-expressing APCs that lack expression of costimulatory molecules. Recognition of such presented peptides will lead to inefficient CD8[+] T cell stimulation and even to induction of peptide tolerance rather than activation.[68] As opposed to short peptides, SLPs require internalization and processing and thus favor presentation by professional APCs such as DCs, leading to optimal T-cell priming and activation. Additionally, SLPs have the advantage of containing both HLA-I- and HLA-II-restricted epitopes and thus have the potential to stimulate both CD4 and

CD8 T-cell responses. Thus long peptide vaccines have more potential to induce sustained and effective antitumor responses.

Multiple peptides targeting different tumor antigens can be combined in the same vaccine to increase the breadth of antitumor responses and avoid immune escape. However, one main disadvantage of this vaccination approach is that peptides alone are not naturally immunogenic. Peptides do not activate pattern recognition receptors (PRRs) or the innate immune system, leading to inefficient and weak T-cell responses. Therefore peptide vaccines need to be coadministered with immune adjuvants to elicit robust immune responses. The main role of adjuvants is to ensure sufficient costimulation by the antigen-presenting cells that prime T cells.[69] Examples of adjuvants employed in cancer vaccines include Montanide incomplete sepping adjuvants (Montanide-ISA), Toll-like receptor (TLR) agonists (polyinosinic-polycytidylic acid-poly-L-lysine carboxymethylcellulose [poly-ICLC]), stimulator of interferon genes (STING) agonists (cyclic dinucleotide [CDN]), or cytokines (GM-CSF). Clinical trials have mostly employed single adjuvants in vaccine formulations, but combination of multiple adjuvants might be necessary to increase immunogenicity of peptide vaccines.

Despite evidence of peptide-specific immune responses in early-phase trials, clinical outcomes in phase III clinical trials with peptide-based vaccines targeting TAAs have overall been disappointing.[69] Examples of phase III clinical trials where peptide vaccination did not result in improved overall survival are the Telovac trial in which the GV1001 vaccine was used to target the telomerase TAA in pancreatic cancer,[19] the START study in which the Tecemotide vaccine was used to target the MUC-1 TAA in NSCLC,[20] and the IMPRINT trial in which the IMA901 vaccine was used to target 10 different TAAs in RCC.[21] In melanoma, patients vaccinated with gp100 peptide showed improved overall survival and progression-free survival in a phase III trial.[70] Efforts to vaccinate against multiple peptides encoding TAAs have continued in other tumor types, including urothelial carcinoma, myeloma, astrocytoma, and glioma. Although these early-phase trials have similarly reported CD8[+] T-cell responses in several patients, clinical benefit will have to be assessed in phase III studies.

Neoantigen peptide vaccines have been brought to the clinic and are still being evaluated in early-phase trials. Preclinical mouse models have shown very strong responses after vaccination with neoantigen peptides, leading to tumor rejection and immunologic protection in both prophylactic and therapeutic settings.[71] Ott et al. published the first clinical trial using personalized peptide vaccines targeting patient-specific neoantigens.[52] In this trial, patients with melanoma were treated with 13 to 20 neoantigen SLPs and poly-ICLC adjuvant with a prime and boost regimen (NeoVax vaccine). Vaccination induced polyfunctional neoantigen-specific CD4[+] and CD8[+] T cells. Interestingly, neoantigen-specific CD4 responses were more abundant than CD8 responses, even though neoantigen selection was based on MHC class I–predicted binding affinities. Four out of six patients had no recurrence up to 25 months after vaccination, and the two patients with recurrence showed complete tumor regression after anti-PD-1 therapy. In these patients, neoantigen-specific T cells persisted long term (4 years) and acquired a memory phenotype. NeoVax was also tested in glioblastoma where, similarly, neoantigen-specific T cells with the ability to infiltrate the intracranial tumor were detected.[53] Given these promising results, the NeoVax vaccine is being currently tested in combination with immune checkpoint blockade (NCT02950766 and NCT03929029). The phase I GAPVAC-101 trial followed a similar approach in glioblastoma, where patients were sequentially vaccinated with APVAC1 (targeting unmutated TAAs) and APVAC2 (targeting neoepitopes) with poly-ICLC and GM-CSF.[53] Unmutated TAAs in APVAC1 elicited memory CD8 responses, whereas neoantigens induced predominantly CD4 T helper 1 (Th1) responses. Additionally, the phase Ib NT-002 represents another promising trial. Here, the NEO-PV-01 vaccine (SLPs targeting patient-specific mutated neoepitopes with the adjuvant poly-ICLC) was used in combination with anti-PD-1 therapy to treat patients with melanoma, NSCLC, or bladder cancer.[55] All patients in all tumor cohorts showed de novo neoantigen-specific CD4 and CD8 T responses. The vaccine-induced T cells showed ability to traffic to the tumor, a cytotoxic phenotype, and induced epitope spread to neoantigens not included in the vaccine. Overall, these early-phase trials of neoantigen peptide vaccines have shown promising results of safety and high immunogenicity and some evidence of clinical response and thus warrant further clinical exploration.

mRNA-BASED VACCINES

Although mRNA has been studied for years as a therapeutic agent and vaccination platform, it is now recognized as one of the most exciting biomedical advances. Interest in mRNA vaccines has dramatically increased because of its rapid response over other vaccine platforms to the COVID-19 pandemic. The FDA has approved two COVID-19 mRNA vaccines (BNT162b2 from BioNTech and Spikevax from Moderna), with BNT162b2 being the first-ever mRNA vaccine approved by the FDA. The 2021 Lasker-DeBakey Clinical Medical Research Award was granted to Katalin Karikó and Drew Weissman for their research in mRNA modifications that enabled the rapid development of these vaccines.

mRNA also represents a promising vaccine platform for cancer. Some of its advantages are high potency, versatility, scalability, speed of development, manufacturing costs, and efficacy. mRNA molecules are used as antigen synthesis templates and can encode multiple antigens in one vaccine. An additional advantage is that mRNA molecules can encode any protein sequence that otherwise could be difficult to synthesize using other platforms such as peptides. mRNA molecules can be produced by in vitro transcription (IVT) using DNA templates. After delivery, the exogenous mRNA enters the cytosol of APCs via endocytosis followed by endosomal escape but does not enter the nucleus, minimizing risk of integration into the host genome. Translation occurs in the cytosol where the protein can be degraded by the proteosome into small peptides for presentation on MHC class I molecules. Additionally, to increase presentation through MHC class II, the translated protein can be routed through lysosomal compartments by fusing it to lysosome-associated membrane proteins (LAMPs) or to the MHC class I cytoplasmatic and transmembrane domain.[72]

In addition to protein translation, the mRNA molecule provides strong intrinsic adjuvanticity by binding to RNA sensors including endosomal TLRs 3, 7, 8, and cytosolic RNA receptors, resulting in the production of type I interferons (IFNs). Though this could theoretically be an advantage to increase immunogenicity, innate immune sensing of RNA can lead to inhibition of translation, increased mRNA degradation, and thus reduced antigen expression. This, combined with the fact that naked mRNA can be quickly degraded by RNases and is poorly internalized by APCs, initially led to the consideration that mRNA was not suitable as a drug. However, new advances in mRNA engineering have resulted in improvements in cellular uptake, intracellular stability, and protein expression efficiency. Examples of modification to prevent mRNA degradation and improve stability and translation efficiency include 5′ cap modifications, optimization of untranslated regions (UTRs), codon optimization of open reading frames (ORFs), use of modified nucleotides, and poly-A tail modification.[73] Additionally, advances in nanoparticle formulations have improved protection of mRNA molecules from extracellular RNases and increased uptake by APCs in vivo. Some of the most commonly employed formulations include lipid nanoparticles (LNPs, which were employed in both Pfizer and Moderna COVID-19 vaccines), lipoplexes (LPX), polymers, or peptides.[73] Finally, investigation of different routes of administration has also provided insight into how mRNA is internalized by APCs. As an example, intravenous and intranodal injections result in the direct uptake by DCs in lymphoid organs, whereas intramuscular or intradermal routes require DC uptake and subsequent transport to draining lymph nodes.[72] Building on these advances, synthetic mRNA has become a highly versatile and efficient gene delivery system and one of the most promising cancer vaccination platforms.

Several mRNA vaccines targeting TAAs have been tested in the clinic in different tumor types. One important study was the phase I Lipo-MERIT trial in which the FixVac (BNT111) vaccine from BioNTech was tested in patients with advanced melanoma. The FixVac vaccine is a nanoparticulate liposomal RNA (RNA-LPX) encoding for four melanoma TAAs including NY-ESO-1, MAGE-A3, tyrosinase, and transmembrane phosphatase with tensin homology (TPTE), that is administered intravenously. It was shown that alone and in combination with PD-1 blockade, FixVac mediates durable objective responses accompanied by the induction of CD4 and CD8 T-cell immunity against the vaccine antigens.[24] FixVac is currently being tested in a phase II trial in combination with cemiplimab (anti-PD-1) in patients with advanced melanoma (NCT04526899). Another important company in the development of mRNA vaccines for cancer is CureVac. CureVac has developed several vaccine candidates for different tumor types including CV9103 and CV9104 for prostate cancer, and CV9201 and CV9202 for NSCLC. These vaccines use the RNActive technology, which employ the nucleotide-binding peptide protamine for RNA complexation and as an adjuvant to activate TLR7/8. The CV9103 vaccine, which encodes for four prostate TAAs (PSA, prostate-specific membrane antigen (PSMA), prostate stem cell antigen (PSCA), six transmembrane epithelial antigen of the prostate (STEAP)), was well tolerated and induced antigen-specific T-cell responses in most patients.[74] However, the CV9104 vaccine, which includes two additional TAAs (PAP and MUC-1), failed to improve survival in a phase II trial.[72] Similarly, CV9201 and CV9202 encode for five and six TAAs, respectively, commonly expressed in NSCLC (NY-ESO-1, MAGEC1, MAGEC2, trophoblast glycoprotein (TPBG), survivin, and MUC1 for CV9202). Although it induced T-cell responses against one or more antigens in most patients, CV9201 did not improve overall survival compared with that usually observed with chemotherapy.[75] CV9202 also elicited vaccine-specific immune responses in the majority of patients and some evidence of clinical efficacy.[76]

mRNA vaccines encoding for mutation-derived tumor neoantigens have also been explored. In different mouse model studies, vaccination with RNA encoding for tumor cell line–specific neoantigens resulted in strong effector and memory neoantigen-specific T-cell responses, which mediate tumor control and rejection.[27] In the clinic, BioNTech and Moderna are leading the development of this vaccine technology. Sahin et al. pioneered the first-in-human study of personalized mRNA neoantigen vaccines with the IVAC MUTANOME trial in 13 patients with advanced melanoma.[56] Patient-specific neoantigens were selected based on whole exome sequencing (WES), RNA sequencing, and predicted binding affinities to HLA-I and HLA-II. Vaccines consisted of two IVT mRNA molecules encoding five 27-mer peptides (pentatopes) with the mutation in position 14, connected by linkers. Vaccines were injected percutaneously into the inguinal lymph node under ultrasound control. Additionally, during personalized vaccine manufacture, patients whose tumors expressed NY-ESO-1 or tyrosinase received a vaccine encoding these TAAs. All patients developed T-cell immunity against vaccine neoantigens including both CD4 and CD8 responses. Eight patients with no detectable tumors before vaccination remained recurrence free for the whole follow-up period (12–23 months). Among patients with metastatic disease at the time of vaccination, two experienced objective responses, one developed a complete response after treatment with PD-1 therapy, and one developed therapy resistance by loss of HLA-I antigen presentation. These promising results have encouraged further investigation of these vaccine strategies into more advanced trials and other tumor types. BioNTech is currently testing Autogen Cevumeran (RO7198457) as a new vaccine candidate through the individualized neoantigen-specific immunotherapy (iNeST) program. Autogen Cevumeran is an intravenously injected, mRNA lipoplex (RNA-LPX) vaccine consisting of two mRNA molecules encoding up to 20 patient-specific neoantigens. Several phase I and phase II clinical trials are testing Autogen Cevumeran as a single therapy or in combination with immune checkpoint blockade in PDAC (NCT04161755), CRC (NCT04486378), melanoma (NCT03815058), and other solid tumors (NCT03289962).

Moderna is also developing several mRNA vaccine candidates. Similar to the approved COVID-19 vaccines, personalized mRNA neoantigen vaccines developed by Moderna use LNPs in their formulation and are injected intramuscularly.[72] mRNA-5671 is a personalized vaccine targeting KRAS neoantigens, and it was tested in a phase I trial enrolling four patients with gastrointestinal (GI) cancer.[57] The vaccine was safe and induced mutation-specific T-cell responses against predicted neoepitopes, although no objective clinical responses were observed in these four patients. mRNA-4157 is another vaccine candidate that encodes for 20 patient-specific neoantigens. The KEYNOTE-603 trial tested the mRNA-4157 vaccine as monotherapy or in combination with anti PD-1 therapy (pembrolizumab) in solid tumors including melanoma, bladder cancer, and NSCLC. The vaccine was safe, elicited CD8 T-cell responses, and showed promising clinical results. Most patients who received monotherapy after resection remained disease free on-study. Complete responses and partial responses were observed with the combination therapy. Clinical response rates compared favorably to published rates for pembrolizumab monotherapy[73] (for an in-depth review, see Miao et al.[73]). This promising vaccine has now moved to phase II trials (KEYNOTE-942, NCT03897881). Overall, mRNA has shown great potential as a vaccination platform and results of clinical trials targeting patient-specific neoantigens are encouraging. Future larger human studies will assess whether they confer any clinical benefit.

Key References

2. Ribas A, Wolchok JD. Cancer immunotherapy using checkpoint blockade. *Science*. 2018;359:1350-1355.
5. Schumacher TN, Scheper W, Kvistborg P. Cancer neoantigens. *Ann Rev Immunol*. 2019;37:173-200.
10. Rizvi NA, et al. Mutational landscape determines sensitivity to PD-1 blockade in non-small cell lung cancer. *Science*. 2015;348:124-128.
23. Kantoff PW, et al. Sipuleucel-T immunotherapy for castration-resistant prostate cancer. *N Engl J Med*. 2010;363:411-422.
24. Sahin U, et al. An RNA vaccine drives immunity in checkpoint-inhibitor-treated melanoma. *Nature*. 2020;585:107-112.
27. Kreiter S, et al. Mutant MHC class II epitopes drive therapeutic immune responses to cancer. *Nature*. 2015;520:692-696.
36. Pearlman AH, et al. Targeting public neoantigens for cancer immunotherapy. *Nat Cancer*. 2021;2:487-497.
37. Rooney MS, Shukla SA, Wu CJ, Getz G, Hacohen N. Molecular and genetic properties of tumors associated with local immune cytolytic activity. *Cell*. 2015;160:48-61.
42. Dunn GP, Bruce AT, Ikeda H, Old LJ, Schreiber RD. Cancer immunoediting: from immunosurveillance to tumor escape. *Nat Immunol*. 2002;3(11):991-998. doi:10.1038/ni1102-991.
51. Carreno BM, et al. Cancer immunotherapy. A dendritic cell vaccine increases the breadth and diversity of melanoma neoantigen-specific T cells. *Science*. 2015;348:803-808.
52. Ott PA, et al. An immunogenic personal neoantigen vaccine for patients with melanoma. *Nature*. 2017;547:217-221.
55. Ott PA, et al. A phase Ib trial of personalized neoantigen therapy plus Anti-PD-1 in patients with advanced melanoma, non-small cell lung cancer, or bladder Cancer. *Cell*. 2020;183:347-362.e24.
56. Sahin U, et al. Personalized RNA mutanome vaccines mobilize poly-specific therapeutic immunity against cancer. *Nature*. 2017;547:222-226.
63. Hu Z, Ott PA, Wu CJ. Towards personalized, tumour-specific, therapeutic vaccines for cancer. *Nat Rev Immunol*. 2018;18:168-182.
64. Sabado RL, Balan S, Bhardwaj N. Dendritic cell-based immunotherapy. *Cell Res*. 2017;27:74-95.
69. Calvo Tardón M, Allard M, Dutoit V, Dietrich PY, Walker PR. Peptides as cancer vaccines. *Curr Opin Pharmacol*. 2019;47:20-26.
71. Castle JC, et al. Exploiting the mutanome for tumor vaccination. *Cancer Res*. 2012;72:1081-1091.
72. Beck JD, et al. mRNA therapeutics in cancer immunotherapy. *Mol Cancer*. 2021;20:1-24.
73. Miao L, Zhang Y, Huang L. mRNA vaccine for cancer immunotherapy. *Mol Cancer*. 2021;20:41.

Visit Elsevier eBooks + (eBooks.Health.Elsevier.com) for complete set of references.

CHAPTER 10

The Major Clinical Components of Cancer Immunotherapy (Modulating Cell-Mediated Immune Mechanisms)

Challice L. Bonifant ■ William R. Burns

SUMMARY OF KEY FACTS

- Immune checkpoints are molecular pathways that blunt the antitumor immune response via limiting the creation of cytotoxic T cells and triggering exhaustion of tumor-reactive immune cells.
- Immune checkpoint inhibitors, especially those targeting the PD-1/PD-L1 pathway, are used to treat patients with a wide range of cancers.
- Adoptive transfer of TILs can result in clinical responses in patients with metastatic melanoma.
- T cells can be engineered to express a CAR targeting a range of cell surface antigens.
- CD19-specific CAR T cells can provide substantial benefit to patients with B-cell malignancies.
- Monoclonal antibodies can treat cancer by inducing antibody-dependent cellular cytotoxicity or complement-dependent cytotoxicity.
- Antibody–drug conjugates allow for antigen-specific delivery of a cancer therapeutic including cytotoxic agents, immunotoxins, and radiopharmaceuticals.
- The success of prophylactic cancer vaccines against human papilloma virus and hepatitis B have fostered interest in using vaccines to prevent other viral-associated malignancies.
- An autologous dendritic cell vaccine targeting prostatic acid phosphatase was the first therapeutic cancer vaccine approved for use in patients with advanced cancer.
- Building on the successes of cancer immunotherapy, trials of combinatorial immunotherapy are underway to assess whether treatment with multiple agents can further augment the antitumor immune response.

The Role and Application of Checkpoint Blockade

INTRODUCTION

Among the clinical successes of cancer immunotherapy, the strategy of immune checkpoint blockade has been adopted most broadly. *Immune checkpoints* refers to the molecular pathways responsible for blunting the antitumor immune response. These include mechanisms that limit

195

the creation of cytotoxic T cells and that result in exhaustion of tumor-reactive immune cells. Though a range of approaches directed toward unique vulnerabilities of a specific cancer hold promise, the targeted manipulation of common molecular pathways that suppress the effector arm of the immune system has demonstrated efficacy across many malignancies. This benefit has been realized through clinical development of monoclonal antibodies that disinhibit the immune system, thereby fueling excitement for pharmacologic manipulation of additional immune checkpoints and for use of checkpoint blockade in combination with other cancer therapeutics.

BACKGROUND

Attempts to generate an immune response against cancer have focused on creation of tumor-reactive T cells and sustained activation of these cytotoxic effector cells. Early efforts were aimed at identification of tumor-associated antigens with the goal of immunizing a host against these peptides. Related work sought to expand the number of cytotoxic T cells capable of recognizing and destroying cancer cells. Through this work, several mechanisms were identified as key mediators by which tumors evade the immune system. Among these, cytotoxic T-lymphocyte antigen 4 (CTLA-4, CD152), an inhibitory signal in the immune synapse, proved to be important. Blockade of the CTLA-4 receptor was shown to induce tumor regression in preclinical models.[1] Furthermore, clinical use of anti-CTLA-4 therapy provided benefit to patients with advanced cancer,[2] thereby leading to U.S. Food and Drug Administration (FDA) approval in 2011. Likewise, development of pharmacologic agents blocking additional immune checkpoints have been successful. Most notable, inhibition of the programmed death 1 (PD-1, CD279) receptor and its primary ligand programmed death ligand-1 (PD-L1, CD274, B7-H1) has shown even greater efficacy across a wide range of malignancies.[3] The success of immune checkpoint blockade was recognized by awarding the 2018 Nobel Prize in Physiology or Medicine to James Allison for work on CTLA-4 and Tasuku Honjo for work on PD-1. Their discoveries have revolutionized the field of immunotherapy, leading to research exploring other immune checkpoint pathways and ways to combine checkpoint blockade with other cancer treatments.

CYTOTOXIC T-LYMPHOCYTE ANTIGEN 4

As outlined in Chapter 7, tumor-reactive T cells are generated when naïve T cells receive two signals from antigen-presenting cells. There must be interaction between the T-cell receptor and its cognate peptide–major histocompatibility complex (MHC; signal 1) and engagement of the costimulatory receptor CD28 with one of its ligands CD80 or CD86 (signal 2), as depicted in Fig. 10.1. Though early efforts in the development of cancer immunotherapies often focused on signal 1, interest in targeting signal 2 was bolstered by the clinical success of inhibiting the negative costimulatory receptor CTLA-4. Compared with CD28, CTLA-4 has a greater affinity for CD80 and CD86 (see Fig. 10.1) and can outcompete CD28 for these costimulatory ligands, thereby impairing T-cell activation.[4] Furthermore, CTLA-4 has the potential to dampen antitumor immune responses, because CTLA-4 is absent on resting memory T cells but becomes rapidly expressed after T-cell activation. This feedback inhibition likely facilitates immune tolerance but also allows tumors to evade the immune system.

The seminal observation that CTLA-4 blockade can potentiate the antitumor immune response came from experiments in which administration of anti-CTLA-4 antibodies led to rejection of transplanted murine colon carcinoma in immunocompetent mice.[1] This preclinical success was followed by clinical development of monoclonal antibodies targeting CTLA-4. Ipilimumab (Yervoy, Bristol-Myers Squibb) was approved by the FDA in 2011 for the treatment of advanced melanoma based on results of two phase III clinical trials.[2,5] Further studies have shown efficacy in subsets of patients with a range of cancers including surgically resected melanoma, renal cell

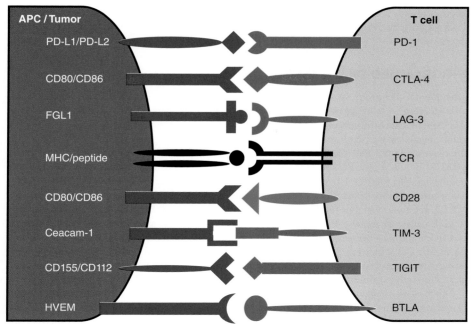

Fig. 10.1   Immune checkpoint molecules. The immune synapse between an antigen-presenting cell (or tumor cell) and a T cell is depicted. A T-cell receptor binds its peptide antigen presented on an MHC molecule (signal 1), as shown in black at the center of the figure. Engagement of the costimulatory receptor CD28 with one of its ligands (CD80 or CD86) is detailed in green (signal 2), and a number of inhibitory immune checkpoint molecules are shown in red, flanking the TCR–MHC complex and interacting with their ligands. Of note, LAG-3 is believed to interact with MHC as well as its ligand FGL1.

carcinoma, colorectal cancer, hepatocellular carcinoma, and non-small cell lung cancer. Though the potential effect of targeting CTLA-4 was clear from these trials, the magnitude of clinical benefit derived from ipilimumab monotherapy was modest. Clinical data pooled from studies of ipilimumab-treated patients with advanced melanoma reported a median overall survival of approximately 1 year (11.4 months) and fewer than 20% of patients had long-term survival.[6] Another CTLA-4-blocking monoclonal antibody tremelimumab (Pfizer, MedImmune, Astra Zeneca) was evaluated in patients with advanced melanoma and demonstrated a similar median overall survival of approximately 1 year (12.6 months); this was compared with standard-of-care chemotherapy, which had a median overall survival of 10.7 months, and the small improvement in survival was not statistically significant (hazard ratio = 0.88, P = .13).[7] Interestingly, the duration of response was substantially longer in patients receiving tremelimumab compared with standard-of-care chemotherapy (35.8 vs 13.7 months, P = .001).

Taken in sum, data from these clinical trials exploring the activity of anti-CTLA-4 therapy led to two fundamental conclusions. First, blockade of an immune checkpoint like CTLA-4 has potential value to patients with a spectrum of human malignancies. Whereas many treatment regimens are only effective against one tumor type, targeting a molecular immune pathway allows broader utility across a range of cancers. Second, despite low response rates with anti-CTLA monotherapy, patients who benefit from this treatment often have favorable long-term outcomes not seen with conventional chemotherapy. This difference seen at the tail of the survival curve is exciting to patients, clinicians, and scientists alike. Therefore it is not surprising that the early experience with CTLA-4 blockade fueled efforts to target other immune checkpoint pathways, to identify predictive biomarkers of response, and to combine CTLA-4 blockade with other cancer therapies.

PROGRAMMED DEATH 1

Subsequent to the promising results from clinical trials using anti-CTLA-4 antibodies, there was rapid development of agents targeting the PD-1 pathway. The PD-1 receptor is similar to CTLA-4 in that both are expressed on activated T cells and can transduce inhibitory signals when engaged with their ligands. However, these immune checkpoint pathways have important differences. For example, the known ligands for PD-1 are PD-L1 (CD274, B7-H1) and PD-L2 (CD273, B7-DC) (see Fig. 10.1). Unlike the CTLA-4 ligands that are expressed on antigen-presenting cells, the PD-1 ligands are found on tumors and other cells within the tumor microenvironment. It is believed that PD-L1 is the dominant ligand present on solid tumors,[8] whereas PD-L2 is found at higher levels on hematologic malignancies.[9] Either ligand can inhibit activated T cells that express PD-1. Whereas the CTLA-4 pathway is generally felt to mediate feedback inhibition between antigen presenting cells and effector T cells in secondary lymphoid tissues, the PD-1 pathway is believed to block tumor-reactive T cells within the tumor microenvironment. Regardless of the precise mechanism(s), PD-1 seems to promote T-cell exhaustion and dampen the antitumor immune response.

Much of our insight into the PD-1 pathway stems from preclinical testing. Notably, PD-L1 expression on tumor cells was shown to confer resistance to host immunity.[10] Furthermore, blockade of the PD-1 ligand inhibited tumor growth in this mouse model of myeloma. Likewise, administration of a monoclonal antibody to PD-L1 in combination with adoptive transfer of tumor-reactive T cells resulted in long-term survival of squamous cell carcinoma-bearing mice.[11] Beyond its promise of clinical benefit, mouse models also suggested that targeting the PD-1 pathway may have less toxicity than targeting other immune checkpoints. Whereas CTLA-4 knockout mice develop uncontrolled lymphoproliferation and have early lethality,[12] PD-1 knockout mice have milder and delayed-onset autoimmunity.[13] Based on these encouraging findings, therapies targeting the PD-1 pathway were advanced into human trials.

Early clinical success was seen with the anti-PD-1 monoclonal antibody nivolumab (Opdivo, Bristol-Myers Squibb). In a Phase I dose escalation study of 39 patients, there were objective responses seen in 3 patients with melanoma, renal cell carcinoma, and colorectal cancer.[14] Subsequent studies with nivolumab have shown durable benefit in patients with non-small cell lung cancer, renal cell carcinoma, and melanoma, as well as efficacy in a number of other cancers; therefore nivolumab received FDA approval in 2014. Of note, pembrolizumab (Keytruda, Merck) was the first monoclonal antibody targeting PD-1 approved by the FDA. This followed impressive results from a large early-phase study in which clinical responses were seen in 52 of 135 patients with advanced melanoma who received the anti-PD-1 antibody (originally named lambrolizumab), including patients previously treated with the anti-CTLA-4 monoclonal antibody ipilimumab.[15]

The efficacy of pembrolizumab was not limited to melanoma, because its use has benefit in the treatment of groups of patients with bladder cancer, breast cancer, cervical cancer, colorectal cancer, gastroesophageal cancers, head and neck squamous cell carcinoma, hepatocellular carcinoma, lymphoma, Merkel cell carcinoma, non-small cell lung cancer, renal cell carcinoma, and tumors with high mutational burden or deficiencies in mismatch repair. Building on the success of nivolumab and pembrolizumab, several other agents targeting the PD-1/PD-L1 pathway have been approved. This includes cemiplimab (Libtayo, Sanofi/Regeneron), which has shown efficacy in the treatment of advanced nonmelanoma skin cancers and PD-L1-expressing non-small cell lung cancer. There has also been clinical success with anti-PD-L1 therapies, including FDA approval of avelumab (Bavencio, Pfizer), atezolizumab (Tecentriq, Genentech), and durvalumab (Imfinzi, Astra Zeneca). With many more trials underway and additional agents in clinical development, blockade of the PD-1 immune checkpoint pathway continues to be a key target in cancer therapy.

LYMPHOCYTE ACTIVATION GENE 3

Subsequent to the clinical success of PD-1 and CTLA-4 pathway blockade, the LAG-3 (CD223) immune checkpoint has become another target of interest in cancer immunotherapy. LAG-3 is a type I transmembrane protein and member of the immunoglobulin superfamily, which is expressed on lymphocytes and binds MHC class II. Early interest in LAG-3 stemmed from its ability to enhance the function of antigen-presenting cells and thereby create a more robust antitumor immune response. Tumor cells engineered to express LAG-3 had impaired growth compared with native tumor cells when implanted into immunocompetent mice, and these mice were protected from future challenge with native tumor cells.[16] This strategy of enhancing host immunity against cancer led to the development of soluble LAG-3 as a vaccine adjuvant. The first agent tested in clinical trials was eftilagimod alpha (IMP321, Immutep), a recombinant protein combining the LAG extracellular domains with the Fc domain of human immunoglobulin (Ig) G1. Patients with metastatic renal cell carcinoma were treated with escalating doses of the compound, which led to activation of CD8 T cells and reduced tumor growth in some patients.[17] Subsequent clinical trials combined eftilagimod alpha and cytotoxic chemotherapy, suggesting modest clinical benefit in patients with metastatic breast cancer. Studies evaluating soluble LAG-3 with cancer vaccines or in combination with PD-1 blockade are ongoing.

In addition to its ability to bind MHC class II, LAG-3 can interact with fibrinogen-like protein 1 (FGL1) (see Fig. 10.1). This distinct function is believed to trigger T-cell exhaustion and blunt T-cell proliferation within the tumor microenvironment,[18] mimicking the interaction between PD-1 and its ligands. Interestingly, LAG-3 and PD-1 are both overexpressed by immune cells in models of chronic infection and LAG-3 expression often parallels PD-1 expression in tumor-reactive T cells. Furthermore, mice deficient in both LAG-3 and PD-1 develop extensive lymphocytic infiltration that results in early death.[19] Based on the clinical success of anti-PD-1 therapy and the potential synergy between the two pathways, preclinical evaluation of LAG-3 blockade has focused on combinatorial approaches with anti-PD-1 agents. Encouragingly, combined anti-PD-1 and anti-LAG-3 treatment has been effective in mouse cancer models. The anti-LAG-3 monoclonal antibody relatlimab (BMS-986016, Bristol-Myers Squibb), which was approved by the FDA in 2022, has been tested in a large phase I/II trial with or without nivolumab in the treatment of patients with advanced cancer. There were encouraging results from this study (NCT01968109) in patients with melanoma, including those previously treated with anti-PD-1/anti-PD-L1 therapy. A subsequent randomized phase II/II trial of nivolumab with or without relatlimab demonstrated greater progression-free survival from dual checkpoint inhibition in patients with previously untreated melanoma.[20] With additional studies ongoing and novel agents in development, it seems that therapies targeting LAG-3 will have a promising role in the treatment of cancer.

OTHER IMMUNE CHECKPOINT PATHWAYS

As the understanding of other immune checkpoints pathways grows, there is interest in clinical development of new agents to expand the armamentarium of cancer therapy. Though a comprehensive summary is beyond the scope of this work, a general overview of additional promising targets is provided in the following sections.

T-Cell Immunoglobulin and Mucin Domain–Containing 3

TIM-3 (CD366) is an immunoglobulin superfamily receptor expressed on the surface of immune cells. Like other immune checkpoint molecules discussed previously, research has focused on its function in T cells. TIM-3 has several known ligands, each seemingly capable of distinct cellular effects. For example, galectin-9 is a soluble ligand that has been shown to induce apoptosis of TIM3[+] T cells[21] and another soluble ligand high-mobility group protein B1 (HMGB1) can interact with TIM-3[+] dendritic cells to dampen antitumor immunity.[22] Nonetheless, it is the interaction between TIM-3 and membrane-bound carcinoembryonic antigen cell adhesion molecule 1 (Ceacam-1) that is believed to trigger T-cell inhibition[23] (see Fig. 10.1). Preclinical models have shown that tumor-infiltrating lymphocytes expressing TIM-3 and PD-1 have reduced ability to proliferate and secrete proinflammatory cytokines; furthermore, dual blockade of TIM-3 and PD-1 had therapeutic benefit in mouse tumor models.[24] Therefore clinical development of monoclonal antibodies blocking TIM-3 has largely focused on combination with anti-PD-1 therapy with some trials even exploring coadministration of agents blocking PD-1, LAG-3, and TIM-3. In addition, bispecific antibodies simultaneously targeting PD-1 and TIM-3 are under investigation.

T-Cell Immunoreceptor and ITIM Domain

Sharing structural domains with other immune checkpoints molecules discussed previously, TIGIT was identified through a genomic search for cell surface proteins containing a conserved immunoreceptor tyrosine-based inhibitory motif (ITIM) domain. TIGIT is expressed on T cells and can trigger the immunosuppressive function of dendritic cells through engagement with its ligand CD155.[25] Further research revealed that TIGIT also serves as an immune checkpoint with the ability to suppress antitumor T-cell function.[26] This can occur through two related mechanisms as (1) TIGIT provides inhibitory signaling upon binding its ligands and (2) TIGIT impairs excitatory signaling from CD226 by outcompeting this costimulatory receptor for the shared ligands CD155 and CD112 (see Fig. 10.1); the relationship between TIGIT and CD226 is akin to that of CTLA-4 and CD28. Likewise, TIGIT blockade can enhance antitumor responses in animal models, and this effect is augmented by combination with other immune checkpoint inhibitors. Based on these encouraging results, clinical evaluation of anti-TIGIT agents is currently underway with several studies targeting TIGIT in addition to other checkpoint pathways.

B- and T-Lymphocyte Attenuator

B- and T-lymphocyte attenuator (BTLA, CD272) is an inhibitory receptor in the CD28 superfamily. As the name suggests, it is expressed on B cells and T cells. However, BTLA can also be found on macrophages and dendritic cells. Herpes virus entry mediator (HVEM) is recognized as the primary ligand for BTLA (see Fig. 10.1); HVEM expression can lead to inhibition of T-cell proliferation and function.[27] Like other immune checkpoint molecules, BTLA has been identified on tumor-infiltrating lymphocytes across a range of malignancies. Given its potential role in dampening the antitumor immune response, clinical development of agents targeting BTLA are proceeding, with phase I clinical trials for patients with advanced cancer now underway.

CONCLUSIONS

Immune checkpoint blockade has rapidly become one of the most exciting cancer treatments. Building on the pioneering work of Nobel laureates James Allison and Tasuku Honjo, scientists continue to develop new agents that can augment the antitumor immune response. Whether through promoting generation of tumor-reactive immune cells or preventing exhaustion of cytotoxic T cells, targeting these molecular pathways has the potential to treat a broad range of malignancies. The clinical success of anti-CTLA-4 therapy provided a glimpse of this promise. However, the broad efficacy of targeting the PD-1 pathway has been transformational. As such, clinicians continue to evaluate these new therapies and explore rational combinations to maximize the clinical benefit for patients with cancer.

The Role and Application of Cell-Based Therapies

CASE VIGNETTE

A 17-year-old male presents in the clinic with subjective fever and easy bruising for the past week. After appropriate workup a diagnosis of t(9;22)/BCR-ABL1 negative pre-B cell acute lymphoblastic leukemia (ALL) is made. Induction therapy with vincristine, anthracycline, asparaginase, and steroids fails to result in complete remission. Additional options for achieving remission to enable hematopoietic cell transplantation (HCT) are discussed with the patient and family, and treatment with tisagenlecleucel, a chimeric antigen receptor (CAR) T-cell product, is scheduled. The patient's lymphocytes are collected, the autologous CAR T cell product is prepared, and infusion is performed after administration of preparative lymphodepleting chemotherapy. On the fourth day postinfusion the patient develops fever (38.9°C), hypotension (BP 73/35), and hypoxia (Sao_2 87%), concerning for cytokine release syndrome (CRS). Intravenous fluids, oxygen, vasopressors, and tocilizumab (interleukin [IL]-6 antagonist) are given, with rapid improvement in the patient's vital signs. Subsequent disease monitoring of the bone marrow and spinal fluid is significant for a lack of detectable disease. This case demonstrates the induction of remission for a poor prognosis malignancy after adoptive transfer of CAR T cells, a revolution in the field of immunotherapy.

TUMOR-INFILTRATING LYMPHOCYTES

The immune system is populated by important effector and supportive cells that react to stressed, infected, or transformed cell types. T lymphocytes are likely the most important, because they quickly traffic to and invade tumor sites and then are able to elicit a specific immune response after T-cell receptor (TCR) recognition of tumor-specific antigens presented in the context of MHC (Fig. 10.2). These infiltrating cells are commonly referred to as *tumor-infiltrating lymphocytes* (TILs). When functional TILs can be identified and directly isolated from a patient's tumor, this is generally considered a favorable prognostic factor. In addition, isolated TILs may be purified and expanded for use in adoptive cell transfer (ACT) as treatment against a variety of solid tumors. Marrow-infiltrating lymphocytes can also be harvested and used against liquid cancers, like multiple myeloma, in which the bone marrow is considered the tumor microenvironment.[28] Rosenberg et al. were the first to investigate the role of TILs as adoptive immunotherapy for cancer in 1986.[29] TILs isolated from tumor-engrafted C57BL/6 mice and cultured in IL-2 for 15 days were 50 to 100 times more potent than lymphokine-activated killer (LAK) cells (widely used in preclinical and clinical studies in 1980s) against various tumor micrometastases in animal models. A year later, Kradin et al. performed the first clinical trial of TILs, showing safety in administration but no responses in seven patients with lung cancer.[30] The first objective clinical responses in TIL treatment were seen in a cohort of 20 patients with metastatic melanoma by Rosenberg et al. in 1989. A single dose of cyclophosphamide followed by infusion of TIL and IL2 led to a reduction of melanoma lesions in 58% of patients, with complete response (CR) in 1 patient and partial response (PR) in 10 patients.[31] This dramatic outcome led to many future clinical trials for metastatic melanoma and other cancers.

    Generation of TIL is a multistep process (Fig. 10.3). First, the tumor lesion is surgically excised and a single-cell suspension is prepared by mechanical or enzymatic separation. This suspension

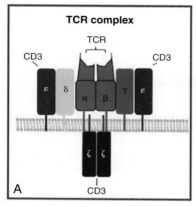
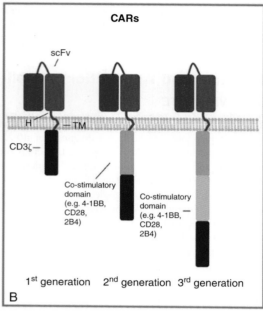

Fig. 10.2   Structure of T-cell receptor (TCR) complex and generations of chimeric antigen receptors (CARs). (A) TCR normally consists of the highly variable α and β chains that possess antigen-binding domains. In the cellular surface the α and β chains associate with adaptor proteins CD3ε, CD3δ, CD3γ, and CD3ζ, which serve as signal transmitters. The stoichiometry of association is TCR αβ - CD3εγ - CD3εδ - CD3ζζ. (B) CARs consist of an extracellular single-chain variable fragment (scFv), a fusion protein of the variable regions of the heavy (VH) and light chains (VL) of immunoglobulins that binds a specific antigen. A hinge domain (H) provides flexibility and the transmembrane portion (TM) anchors the molecule in the surface. The intracellular domains of the CAR transmit the signaling after antigen binding. First-generation CAR consists solely of the CD3ζ intracellular domain, whereas second- and third-generation CARs contain additionally intracellular costimulatory receptors.

is cultured with IL-2 for approximately 2 weeks, leading to survival and proliferation of TILs but death of tumor cells. Next, TILs are rapidly expanded using IL-2, anti-CD3 antibody, and irradiated feeder cells. Once the necessary yield for immunotherapeutic infusion is achieved (commonly 1×10^{10} to 2×10^{11} cells), the TIL product consists of a heterogeneous population of T cells. Activated lymphocytes can be purified via flow cytometric or magnetic bead sorting if specific T-cell subsets are desired. Additional studies are needed to define the clinical benefit of TIL therapy and to identify the optimal T-cell population for sustained antitumor activity.

Since 1989, TIL therapy has been investigated in more than 15 clinical trials of patients with metastatic melanoma. Most of these studies have evaluated TILs as monotherapy in patients not previously treated with PD-1 blockade. Overall, an objective clinical response and a complete remission have been documented in approximately 50% and 10% to 15% of treated patients, respectively. As immune checkpoint inhibition has evolved to become first-line treatment, these encouraging results led several groups to investigate the potentially additional benefit of TILs as a combinational therapy with or as an alternative treatment. Sarnaik et al. investigated the role of the Lifileucel TIL product in the treatment of 66 patients with advanced melanoma (metastatic or unresectable) that progressed after immune checkpoint inhibition (anti-PD-1, anti-PD-L1, anti-CTLA-4) and targeted therapies (BRAF ± MEK inhibitors if *BRAF* V600 mutated

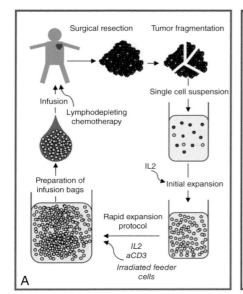
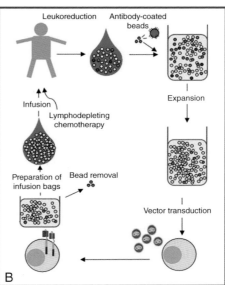

Fig. 10.3 **Generation of tumor-infiltrating lymphocytes (TILs) and chimeric antigen receptor (CAR) T-cell adoptive therapies.** (A) Preparation of TILs. Tumor is isolated from the patients and fragmented and a single-cell suspension is enzymatically prepared. This suspension is cultured with IL-2 during initial expansion and with IL-2, anti-CD3 antibodies, and irradiated feeder cells during the rapid expansion protocol, leading to clinical-grade cell counts. The product is prepared for infusion to the patient after they receive lymphodepleting chemotherapy. (B) Preparation of CAR T cells. Collection of patient lymphocytes, enrichment, and activation with anti-CD3/anti-CD28 antibodies is followed by transduction with CAR transgene encoding vectors. The resultant CAR T cells are further expanded and prepared for autologous infusion.

tumors). An objective response was seen in 36% of patients (22 PR and 2 CR), and 44% had stable disease. Objective response was observed to be 41% in the cohort of patients with cancer refractory to anti-PD-1 or anti-PD-L1 therapies. Rates of survival greater than 1 year were 92% in patients who had an objective response to treatment and 38% in patients with stable disease.[32] These encouraging results hold promise for the use of TILs in patients with treatment-refractory melanoma in whom therapeutic options are limited. Nonetheless, there are no TIL therapies approved by the FDA for melanoma.

TILs have been isolated and expanded from solid tumors other than melanoma; these include breast cancer, renal cell carcinoma, and gastrointestinal malignancies. In contrast to TILs isolated from melanoma, these products have shown variable antitumor efficacy in preclinical models. There are limited clinical studies of TIL monotherapy as treatment for nonmelanoma solid tumors and only one trial reporting objective responses. Stevanović et al. investigated the infusion of TILs selected for human papillomavirus (HPV) oncoprotein reactivity in nine patients with refractory, metastatic cervical cancer. Two patients achieved a CR (lasting 15 and 22 months) and one patient had a short-lived PR.[33] The disparity in antitumor responsiveness of melanoma-derived TILs versus those obtained from other tumors may be explained by differences in (1) disease-associated mutational burden that ultimately drives immunogenicity, (2) the variable immunosuppressive tumor microenvironment, (3) differences in cellular composition within the harvested TILs, and (4) the differentiation state of infiltrative CD4$^+$ and CD8$^+$ T lymphocytes. Melanoma is characterized by high tumor mutational burden (TMB) and neoantigen expression, which correlates with clinical benefit of TIL immunotherapy.[34] Furthermore, melanoma TILs are less differentiated and possess high proliferative capacity. Continued research efforts are imperative to overcome the limitations of TIL therapy and improve clinical responses in tumors other than melanoma.

Preconditioning with lymphodepleting (LD) chemotherapy prior to TIL infusion is crucial for optimal activity. Induction of lymphopenia creates "physical space" for the transferred TILs, depletes immunosuppressive regulatory T cells, and reduces competition for homeostatic cytokines (e.g., IL-7 and IL-15). One standard nonmyeloablative LD chemotherapy regimen includes cyclophosphamide (Cy, 60 mg/kg for 2 days, 120 mg/kg) and fludarabine (Flu; 25 mg/m^2 for 5 days, 125 mg/m^2) administered 24 hours before cell infusion. Nissani et al. investigated the efficacy and safety of different LD regimens including Cy, Flu, and/or total body irradiation (TBI) in patients with stage IV melanoma receiving TILs (NCT03166397). In this study, 60 mg/kg Cy/125 mg/m^2 Flu was the most optimal regimen to stimulate TIL expansion with a tolerable toxicity profile.[35] LD is followed by TIL infusion and then commonly by systemic cytokine administration to support infused T-cell proliferation and survival. High-dose IL-2 is most frequently infused as a bolus of 720,000 IU/kg three times a day for 5 days, as tolerated. Lower doses of cytokine have been tested in small numbers of patients, but the potential to sustain satisfactory TIL responses requires investigation in larger cohorts of patients. Common toxicities observed with TIL treatment include febrile neutropenia, pancytopenia, high fever, chills, pulmonary congestion, and hypotension.[36] These are likely associated with LD chemotherapy and/or IL-2 infusion. An uncommon, but significant, potential side effect of TIL therapy is the development of autoimmune-like side effects (e.g., vitiligo, uveitis, and rash).

The major advantage of TIL therapy over other forms of ACT is the capability of specific recognition and targeting of patient's unique tumor-associated antigens. Exomic or whole-genome DNA sequencing with subsequent RNA sequencing have enabled identification of thousands of tumor-specific mutations and expression of neoantigens. Enrichment of the TIL product with neoantigen-directed populations can further enhance antitumor efficacy. This approach is possible by culturing TIL with autologous antigen-presenting cells that have been transduced with minigenes or peptides encoding these neoantigens. Despite its therapeutic promise, there are several challenges to widespread utilization of this technology. First, development of TIL therapy is personalized to a specific patient with high production costs and the need for specialized personnel and production facilities. Second, patients must undergo a procedure to obtain the tumor for TIL production. Third, long manufacturing time may limit its use in patients who experience tumor growth prior to administration of TIL therapy. For these reasons, the current focus of clinical development is centered on decreasing production time, improving patient selection, and simplifying manufacturing methods. Overcoming these limitations will help realize the promise of TIL therapy in the treatment of cancer.

CHIMERIC ANTIGEN RECEPTOR–ENGINEERED T CELLS

Adoptive transfer of T cells engineered to express a chimeric antigen receptor (CAR) has revolutionized the field of immunotherapy. Treatment with CAR T cells, which possess artificial receptors that enable robust, antigen-dependent T-cell activation, has resulted in clinical success of high-risk leukemia. CARs are synthetic molecules comprising an extracellular target-binding single-chain variable fragment (scFv) fused to a hinge, transmembrane, and intracellular domains that transmit downstream signaling (see Fig. 10.2B). Eshhar et al.[37] first engineered T cells with a chimeric molecule comprising a, scFV fused with the TCRζ chain. This molecule would later be described as a first-generation CAR (see Fig. 10.2B). Despite antitumor specificity, T cells engineered with first-generation CARs did not expand in vivo or result in objective clinical responses after CAR-T cell infusion. Krause et al.[38] first designed and tested a costimulatory-only CAR, using the CD28 intracellular domain. These CAR T cells effectively proliferated, produced IL-2, and exhibited antitumor killing in an antigen-specific manner.[39] Savoldo et al. showed the positive clinical effect of including CD28 costimulation with TCRζ activation (signal 1 and signal 2) in CAR T cells infused to human patients.[40] Use of costimulatory 4-1BB has also proven successful in amplifying CAR T-cell activation and survival.[41] To date, CD28 and 4-1BB are the most well-studied costimulatory domains of T-cell CARs. Others, such as OX40 and ICOS, are also being tested.

Among all antigens targeted by CAR T cells, CD19 has thus far been most effectively targeted. CD19 is a molecule present on the surface of B-lineage malignant cells and is an optimal target because of its restricted expression in B cells (and no other healthy tissue) and lack of expression on hematopoietic stem cells and plasma cells. Kochenderfer et al. described the first report of a patient with relapsed stage IVB follicular lymphoma treated with a CD19.CD28.ζ CAR T-cells, showing lymphoma regression lasting 32 weeks.[42] This report was followed by several clinical trials investigating the use of CD19 CAR T cells as treatment for relapsed or refractory pre-B cell ALL and non-Hodgkin lymphoma. Immunotherapy for relapsed or refractory pre-B cell ALL with CD19 CAR T-cells manufactured at a number of different academic centers led to complete disease remissions in 67% to 90% of patients.[43] In non-Hodgkin lymphoma, Schuster et al. first showed impressive clinical outcomes in 28 patients with relapsed or refractory diffuse large B-cell lymphoma (DLBCL) and follicular lymphoma, with 64% achieving objective responses.[44] This clinical success has quickly led to the development of commercially available CD19 CAR T cells for patients with CD19-positive malignancies.

In 2017, the FDA approved tisagenlecleucel, a CAR T-cell therapy that uses an anti-CD19.4-1BB.CD3ζ CAR (19.4-1BB.ζ), for the treatment of pediatric/young adult (≤25 years old) relapsed or refractory pre-B cell ALL. Tisagenlecleucel is the first cell-based gene therapy to gain commercial approval from the FDA, and its application was further expanded to include adult patients with relapsed or refractory DLBCL in 2018. To date, additional autologous CAR T-cell products have received FDA approval. Brexucabtagene autoleucel (19.CD28.ζ) is approved for use in adult patients with relapsed or refractory mantle cell lymphoma and ALL. Axicabtagene ciloleucel (19.CD28.ζ) and lisocabtagene maraleucel (19.4-1BB.ζ) are approved for adult relapsed or refractory B-cell lymphomas including DLBCL (not otherwise specified or arising from follicular lymphoma), primary mediastinal large B-cell lymphoma, and high-grade B-cell lymphoma. Lisocabtagene maraleucel is also used in adult relapsed or refractory grade 3B follicular lymphoma. Idecabtagene vicleucel is the first FDA-approved CAR T-cell product directed against a non-CD19 target: B-cell maturation antigen (BCMA). This BCMA.4-1BB.ζ CAR T-cell therapy is approved for the use in adult relapsed or refractory multiple myeloma, after treatment with four or more lines of therapies, to include an immunomodulatory agent, a proteasome inhibitor, and an anti-CD38 monoclonal antibody.

All of the FDA-approved CAR T-cell products use autologous patient-derived starting material. The use of autologous products is currently necessary to avoid the risk of graft-vs-host disease (GvHD), a potential severe side effect of allogeneic T-cell ACT. For CAR T-cell manufacturing, patient lymphocytes are collected and then enriched and activated, typically with anti-CD3/anti-CD28 antibody coated beads. T-cell activation is followed by cell modification, most often by viral transduction with vectors encoding the CAR transgene. After transduction, the cells are further expanded ex vivo to the desired cell number (i.e., $1-3 \times 10^6$ CAR T cells/kg), washed, and frozen for shipment and patient infusion (see Fig. 10.3B). Similar to adoptive transfer of TILs, lymphodepleting chemotherapy is a pivotal component of CAR T-cell therapy, because this promotes in vivo expansion, long-term persistence, and antitumor effects. Lymphodepleting chemotherapy may also prevent CAR T-cell rejection due to immune responses against CAR epitopes. After completion of chemotherapy, patients are given intravenous CAR T-cell infusion and monitored daily for clinical signs of toxicity during the first 7 to 10 days.

CAR T-cell therapy is often associated with severe systemic toxicities that require a high level of clinical preparedness for prompt recognition and management.[45] The most prevalent and often catastrophic side effect is cytokine release syndrome (CRS).[46] CRS is characterized by systemic elevation of inflammatory cytokines resultant from CAR T-cell expansion and monocyte activation, including tumor necrosis factor alpha (TNF-α), IL-6, IL-1β, IL-10, and interferon gamma (IFN-γ). Clinical findings of CRS include high fever, flu-like symptoms, gastrointestinal (GI) disturbances, hypotension, tachycardia, hypoxia, capillary leak, organ failure, and death. Management is per CRS grade, defined by temperature elevation, severity of hypotension, and degree of hypoxia. With supportive measures, high-grade CRS (≥3) can usually be reversed with tocilizumab, a humanized monoclonal antibody against the IL-6 receptor. The use of high-dose corticosteroids is typically reserved for nonresponders to tocilizumab. Another serious complication of CAR T-cell therapy is immune effector cell–associated neurotoxicity syndrome (ICANS), most likely caused by blood–brain barrier (BBB) dysfunction in concert with T-cell activation.[46] ICANS symptoms include headache, altered consciousness and delirium, expressive aphasia, seizure, and coma. Corticosteroids are the cornerstone of ICANS management, because blockade of the IL-6 receptor using tocilizumab is not effective because of limited pharmacologic distribution. Patients infused with CAR T cells at a higher disease burden are more likely to develop CRS or ICANS. Early intervention is important for resolution of these toxicities. However, these interventions to mitigate CRS or ICANS can also abrogate CAR T-cell function. A hemophagocytic lymphohistiocytosis-like toxicity has also been reported after CAR T-cell treatment associated with prominent hyperferritinemia and multiorgan failure.[47] Other, less severe potential side effects of CAR T-cell treatment include hypogammaglobinemia due to B-cell aplasia (CD19 CARs), prolonged cytopenias, hypersensitivity reactions, serious infections, and, less commonly, second malignancies.[45]

There are several areas in which clinical application of CAR T-cell immunotherapy that can be improved. The median time required for autologous CAR T-cell production is 23 days, a time frame that could be reduced through optimization of the manufacturing process. Moreover, per patient manufacturing costs are quite high, which is an important consideration that should stimulate efforts to automate and decrease cost so that all patients have access to this novel technology when it is needed. Continued research is also focused on strategies to mitigate observed toxicities, such as inclusion of safety switches that can be deployed when toxicity is anticipated. Improved CRS-directed therapies, such as with cytokine-directed monoclonal antibodies, is also an area of active clinical investigation. CAR T-cell application will ideally extend to solid tumors and other hematologic cancers (T-ALL, acute myeloid leukemia). Identification of novel tumor-specific antigens and modulation of interactions between T cells and the tumor microenvironment are specific areas under investigation in preclinical and clinical trials. With these advances, CAR T-cell technology is poised to expand the therapeutic options for patients with a range of cancer types.

The Role and Application of Antibody-Based Therapies

CASE VIGNETTE

A 13-year-old male presents to the emergency department with sore throat and fatigue. His CBC shows blasts on the differential and a comprehensive workup leads to the diagnosis of p53 mutated, complex karyotype acute myeloid leukemia (AML). He receives induction therapy with cytarabine, daunorubicin, and gemtuzumab ozogamicin, a CD33-targeting antibody–drug conjugate. His disease remains refractory to upfront treatment and salvage options are discussed with the family. He enrolls in a phase I clinical trial investigating the use of flotetuzumab, a CD123xCD3 dual-affinity retargeting protein (DART), for the treatment of pediatric recurrent or refractory AML. His treatment course is complicated by cytokine release syndrome requiring intensive care unit (ICU) admission for cardiorespiratory support. Disease assessment after one cycle of treatment demonstrated partial response with reduction in percentage of marrow blasts and negative CNS status. This case demonstrates the role of antibody-based therapies in the treatment of cancer, including monoclonal antibodies, antibody–drug conjugates, and novel application of bi- or trispecific engagers.

BACKGROUND

Antibodies are a key component of the adaptive immune system. They are produced by mature B cells in a highly regulated way to diversify the immune response. B cells develop from lymphoid precursors in the bone marrow and through a series of maturation steps assemble unique antibodies on their cell surface. Antibodies are composed of two heavy chains and two light chains connected through disulfide bonds. The constant domains of the heavy chains form the Fc portion of the antibody. The variable regions of the heavy and light chain undergo a genetic process known as VDJ recombination to confer unique antigen specificity to each antibody. Mature B cells traffic to lymph nodes where, under antigen stimulation, they are selected to undergo class switching and further differentiate into plasma cells that release soluble antibodies into circulation. An antibody response is activated when the immune system recognizes a foreign antigen. This remarkable antigen specificity and diversity can be harnessed as immunotherapy to target tumor-specific surface antigens.

Monoclonal antibodies (mAbs) targeting tumor-specific antigens can be isolated for further design and translation for clinical use. Two primary platforms exist for the generation of mAbs with high antigen-specific recognition. One technology comprises injection of a tumor antigen into a nonhuman species and isolation of antibodies specific to the foreign antigen. These antibodies can then be engineered to create chimeric or humanized antibodies to minimize immunogenicity by incorporation of the nonhuman variable regions into a human Fc domain.[48-50] Fully human antibodies can be created using hybridoma technology in transgenic mouse models.[51] A more contemporary platform known as *antibody phage display* allows for in vitro selection of human antibodies through isolation of high-affinity ligands. In this system, human immunoglobin gene libraries are displayed on the surface of bacteriophages and probed against antigens of interest to isolate a specific high-affinity antibody.[52-55] Isolated mAbs can be further modified to improve functionality. Single-chain fragment variables (scFvs) consist of only the variable regions of the light and heavy chain and are connected through a peptide linker. In addition to scFvs, other formulations of the antibody heavy and light chain domains are possible.[56] mAbs can further be conjugated to cytotoxic drugs for targeted delivery. Additional engineering to generate bispecific and trispecific molecules can also extend functionality (Fig. 10.4). The following sections will review antibody-based therapies in further detail.

MONOCLONAL ANTIBODIES

Antibody-based therapies are among the most important and successful treatments for a rising number of cancer diagnoses. The general mechanism of action of most mAbs includes immune system redirection toward antibody-dependent cellular cytotoxicity (ADCC) or complement-dependent cytotoxicity (CDC) for specific action against malignant cells.[57] Many mAbs alter signal transduction via interaction with growth factor receptors at the target or downregulate expression or accessibility of key surface antigens.[57] Their actions can further be combined with

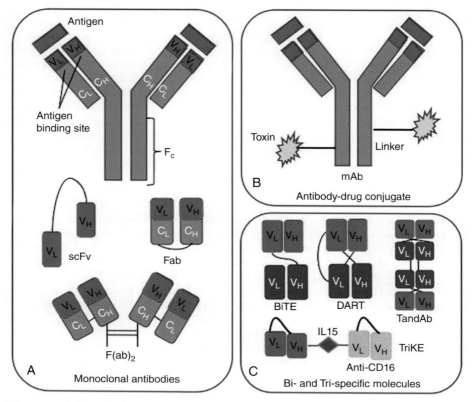

Fig. 10.4 Summary of antibody-based therapies. (A) Monoclonal antibody (mAb) structure with the variable portions of light chain and heavy chain conferring antigen specificity. Variations in mAb structure include the single-chain variable fragments (scFv), fragment antigen-binding (Fab), and F(ab)₂. (B) Antibody–drug conjugates (ADCs) consist of an mAb linked to a cytotoxic, immunotoxic, or radiotoxic agent. (C) Bispecific and trispecific molecules incorporate multiple antigen-binding sites. Bispecific T-cell engagers (BiTEs), dual-affinity retargeting bispecific antibodies (DARTs), and tandem diabodies (TandAbs) are types of bispecific molecules. Trispecific killer cell engagers (TriKEs) are a type of trispecific molecule that engages natural killer (NK) cells through CD16 and produces IL-15 to enhance NK cell function for targeted activity against tumor cells.

chemotherapy for synergistic effect.[57] Of note, checkpoint inhibitors including ipilimumab (CTLA-4 inhibitor) and nivolumab and pembrolizumab (PD-1 inhibitors) represent a key category of monoclonal antibody therapy that has changed the treatment landscape for solid tumors, and are discussed in more detail in **The role and application of checkpoint blockade**. Table 10.1 provides a comprehensive overview of FDA-approved monoclonal antibodies for use in clinical practice. Notable monoclonal antibody therapies that have significantly advanced treatment of solid tumors and hematologic malignancies are highlighted in the following paragraphs.

Rituximab is a human/murine chimeric mAb targeting CD20,[58-60] a cell surface antigen expressed on the surface of healthy and most malignant B cells. This mAb was FDA approved for the treatment of relapsed or refractory indolent non-Hodgkin lymphoma (NHL) in 1997 based on data from a phase II trial of rituximab monotherapy in 166 patients with relapsed or refractory low-grade NHL, with an overall response rate in the intent-to-treat group of 48% and a projected median time to progression of 13 months.[61] Approvals for other B cell–derived hematologic malignancies followed in subsequent years. Rituximab is now standard of care for numerous diagnoses including follicular lymphoma (FL), diffuse large B-cell lymphoma (DLBCL), and

TABLE 10.1 ■ **FDA-Approved Monoclonal Antibodies**

Name	Format	Target Antigen	Indication
Hematologic Malignancies			
Alemtuzumab	Humanized IgG1	CD52	B-cell chronic lymphocytic leukemia
Daratumumab	Human IgG1	CD38	Multiple myeloma
Elotuzumab	Humanized IgG1	SLAMF7	Multiple myeloma
Isatuximab	Chimeric IgG1	CD38	Multiple myeloma
Mogamulizumab	Humanized IgG1	CCR4	Cutaneous T-cell lymphoma
Obinutuzumab	Humanized IgG2	CD20	Chronic lymphocytic leukemia, follicular lymphoma
Ofatumumab	Human IgG1	CD20	Chronic lymphocytic leukemia
Rituximab	Chimeric IgG1	CD20	B-cell lymphoma
Solid Tumors			
Atezolizumab	Humanized IgG1	PD-L1	Bladder cancer, non-small cell lung cancer, triple-negative breast cancer, small cell lung cancer, hepatocellular carcinoma, melanoma
Avelumab	Human IgG1	PD-L1	Urothelial carcinoma, Merkel cell carcinoma, renal cell carcinoma
Bevacizumab	Humanized IgG1	VEGF	Colorectal cancer, non-small cell lung cancer, renal cancer, glioblastoma, cervical cancer
Cemiplimab	Human IgG4	PD-1	Cutaneous squamous cell carcinoma, basal cell carcinoma, non-small cell lung cancer
Cetuximab	Chimeric IgG1	EGFR	Colorectal cancer, head and neck squamous cell carcinoma
Dinutuximab	Chimeric IgG1	GD2	Neuroblastoma
Durvalumab	Human IgG1	PD-L1	Bladder cancer, non-small cell lung cancer, small cell lung cancer
Ipilimumab	Human IgG1	CTLA-4	Melanoma, renal cell carcinoma, colorectal cancer, hepatocellular carcinoma, non-small cell lung cancer, malignant pleural mesothelioma
Necitumumab	Human IgG1	EGFR	Non-small cell lung cancer
Nivolumab	Human IgG4	PD-1	Melanoma, non-small cell lung cancer, renal cancer, classical Hodgkin lymphoma, head and neck cancer, urothelial carcinoma, colorectal cancer, hepatocellular carcinoma, esophageal carcinoma, malignant pleural mesothelioma, gastric cancer
Panitumumab	Human IgG2	EGFR	Colorectal cancer
Pembrolizumab	Humanized IgG4	PD-1	Melanoma, triple-negative breast cancer, non-small cell lung cancer, head and neck squamous cell cancer, classical Hodgkin lymphoma, primary mediastinal B-cell lymphoma, urothelial carcinoma, microsatellite instability-high or mismatch repair–deficient solid tumors, colorectal cancer, gastroesophageal junction adenocarcinoma, cervical cancer, hepatocellular carcinoma, Merkel cell carcinoma, renal cell carcinoma, cutaneous squamous cell carcinoma
Pertuzumab	Humanized IgG1	HER2	Breast cancer
Ramucirumab	Human IgG1	VEGFR2	Gastric cancer, non-small cell lung cancer, colorectal cancer, hepatocellular carcinoma
Trastuzumab	Humanized IgG1	HER2	Breast cancer

chronic lymphocytic lymphoma (CLL) and is routinely used off-label for treatment of mantle cell lymphoma (MCL), marginal zone lymphoma, Hodgkin lymphoma, Burkitt lymphoma, and B-lineage acute lymphoblastic leukemia.[62]

Bevacizumab is another mAb whose clinical use advanced the application of this class of drugs for the treatment of cancer. Bevacizumab targets VEGF-A, a key signaling protein secreted by tumor cells that induces blood vessel formation.[63] Once soluble VEGF-A is bound, its interaction with the VEFGR is sterically inhibited and angiogenesis blocked.[63] Bevacizumab was first studied in solid tumors dependent on angiogenesis for growth and metastasis. These included metastatic colorectal cancer (mCRC), non-small cell lung cancer (NSCLC), metastatic breast cancer (mBC), glioblastoma multiforme (GBM), ovarian cancer (OC), and renal cell carcinoma (RCC).[63] The drug was FDA approved in 2004 for the treatment of mCRC based on a phase III clinical trial, AVF2107g, evaluating bevacizumab as first-line treatment for mCRC in combination with irinotecan, fluorouracil, and leucovorin versus chemotherapy alone. The addition of bevacizumab to this regimen lead to an increased median duration of survival (20.3 months in the bevacizumab group vs 15.6 months in the control group; hazard ratio (HR) = 0.66, $P < .001$), with grade 3 hypertension as the most common adverse effect.[64] In the intervening years since initial FDA approval, bevacizumab has been approved for use in a wide spectrum of solid tumors. The role of bevacizumab in modulating the immunosuppressive tumor microenvironment highlights the potential for use as a combination regimen, particularly with immune checkpoint inhibitors.[63]

Finally, trastuzumab is a recombinant humanized mAb that has revolutionized the treatment of human epidermal growth factor 2 (HER2)-positive breast cancer. Approximately 20% of women diagnosed with invasive breast cancer have HER2 oncogenic amplification.[65] HER2 is a cell surface glycoprotein that contains extracellular ligand-binding domains linked to intracellular domains with tyrosine kinase activity. Downstream signaling events drive cell growth and proliferation. Trastuzumab binds the extracellular domain of HER2 and prevents downstream signaling events.[66] Its binding causes both cell cycle arrest and induced ADCC by immune effector cell recruitment.[67] Trastuzumab is now an FDA-approved and standard-of-care treatment for patients with early and advanced HER2-positive breast cancer either simultaneously or in sequence with chemotherapy.[68] A 2012 Cochrane Review evaluated eight randomized controlled trials comparing the efficacy and safety profile of trastuzumab alone or together with chemotherapy compared with no treatment or standard chemotherapy alone. The analysis of 11,991 patients resulted in a combined HR for overall survival (OS) of 0.66 (95% confidence interval [CI], 0.57–0.77; $P < .00001$) and disease-free survival of 0.60 (95% CI, 0.50–0.71; $P < .00001$), strongly favoring trastuzumab-containing regimens.[69] Trastuzumab treatment is associated with a risk of cardiac toxicity to include congestive heart failure and left ventricular ejection fraction decline.[69] Newer derivations of trastuzumab are aimed at enhancing tumor-specific cytotoxicity through conjugation to either emtansine (T-DM1) or deruxtecan (DS-8201), both of which have shown clinical benefit.[70,71] mAbs represent a major advance in the field of immunotherapy, but despite the notable exceptions reviewed here, the antitumor activity of mAbs alone is often limited, necessitating further modification to enhance efficacy.

ANTIBODY–DRUG CONJUGATES

An antibody–drug conjugate (ADCs) combines the antigen specificity of mAbs with the targeted release of cytotoxic drugs. Linking mAbs to cytotoxic agents, immunotoxins, and radiopharmaceutical agents allows for specific delivery to tumor cells through antibody binding and internalization.[72] Early iterations of ADCs involved the use of murine monoclonal antibodies conjugated to chemotherapeutic agents such as doxorubicin and methotrexate. These were not clinically useful owing to high immunogenicity and low drug potency. Newer ADCs use humanized mAbs, drugs that are 100 to 1000 times more potent, and incorporate improved target selection and binding and internalization efficiency.[72] Table 10.2 provides a comprehensive overview of FDA-approved ADCs for use in clinical practice with two agents highlighted whose use is now standard.

Gemtuzumab ozogamicin (GO) is an ADC consisting of a recombinant humanized CD33-targeting mAb (gemtuzumab) linked to a cytotoxic derivative of calicheamicin (ozogamicin), a powerful DNA-damaging agent.[73] CD33 is expressed on the surface of AML cells in >80% of patients and is rapidly internalized.[73,74] GO binds CD33 with high affinity followed by internalization and lysosomal processing with release of ozogamicin, which then causes DNA damage and cell cycle arrest.[75] The clinical efficacy and safety of GO monotherapy were initially evaluated through three open-label, single-arm, phase II studies of AML in first relapse. Two hundred seventy-seven patients with a median age 61 received treatment with GO.[76] Of these patients, 26% achieved remission with a median OS of 12.6 months. Primary side effects included grade 3 or 4 neutropenia (98%), thrombocytopenia (99%), grade 3 or 4 sepsis (17%), pneumonia (8%), grade 3 or 4 hyperbilirubinemia (29%), AST elevation (18%), and ALT elevation (9%). These findings led to an accelerated FDA approval for GO as treatment for relapsed AML in 2000. Postmarketing studies, however, failed to confirm efficacy in a follow-up phase III randomized controlled trial (SWOG-S0106) of GO dosed at 6 mg/m² combined with induction therapy versus induction therapy alone. This, in addition to relatively higher toxicity, led to the voluntary removal of GO from U.S. commercial markets in 2010.[77] A subsequent multicenter, randomized, open-label phase III clinical trial, ALFA-0701, evaluated fractionated GO dosing in combination with upfront induction and consolidation therapy for newly diagnosed CD33+ AML versus chemotherapy alone. Results from 278 patients reconfirmed the clinical benefit of GO with median event-free survival of 15.6 months in the GO + chemotherapy arm vs 9.7 months in the control arm (HR = 0.58; 95% CI, 0.43–0.73; P = .0003), without a significant difference in induction mortality between each arm.[78] The findings from this trial reinstated the FDA approval for GO in the upfront setting in combination with standard induction chemotherapy. Though this approval is accompanied by a black box warning for hepatotoxicity, including the risk of

TABLE 10.2 ■ **FDA-Approved Antibody–Drug Conjugates**

Name	Format	Target Antigen	Indication
Hematologic Malignancies			
Belantamab mafodotin-blmf		BCMA	Multiple myeloma
Brentuximab vedotin	Chimeric ADC	CD30	Hodgkin lymphoma, anaplastic large cell lymphoma
Gemtuzumab ozogamicin	Humanized ADC	CD33	Acute myeloid leukemia
Ibritumomab tiuxetan	Murine IgG1	CD20	Non-Hodgkin lymphoma
Inotuzumab ozogamicin	Humanized ADC	CD22	Acute lymphoblastic leukemia
Iodine tositumomab	Murine IgG2	CD20	Non-Hodgkin lymphoma
Loncastuximab tesirine-lpyl	Humanized IgG1	CD19	Large B-cell lymphoma
Moxetumomab pasudodox	Murine IgG1 dsFv	CD22	Hairy cell leukemia
Polatuzumab vedotin	Humanized ADC	CD79B	B-cell lymphoma
Solid Tumors			
Enfortumab vedotin	Human ADC	Nectin-4	Bladder cancer
Sacituzumab govitecan	Humanized ADC	TROP2	Triple-negative breast cancer
Tisotumab vedotin-tftv	Human ADC	Tissue Factor	Cervical cancer
Trastuzumab emtansine	Humanized ADC	HER2	Breast cancer
Trastuzumab deruxtecan	Humanized ADC	HER2	Breast cancer

developing severe or fatal sinusoidal obstructive syndrome (SOS), the GO dosing fractionation decreased the incidence of SOS from 20% to 40% to 0% to 5%.[78-81] Fractionated GO is now standard of care as monotherapy in CD33+ relapsed or refractory AML for patients aged 2 years and older, as combination therapy with standard induction and consolidation chemotherapy in newly diagnosed de novo CD33+ AML, and as single-agent therapy in CD33+ AML for adult patients who are unable to tolerate intensive chemotherapy.[82]

Brentuximab vedotin is another ADC that is a powerful targeted therapy for hematologic malignancies. It is a chimeric anti-CD30 mAb conjugated to monomethyl auristatin E (MMAE), a potent antitubulin. Release of the MMAE effector molecule disrupts the microtubule network necessary for mitosis and cell cycle progression.[83,84] Similar to all ADCs, binding of brentuximab vedotin can induce tumor killing through ADCC.[85] CD30 is expressed on the cell surface of normal activated T cell, B cells, and natural killer (NK) cells, as well as several malignant tumors, including Hodgkin lymphoma (HL), anaplastic large cell lymphoma (ALCL), certain types of B cell–derived NHL, mature T-cell lymphomas, and germ-line malignancies.[85] A phase I study of 45 patients, of which 42 had relapsed/refractory classical HL, 2 had systemic ALCL, and 1 had CD30+ angioimmunoblastic T-cell lymphoma, who received brentuximab vedotin at doses of 0.1 to 3.6 mg/kg every 3 weeks demonstrated complete response (CR) in 11 patients (25%), partial response (PR) in 6 patients (14%), and stable disease in 19 patients of 44 evaluable (43%). The median duration of response was at least 9.7 months.[86] Primary adverse events included fatigue, pyrexia, diarrhea, nausea, neutropenia, and peripheral neuropathy. An additional phase I study evaluated brentuximab vedotin using a more frequent dosing regimen and showed similar promising results.[87] This led to a pivotal phase II study for patients with relapse/refractory classical HL after failed hematopoietic autologous stem cell transplantation who were treated with brentuximab vedotin at the maximum tolerated dose of 1.8 mg/kg every 3 weeks for up to 16 cycles.[88] For the 102 patients included in the study, the estimated OS was 41% (95% CI, 31–51) and the progression-free survival (PFS) was 22% (95% CI, 13–31). These rates were even higher in the 34 patients who achieved CR after brentuximab vedotin, with 64% OS (95% CI, 48–80) and 52% PFS (95% CI, 34–69). Brentuximab is now FDA approved for use against multiple CD30-expressing tumors with a generally well-tolerated side effect profile, though peripheral neuropathy remains a significant potential toxicity.

BISPECIFIC AND TRISPECIFIC MOLECULES

A further enhancement to antibody-based therapies includes engineering to generate bi- and trispecific molecules designed to bind two or three distinct antigens. The specificity of these small molecules can bridge target and effector cells or can modulate cell signaling pathways through binding of two epitopes on the same cell.[89] Numerous variations on this general mechanistic principle have been translated into clinical practice. Bispecific T-cell engagers (BiTEs) comprise two scFvs combined into a single protein chain with a peptide linker. BiTEs target a cell surface target antigen and CD3 in the T-cell receptor complex to specifically direct T-cell effector function.[89] Dual-affinity retargeting (DART) bispecific antibodies are composed of an antibody heavy chain covalently linked to its light chain to mimic the structure of endogenous IgG. DARTs can similarly target cell surface tumor antigens and CD3 on T cells for directed cytotoxicity.[89] Tandem diabodies (TandAbs) incorporate two binding sites for each antigen and have a larger molecular weight, thus avoiding first-pass renal clearance[89] and extending their circulating half-life.[90] Finally, bispecific and trispecific killer cell engagers are small molecules containing two (BiKE) or three (TriKE) scFvs targeting target surface antigen and CD16 to induce formation of a target cell/NK cell immunologic synapse.[91] Table 10.3 provides a comprehensive overview of FDA-approved or late-stage clinical bispecific molecules. Trispecific agents are primarily in preclinical or early clinical stages. Blinatumomab, now approved for relapsed/refractory B-cell ALL;

TABLE 10.3 ■ FDA-Approved, In Review, or Late-Stage Clinical Bispecific Molecules

Name	Format	Target Antigen	Indication
Approved			
Amivantamab-vmjw	Bispecific	EGFRxMET	Non-small cell lung cancer
Blinatumomab	Bispecific	CD19 x CD3	B-cell precursor acute lymphoblastic leukemia
Priority Review, Expedited Designations, or Late-Phase Clinical Trial			
Glofitamab	Bispecific	CD20 x CD3	Diffuse large B-cell lymphoma
KN046	Bispecific	PD-L1 x CTLA4	Non-small cell lung cancer
IBI318	Bispecific	PD-1 x PD-L1	Non-small cell lung cancer
Epcoritamab	Bispecific	CD20 x CD3	Diffuse large B-cell lymphoma
Tebotelimab	Bispecific	PD-1 x LAG-3	Gastric and gastroesophageal junction carcinoma
Tebentafusp	Bispecific	TCR x CD3	Melanoma
Mosunetuzumab	Bispecific	CD20 x CD3	Follicular lymphoma
Zanidatamb	Bispecific	HER2 ECD2 x ECD4	Biliary tract cancers
Flotetuzumab	Bispecific	CD123 x CD3	Acute myeloid leukemia
APVO436	Bispecific	CD123 x CD3	Acute myeloid leukemia
Zenocutuzumab	Bispecific	HER2 x HER3	Pancreatic cancer
TNB383B	Bispecific	BCMA x CD3	Multiple myeloma

flotetuzumab, in late clinical trials for AML; and GTB-3550, a TriKE in early clinical development, are reviewed.

Blinatumomab is a BiTE that targets CD19 on B cells and CD3 on T cells to induce targeted killing of B-lymphocyte blasts through release of cytotoxic granules. Blinatumomab is FDA approved for the treatment of relapsed or refractory B-cell ALL and is currently being investigated in pediatric clinical trials as an upfront agent for the initial treatment of standard risk ALL. A multicenter phase II study of 189 adults with Philadelphia chromosome–negative (Ph−) relapsed/refractory disease demonstrated CR or CR with partial hematologic recovery (CRh) in 43% of patients within two treatment cycles.[92] A subsequent randomized phase III clinical trial in pediatric patients (age >28 days to <18 years) with Ph−high-risk B-cell ALL in first relapse in morphologic CR (M1 marrow, <5% blasts) or with M2 marrow (blasts >5%, <25%) at randomization received one cycle of continuous blinatumomab versus chemotherapy for consolidative therapy.[93] This clinical trial aimed to investigate the efficacy of blinatumomab compared with conventional chemotherapy in reducing residual leukemia burden prior to planned HSCT. The estimated event-free survival (EFS) at 24 months was 66.2% (95% CI, 50.1–78.2) in the blinatumomab group compared with 27.1% (95% CI, 13.2–43) in the chemotherapy group. Minimal residual disease (MRD) remission was observed in 90% of patients in the blinatumomab group compared with 54% in the chemotherapy group. Enrollment in this trial was terminated early because of clear benefit in patients randomized to receive blinatumomab. Blinatumomab is FDA approved for the treatment of B-cell ALL in first or second CR with MRD ≥0.1% and for relapsed or refractory B-cell ALL in children and adults. Due to the very short life of blinatumomab, it requires administration through continuous infusion, which poses logistical challenges. Primary adverse effects of blinatumomab include cytokine release syndrome and neurotoxicity.

Flotetuzumab, a DART, targets CD123 on myeloid blasts and CD3 on T cells to induce targeted killing of AML. Approximately 50% of patients diagnosed with AML do not respond to conventional induction therapy or relapse within 6 months after achieving remission.[94,95] Poor outcomes in patients with induction failure or early relapse of AML have been linked to subtype-specific immune transcriptomic profiles, highlighting the benefit of considering immunotherapy in this subset.[96] A multicenter phase I/II dose escalation study of flotetuzumab in relapsed/refractory AML or intermediate-2/high-risk MDS with a standard 3 + 3 dose escalation design identified a recommended dose of 500 ng/kg per day.[97] Among 30 patients with primary induction failure or early relapse treated at this recommended dose, the rate of CR or CRh was 26.7% with a median OS of 10.2 months (range, 1.87–27.27) and 6- and 12-month survival rates of 75% (95% CI, 0.45–1.05) and 50% (95% CI, 0.154–0.846), respectively. Immunoprofiling of bone marrow samples identified a 10-gene signature panel that could be used to predict CR to flotetuzumab, reflective of higher immune infiltration and production of inflammatory cytokines in the bone marrow microenvironment. Infusion reactions and CRS were the primary adverse events and were effectively mitigated through premedication, stepwise dosing, early treatment with the IL-6R blocking agent tocilizumab, and temporary dose reductions and holds to prevent progression to severe grading. Flotetzumab has shown particular promise in high-risk subpopulations including patients with TP53 mutated AML. It represents a key advance in the field of immunotherapy for AML.

As a final example, TriKEs have been designed to augment ADCC by coengaging CD16 on NK cells and tumor specific antigens.[98] One class of TriKEs incorporates the IL-15 cytokine as a structural component to enhance NK cell function. Preclinical investigation comparing an anti-CD16 x IL-15 x anti-CD33 TriKE to an anti-CD16 x anti-CD33 BiKE demonstrated enhanced NK cell cytotoxicity and tumor control as well as improved NK cell survival and expansion of the TriKE in a mouse model.[97,99] Consequently, an anti-CD16 x IL-15 x anti-CD33 TriKE, GTB-3550, is now being studied in a multicenter phase I/II clinical trial (NCT03214666) for the treatment of CD33+ high-risk myelodysplastic syndromes, relapsed or refractory AML, or advanced systemic mastocytosis. Preliminary data from four enrolled patients confirmed safety of the treatment without significantly toxicity and NK cell proliferation, though no objective responses were seen at the tested dose.[100] These novel trispecific pharmacologics represent a new frontier in targeted therapy that not only incorporates colocalization of immune effector cells and tumor cells but also that delivers localized cytokine to promote robust effector cell expansion and activation.

CONCLUSIONS

Antibody-based therapies have revolutionized the treatment landscape for many solid tumors and hematologic malignancies. In monoclonal, bispecific, or trispecific formats, they are able to reorient immune surveillance and cytotoxicity in a targeted manner. Antibody-based therapies have seen greater success in hematologic malignancies compared with solid tumors because of greater antigen accessibility and challenges with effective penetration of the tumor microenvironment. The target specificity that comes with antibody-based therapies can be harnessed for drug delivery for more powerful antitumor activity. Combination of antibody-based therapies with cellular therapies or other treatment modalities represents an active area of study that has the potential to solve some significant limitations in drug trafficking and duration of action.

The Role and Application of Cancer Vaccines

INTRODUCTION

Vaccines are created to stimulate the immune system against disease. This approach has been very effective in protecting humans from a broad range of microbial pathogens. By training the immune system to recognize these infectious diseases, the clinical manifestations of illness may be reduced or even avoided altogether. Furthermore, vaccinations tend to have only mild, short-term side effects while offering robust, long-lasting protection. This promise of safety and efficacy has led to clinical development of cancer vaccines. Please refer to Chapter 9: Vaccines and Active Immunization Against Cancer for an overview of vaccine technologies and emerging approaches to achieve anticancer immunity. This section focuses on cancer vaccines currently used in clinical practice.

BACKGROUND

Despite the popularization of cancer immunotherapy, the concept of immunizing a host against cancer is quite old. Even the scientific basis of cancer vaccines began over 150 years ago, when Busch and Fehleisen both noted that erysipelas infection could lead to tumor regression in patients with cancer. Fehleisen later identified that *Streptococcus pyogenes* caused these erysipelas-induced tumor responses. At the end of the 19th century, William Coley administered heat-inactivated bacteria, termed *Coley's toxins*, into patients with advanced cancer and reported clinical successes. Though Coley's toxins later fell out of favor, Lloyd Old demonstrated that bacillus Calmette-Guerin (BCG) could immunize mice against transplanted tumors.[101] This led to clinical studies of BCG in patients with superficial bladder cancer.[102] As knowledge about the fundamentals of immunology has grown since the later half of the 20th century, so has interest in cancer vaccines.

Just as vaccines can reduce the risk of microbial infection, immunization can also prevent long-term health problems (including development of some cancers) that are the sequelae of these infections. As such, there has been interest in the clinical development of several prophylactic cancer vaccines. Vaccines against human papilloma virus, for example, have been effective in reducing the risk of cervical cancer. Likewise, efforts to immunize patients against hepatitis B have resulted in fewer cases of hepatocellular carcinoma caused by this virus. These successes have fostered interest in using vaccines to prevent other viral-associated malignancies.

Unfortunately, most cancer vaccines have not resulted in regression of established tumors or prevented recurrence of treated malignancies. After decades of underwhelming efficacy, however, there is renewed enthusiasm in the clinical development of therapeutic cancer vaccines. This is bolstered by a growing understanding of tumor-induced immunosuppression and an expanding repertoire of cancer antigens. Furthermore, novel vaccine platforms and combinatorial approaches (such as use of immune checkpoint blockade) have rekindled the promise of cancer vaccines.

PREVENTATIVE CANCER VACCINES

Because viral infections have been shown to factor in the pathogenesis of several malignancies, investigators have developed prophylactic cancer vaccines to protect individuals from these tumors. Human papilloma virus (HPV), for example, is the primary cause of cervical cancer, anal cancer, and other HPV-induced malignancies. Likewise, chronic viral infection with hepatitis B increases the risk of hepatocellular carcinoma. Vaccines against these viruses have shown efficacy in reducing the risk of cancer and encouraged development of vaccines to prevent infection with other cancer-causing viruses.

Human Papilloma Virus

HPV is the most common sexually transmitted pathogen in the United States, causing both anogenital and oropharyngeal diseases. Persistent viral infection contributes to the majority of cervical, anal, and oropharyngeal cancers. Of the many HPV genotypes, several have been identified as most contributory to the development of these cancers. The high-risk genotypes HPV type 16 and HPV type 18 lead to approximately 70% of cervical cancers, 90% of anal cancers, and most viral-induced head and neck cancers. Therefore vaccine development has focused on these two high-risk HPV genotypes.

A recombinant HPV bivalent (types 16 and 18) vaccine (Cervarix, GlaxoSmithKline) was approved by the FDA in 2009 for the prevention of cervical cancer. This vaccine uses the adjuvant AS04, consisting of aluminum hydroxide and 3-O-desacyl-4'-monophosphoryl lipid A, to enhance immunogenicity. The randomized, double-blind phase III Papilloma TRIal against Cancer In young Adults (PATRICIA) study revealed 92% efficacy against cervical intraepithelial neoplasia associated with these two high-risk HPV genotypes.[103] These results led to approval of Cervarix to protect females between the ages of 9 to 25 from cervical intraepithelial neoplasia. The vaccine can also help in the prevention of other cancers induced by HPV types 16 and 18, such as anal, head and neck, penile, vulval, and vaginal cancers.

Other HPV vaccines have been developed to provide broader protection beyond the high-risk genotypes. HPV types 6 and 11 are felt to account for most anogenital warts, leading to the expanded coverage of a recombinant HPV quadrivalent (types 6, 11, 16, and 18) vaccine (Gardasil, Merck). In addition to prevention of cervical cancer, Gardasil is FDA approved for prevention of vulvar cancer, vaginal cancer, and anal cancer, as well as precancerous lesions caused by these four HPV genotypes. A nine-valent HPV vaccine (Gardasil 9, Merck) has been developed to target HPV types, 6, 11, 16, 18, 31, 33, 45, 52, and 58. These additional five HPV genotypes (31, 33, 45, 52, and 58) not included in the quadrivalent vaccine are associated with an additional 20% of cervical cancers worldwide. Furthermore, HPV types 31 and 33 are considered high risk for head and neck cancers. In light of new HPV vaccines and emerging clinical data, guidelines for HPV vaccination continue to evolve.[104]

Hepatitis B

Viral hepatitis is a major risk factor for the development of hepatocellular carcinoma. This is most common in patients with progressive liver injury leading to cirrhosis. However, chronic infection with either the hepatitis B virus (HBV) or the hepatitis C virus can also cause cancer in patients without cirrhosis. Though treatment of chronic viral hepatitis can reduce a patient's risk of hepatocellular carcinoma, vaccination to prevent viral infection is a more effective approach. Fortunately, several HBV vaccines are available to patients throughout the world. First-generation vaccines derived from plasma have been replaced with recombinant vaccines derived from yeast or mammalian cells. Two conventional recombinant vaccines, Recombivax HB (Merck) and Engerix-B (GlaxoSmithKline), have been available since the 1980s. These vaccines are derived from yeast and use an alum adjuvant. Both are approved by the FDA for prevention of HBV infection but have reduced efficacy in patients with several health conditions including diabetes mellitus. Another yeast-derived recombinant HBV vaccine was developed using a Toll-like receptor 9 adjuvant (Heplisav-B, Dynavax). Compared with Engerix-B in a cohort of patients with diabetes, Heplisav-B was found to have better seroprotection.[105] Lastly, a trivalent vaccine derived from mammalian cells (Prehevbrio, VBI Vaccines) targets multiple HBV surface antigens and was approved by the FDA in 2021. This vaccine also seems to have superior immunogenicity for adults ≥45 years old who have diminished response to conventional monovalent vaccines[106] and may reduce vaccine escape from the HBV surface antigen. Efforts to improve HBV vaccines are focused on simplifying the dosing schedule and improving the efficacy in patients without seroprotection.

THERAPEUTIC CANCER VACCINES

Following in the footsteps of William Coley's attempts to immunize patients with advanced cancer, many groups have worked to develop therapeutic cancer vaccines since the early 20th century. This is an attractive approach given the promise of safety, ease of use, lack of side effects, and durability. These efforts have often led to favorable surrogate endpoints (e.g., detection of circulating tumor-reactive T cells or lymphocyte infiltration within the tumor), but patients have rarely experienced measurable clinical benefit.[107] In fact, Lloyd Old's discovery that bacillus Calmette-Guerin (BCG) can generate an antitumor immune response remains one of the few successes; BCG (TICE BCG, Organon Teknika) is still used, but its therapeutic effect seems limited to patients with early-stage bladder cancer. Nonetheless, attempts to develop cancer vaccines have continued. One approach involves generating a personalized vaccine through modification of a patient's cells within a clinical laboratory. These autologous cancer vaccines may be generated from a patient's actual tumor or via ex vivo stimulation of a patient's own antigen-presenting cells. The first cancer vaccine of this type approved by the FDA was sipuleucel-T (Provenge, Dendreon), an autologous dendritic cell vaccine targeting prostatic acid phosphatase (PAP). This treatment, which is prepared from peripheral blood mononuclear cells exposed to the PAP tumor antigen and an immune cell growth factor, has shown benefit in patients with metastatic prostate cancer. Another common approach has been in vivo stimulation of the adaptive immune system to recognize a tumor-associated antigen, which may be found in some normal cells but is highly overexpressed in specific cancer cells, or to target a tumor-specific antigen such as mutated neoantigens found in cancer cells but not normal cells. With discovery of promising tumor antigens and improvement in adjuvant technologies, there are numerous therapeutic vaccines in clinical development. Many in the pipeline will be evaluated in combination with immune checkpoint blockade to best treat established cancers or to prevent recurrence of treated malignancies.

Bacillus Calmette-Guerin

BCG is a live, attenuated form of *Mycobacterium bovis*. Beyond its use as a tuberculosis vaccine, BCG plays an important role in the treatment of patients with early-stage bladder cancer. As mentioned previously in this section, there has been long-standing interest in the ability of microbes to treat cancer dating back to Coley's toxins. Though work had suggested that tuberculin may prevent the development of cancer,[108] it was a randomized trial by the Southwest Oncology Group that clearly demonstrated that BCG immunotherapy was beneficial in patients with non-muscle-invasive bladder cancer.[109] Subsequent trials have evaluated BCG with either cytokine therapy or immune checkpoint blockade, although it is unclear whether there is synergy in these combinatorial immunotherapy approaches. Despite its common clinical use, the mechanism of action by which BCG leads to antitumor immunity is incompletely understood. One prevailing model begins with BCG attaching to and invading the urothelium, where it triggers an innate immune response and ultimately activates the adaptive immune system. Lastly, there continues to be interest in exploring vaccination with BCG in the prevention of and treatment for other malignancies.

Sipuleucel-T

Sipuleucel-T, which was approved by the FDA in 2010, has demonstrated that a therapeutic cancer vaccine can be effective in patients with advanced cancer. This autologous vaccine targets PAP, a tumor-associated antigen expressed on prostate cancer. The treatment consists of leukapheresis to isolate a patient's peripheral blood mononuclear cells. These cells then undergo ex vivo exposure with PA2024, a fusion protein combining the tumor antigen PAP with granulocyte-macrophage colony-stimulating factor (GM-CSF) before the resultant dendritic cell vaccine is administered back to the patient. Studies have demonstrated safety and efficacy of sipuleucel-T in patients with metastatic prostate cancer. Interestingly, early-stage clinical trials demonstrated prolonged overall survival in patients receiving treatment, although the primary endpoint of progression-free survival was not met. In the IMPACT study, a multicenter phase III randomized controlled trial, 512 patients with castration-resistant prostate cancer were assigned in a 2:1 ratio to receive sipuleucel-T or placebo.[110] The sipuleucel-T group had prolonged median overall survival, reduced risk of death, and improved 36-month survival, which were all statistically significant. Similar to previous trials, however, there did not appear to be objective responses in the treatment arm and time to progression was comparable in both groups. The role of sipuleucel-T in the treatment of prostate cancer continues to evolve as new therapies emerge, but a randomized phase II trial of sipuleucel-T with or without radium-223 in patients with bone-predominant metastatic prostate cancer suggested a more robust therapeutic effect of combinatorial therapy.[111]

CONCLUSIONS

Though vaccines are a cornerstone in the defense against infectious diseases, their role in the management of cancer is frustratingly mixed. One notable breakthrough has been the development of preventative cancer vaccines. These not only protect a patient from the short-term sequelae of microbial pathogens but also reduce a patient's long-term risk of developing cancer. Furthermore, widespread vaccination across a population can benefit individuals who have not been immunized because of a reduction in transmission rates. As we continue to understand the part that viruses (and other microbes) play in the pathogenesis of cancer, it seems clear that our armamentarium of prophylactic cancer vaccines will expand accordingly. On the other hand, therapeutic cancer vaccines continue to have limited clinical benefit. Though the rationale for this approach is sound and there have been some therapeutic successes in specific cancer types, the full potential of therapeutic cancer vaccines has not been realized. Nonetheless, active research in the areas of antigen discovery, tumor-induced immunosuppression, vaccine delivery, and combinatorial immunotherapy has bolstered ongoing clinical development. For those reasons, there is optimism that novel vaccines may yet play a role in eradicating malignancies.

Combination Immunotherapies in Practice and Clinical Research Trials

INTRODUCTION

Though the preceding sections illustrate the clinical advances made using primarily single agent immunotherapies, there is powerful biologic rationale to combine the described cancer treatment modalities. Immune checkpoint inhibition can fail owing to lack of T-cell infiltration, effector cell anergy, or iatrogenic T-cell dysfunction, such as occurs after the administration of intensive chemotherapy. Though adoptive cell therapy (ACT) can be effective, remissions are not always durable. Outcomes after the use of CAR T-cell therapy for the treatment of B-cell hematologic malignancies are surprisingly good, with remission achievable ~70% to 80% of the time. CAR T-cell therapy as treatment for solid tumors is less effective. Though short-term responses can be quite impressive, CAR T and ACT durable activity can be subverted by immunologic evasion, including via T cell PD-1 upregulation and tumor cell PD-L1 expression, among others. Antibody therapy is challenged by pharmacologic restriction that limits tissue and CNS penetration of drug as well as relatively rapid metabolism and clearance. Vaccines depend on host immunologic responsiveness for efficacy.

IMMUNE CHECKPOINT BLOCKADE + ADOPTIVE CELL THERAPY

Activated T cells upregulate PD-1 expression, and it is well established that tumor and dendritic cells exposed to inflammatory cytokine in the tumor microenvironment (TME) upregulate PD-L1. This biologic understanding has prompted preclinical and clinical study combining infusion of activated T cells and PD-1 or PD-L1 inhibitory antibodies (immune checkpoint inhibition, ICI). For engineered CAR T cells specifically, preclinical study using in vitro cell culture and immunocompetent mouse modeling has established that circumventing this mechanism of immune suppression can improve effector cell function.[112] To additionally support the previously mentioned premise, analysis of infusion products from nonresponders of ACT has shown activation of the checkpoint molecules PD-1, TIM-3, and LAG-3 compared with T-cell products of responding patients, suggesting that T-cell exhaustion is an important modifiable feature of cell therapy inefficacy.[113] There is at present an emerging, but limited, clinical experience reporting the safety and efficacy of combination ICI and CAR T-cell therapy. The combination of CD19-targeted CAR T cells and pembrolizumab has been described in a case report of a patient found refractory to CAR T cell infusion with high PD-L1 expression on their lymphoma. Treatment with the PD-1-blocking agent was followed by CAR T-cell expansion and tumor regression, with no severe toxicity described.[114] ICI was subsequently trialed in a larger, heterogenous cohort of patients with either B-cell ALL or B-cell lymphoma who were refractory to CD19-targeted CAR T-cell infusion or who had return of circulating CD19+ B cells noted after initial loss.[115] Patients with initial tumor response were noted to have augmented CAR T cell functionality after PD-1 blockade; however, these data have yet only been presented in abstract form.[115] In solid tumors, a phase I study investigated GD2-directed CAR T cells alone, lymphodepleting (LD) chemotherapy (fludarabine, cyclophosphamide) plus GD2-CAR T cells, and LD, GD2-CAR T cells, and the PD-1-blocking agent pembrolizumab for the treatment of neuroblastoma in pediatric patients.[116] Though LD improved CAR T-cell expansion in infused patients, the addition of ICI in this trial did not have additional therapeutic benefit. All patient cohorts were safely treated without any reported severe toxicities attributable to the treatments administered. A second experience has been reported in a subset of patients who received regionally infused mesothelin-targeted CAR T cells in combination with pembrolizumab as treatment for mesothelioma as a subcohort of treated patients in a phase I trial. Eighteen patients participating in this trial subsequently were administered anti-PD1 ICI, with two patients achieving a complete metabolic response and eight having sustained stable disease ≥6 months.[117]

IMMUNE CHECKPOINT BLOCKADE + ANTIBODY-BASED THERAPY

The utility of antibody-based therapy, including the use of bispecific agents designed to activate T-cell function, is restricted by their pharmacologic distribution and drug half-life. The ultimate antitumor efficacy of these agents also hinges on the presence of a functional effector cell population that can be stimulated toward targeted cytotoxicity. As such, when host T-cell function is hampered by immune checkpoint blockade because of tumor expression of PD-L1, consideration of combination ICI and antibody-based therapies is warranted.

The CD19xCD3 bispecific small molecule blinatumomab has been studied in this context, with stimulatory PD-1 upregulation on T cells and PD-L1 expression on CD19+ target cells observed.[118] In small numbers of patient samples, a greater degree of PD-1 upregulation may be associated with nonresponse to therapy with the bispecific agent.[118] A report of a single patient with refractory ALL administered nivolumab + blinatumomab details expected inflammatory toxicity and a complete response to therapy but with relapse noted <2 months after cessation of treatment.[118] The clinical data have encouraged recruitment in open clinical trials testing the combination of blinatumomab and ICI for relapsed and refractory disease in adult and pediatric patients (NCT02879695, NCT045463990). Bispecific agents for other hematologic malignancies, such as AML and multiple myeloma, have also been studied together with ICI, though there are no data available yet from patients treated with combination therapy in these diseases. Antibody-based and ICI combination therapy used for solid tumor treatment is equally promising, with a phase I clinical trial testing a T-cell/tumor cell–engaging molecule, CEAxCD3, in combination with the anti-PD-L1 antibody atezolizumab, for the treatment of metastatic colon cancer completed enrollment in 2020. Early data presented in abstract form suggest treatment-induced inflammation and a need for continued data analysis (NCT02650713).

IMMUNE CHECKPOINT BLOCKADE + VACCINES

Though one of the earliest immune-based therapies developed against cancer, vaccination as monotherapy has not had dramatic clinical success. Immune escape mechanisms evolved by advanced and progressive tumors include immune inhibitory molecule overexpression that, when combined with T-cell exhaustion secondary to chronic antigen exposure, leads to a lackluster immunologic response. There is therefore clear rationale to strengthen the available number and quality of T cells with specificity for tumor antigens with vaccination and to then enhance their functionality with ICI.

The combination of cancer vaccination and ICI has been tested thus far primarily as treatment for refractory solid tumors. In one phase IIB trial, the anti-CTLA-4 agent ipilimumab was given alone or together with a GM-CSF gene–transfected, lethally irradiated pancreatic adenocarcinoma vaccine (GVAX) to 30 randomized patients with advanced pancreatic cancer.[119] This combination therapy led to improved overall survival at 1 year compared with the CTLA-4 antibody alone (27% vs 7%), though it was not directly compared in this study to GVAX monotherapy.[119] Similarly, CTLA-4 blockade has been combined with dendritic cell vaccination as treatment for metastatic melanoma with good outcomes and tolerable expected toxicities.[120,121] The overall number of patients with any cancer treated with the combination of a cancer-directed vaccine and a CTLA-4 inhibitory antibody remains small, with even more restricted correlative biologic study. This and the heterogeneity of treatment regimens, vaccine formulations, and disease processes precludes drawing of solid conclusions regarding universal safety or efficacy.

The use of PD-1 blockade and cancer vaccines has also been considered in combination. Pembrolizumab and a p53-expressing vaccinia vaccine have been studied together as treatment for advanced solid tumors in 11 patients.[122] Patients in this trial received triweekly infusions of the vaccine and pembrolizumab for 1 week and then weekly vaccine every 3 weeks until disease progression. Encouragingly, three patients showed clinical responses to combination therapy, with detectable and persistent circulating p53-specific CTLs able to be isolated. PD-1 ICI in combination with vaccination has also been trialed for HPV-associated cancer[123] and melanoma[124,125] with promising clinical responsiveness and a tolerable safety profile.

ADOPTIVE CELL THERAPY + VACCINES

Though adoptive cell therapy is clearly effective in specific clinical scenarios, infusion of unselected T or NK cells can be nonspecific and cause toxicity with no clinical benefit. Directing this powerful antitumor effector cell response specifically to tumor cells is possible by combining ACT with vaccination. In contrast, in situations in which vaccine monotherapy is ineffective, provision of a healthy and activated effector cell population may be a solution to strengthen vaccine-mediated anticancer activity. To this end, ACT and vaccination combined to specifically boost the population of infused anticancer T cells is a strategy that is now being studied in patients, though there are no readily available efficacy or safety data yet. Preclinical study has shown in immunocompetent mouse models that T cells genetically engineered to express T-cell receptors specific for bacterial or cancer-associated antigens can be employed together with targeted vaccination to stimulate specific T-cell proliferation.[126,127] A particularly promising approach to support ACT persistence and late expansion is the engineering of viral-specific T cells (VSTs) isolated via ex vivo culture to express cancer-specific CARs.[128] These CAR-VSTs can be boosted with subsequent vaccination, as detailed for GD2-VZV-specific CAR T cells.[128] This cell therapy product is the subject of an active phase I trial, with results highly anticipated (NCT01953900).

CONCLUSIONS

It is evident that combination immunotherapy is rational, with consideration of the use of multiple agents likely necessary to amplify antitumor efficacy. The immune response and tumor microenvironment (whether hematologic or solid malignancy) are both uniquely complex, with tumor evasion possible via a variety of biologic mechanisms. Focus on (1) antigen specificity, (2) T-cell activation, (3) prevention of exhaustion, and (4) pharmacologic distribution and durability is critical when developing and choosing therapy for patients with advanced disease. Nevertheless, while testing strategies designed for powerful immune activation and tumor killing, local and systemic toxicity must be expected and monitored. Novel agents should ultimately be developed to refine antitumor directed cytotoxicity while minimizing unspecific inflammation.

Acknowledgment

The authors gratefully acknowledge the contributions of Ilias Christodoulou, MD, and Ruyan Rahnama, MD.

Disclosure

CB has pending patent applications in the field of engineered effector cell therapies and has received research funding from Merck, Sharpe, Dohme, Inc, Bristol Myers Squibb, and Kiadis Pharma.

Key References

1. Leach DR, Krummel MF, Allison JP. Enhancement of antitumor immunity by CTLA-4 blockade. *Science*. 1996;271(5256):1734-1736.
2. Hodi FS, O'Day SJ, McDermott DF, et al. Improved survival with ipilimumab in patients with metastatic melanoma. *N Engl J Med*. 2010;363(8):711-723.
15. Hamid O, Robert C, Daud A, et al. Safety and tumor responses with lambrolizumab (anti-PD-1) in melanoma. *N Engl J Med*. 2013;369(2):134-144.
20. Tawbi HA, Schadendorf D, Lipson EJ, et al. Relatlimab and Nivolumab versus Nivolumab in untreated advanced melanoma. *N Engl J Med*. 2022;386(1):24-34.
31. Rosenberg SA, Packard BS, Aebersold PM, et al. Use of tumor-infiltrating lymphocytes and interleukin-2 in the immunotherapy of patients with metastatic melanoma. *N Engl J Med*. 1988;319(25):1676-1680.
32. Sarnaik AA, Hamid O, Khushalani NI, et al. Lifileucel, a tumor-infiltrating lymphocyte therapy, in metastatic melanoma. *J Clin Oncol*. 2021;39(24):2656-2666.
37. Eshhar Z, Waks T, Gross G, Schindler DG. Specific activation and targeting of cytotoxic lymphocytes through chimeric single chains consisting of antibody-binding domains and the gamma or zeta subunits of the immunoglobulin and T-cell receptors. *Proc Natl Acad Sci U S A*. 1993;90(2):720-724.
40. Savoldo B, Ramos CA, Liu E, et al. CD28 costimulation improves expansion and persistence of chimeric antigen receptor-modified T cells in lymphoma patients. *J Clin Invest*. 2011;121(5):1822-1826. doi:10.1172/JCI46110.
41. Imai C, Mihara K, Andreansky M, et al. Chimeric receptors with 4-1BB signaling capacity provoke potent cytotoxicity against acute lymphoblastic leukemia. *Leukemia*. 2004;18(4):676-684. doi:10.1038/sj.leu.2403302.
42. Kochenderfer JN, Wilson WH, Janik JE, et al. Eradication of B-lineage cells and regression of lymphoma in a patient treated with autologous T cells genetically engineered to recognize CD19. *Blood*. 2010;116(20):4099-4102. doi:10.1182/blood-2010-04-281931.

61. McLaughlin P, Grillo-Lopez AJ, Link BK, et al. Rituximab chimeric anti-CD20 monoclonal antibody therapy for relapsed indolent lymphoma: half of patients respond to a four-dose treatment program. *J Clin Oncol.* 1998;16(8):2825-2833.

64. Hurwitz H, Fehrenbacher L, Novotny W, et al. Bevacizumab plus irinotecan, fluorouracil, and leucovorin for metastatic colorectal cancer. *N Engl J Med.* 2004;350(23):2335-2342.

69. Moja L, Tagliabue L, Balduzzi S, et al. Trastuzumab containing regimens for early breast cancer. *Cochrane Database Syst Rev.* 2012;2012(4):CD006243.

76. Larson RA, Sievers EL, Stadtmauer EA, et al. Final report of the efficacy and safety of gemtuzumab ozogamicin (Mylotarg) in patients with CD33-positive acute myeloid leukemia in first recurrence. *Cancer.* 2005;104(7):1442-1452.

92. Topp MS, Gokbuget N, Stein AS, et al. Safety and activity of blinatumomab for adult patients with relapsed or refractory B-precursor acute lymphoblastic leukaemia: a multicentre, single-arm, phase 2 study. *Lancet Oncol.* 2015;16(1):57-66.

101. Old LJ, Clarke DA, Benacerraf B. Effect of Bacillus Calmette-Guerin infection on transplanted tumours in the mouse. *Nature.* 1959;184(suppl 5):291-292.

103. Paavonen J, Naud P, Salmeron J, et al. Efficacy of human papillomavirus (HPV)-16/18 AS04-adjuvanted vaccine against cervical infection and precancer caused by oncogenic HPV types (PATRICIA): final analysis of a double-blind, randomised study in young women. *Lancet.* 2009;374(9686):301-314. doi:10.1016/S0140-6736(09)61248-4.

110. Kantoff PW, Higano CS, Shore ND, et al. Sipuleucel-T immunotherapy for castration-resistant prostate cancer. *N Engl J Med.* 2010;363(5):411-422.

Visit Elsevier eBooks + (eBooks.Health.Elsevier.com) for complete set of references.

CHAPTER 11

The Microbiome and Cancer Immunotherapy

John E. Niederhuber

SUMMARY OF KEY FACTS

- The human microbiota is composed of bacteria, viruses, fungi, yeast, protozoa, and archaea. Because of its commensal relationship with the host, it is identified as a functioning organ system.
- The gut microbiota has been shown to have a critical role in immunotherapy outcomes.
- Colonies of the microbiota are found on the surfaces of the digestive tract, respiratory system, urogenital tracts, and skin.
- The human microbiota has more than 1000 different microbial species.
- An estimated 3.8×10^{13} actual microorganisms can be found in the human gastrointestinal tract. More important, the varied microbiota of the gut express more than 3 million genes.
- Bacteroidetes and Firmicutes phyla account for an estimated 90% of the bacterial colonies in the gastrointestinal tract. Actinobacteria, Cyanobacteria, Fusobacteria, Proteobacteria, and Verrucomicrobia phyla constitute the remaining 10%.
- The initial microbiota of the neonate is acquired by vertical transmission from the mother and is thus accompanied by an inherited tolerogenic immunity to the colonizing microbiota.
- The early seeding and maturation of the newborn microbiota is critical to the development of a healthy, robust immune response system.
- The commensal relationship and integrity of the immune system goes on throughout life and is especially subject to any dysbiosis within the gut microbiome.
- Certain gut microbes and their metabolites have the ability to alter somatic cell DNA, resulting in cells with a malignant potential. An estimated 15% to 20% of human cancers have microbial and viral origins.
- Clinical studies have demonstrated that patients with lung cancer and kidney cancer having a poor response to treatment with PD-1 blockade had low levels of the gut bacterium *Akkermansia muciniphila.*
- Responders to anti-PD-1 blockade in this study had more abundant gut *Bifidobacterium longum*, *Collinsella aerofaciens*, and *Enterococcus faecium* than nonresponders.
- Clinical observations concerning the importance of the gut microbiome to achieving an effective ICI response have been supported by experiments in a number of ICI murine tumor models.
- Adoptive T-cell transfer anticancer immunotherapies, including CAR T cells, involve pretreatment lymphodepletion and the use of broad-spectrum antibiotics. Such additions to the therapeutic regimen are disruptive to the gut microbiome.

Continued on following page

Introduction

I recall during my directorship of the National Cancer Institute (2006–2010) being appointed as one of several National Institutes of Health (NIH) institute directors to serve on an NIH external advisory committee charged with advising the NIH director regarding areas of science ready for prioritization. Consensus was quickly reached that the microbiome and its relationship to health and disease was primed for a significant research investment.[1,2] Discussion by those participating recognized that the organisms residing in the body such as bacteria, viruses, fungi, yeast, protozoa, and archaea, along with their genomes and metabolic products, actually can be considered an organ system in their own right.[3] Though these varied organisms comprising the microbiota may be found virtually anywhere on the body, focus has been on sites such as skin and mucous membranes of the body's external facing structures and the epithelial linings of the lungs, genitourinary tract, and gastrointestinal system.[4]

As a result, in 2007 the NIH launched the Human Microbiome Project (HMP). The first phase of HMP (2007–2012) was focused on identifying and characterizing the human microbiota.[5,6] The second phase was launched in 2014 as the Integrative HMP (iHMP; http://ihmpdcc.org) with the goal of generating integrated longitudinal data sets of microbiota biologic properties in association with disease conditions. An emphasis was placed on establishing the technologies of 16S rRNA gene profiling, whole metagenomic shotgun sequencing, whole genome sequencing, metatranscriptomics, metabolomics, and immunoproteomics as tools to study the human microbiota and how this complex system integrates as a functioning organ with the host.[7] Current science in this field is greatly enabled by advances in computational biology, artificial intelligence, machine learning, and powerful computer systems capable of integrating large data sets.

The technologies originally developed to accomplish the Human Genome Project, as one can readily understand, were enabling to the iHMP. The iHMP was designed to be an interdisciplinary effort of disease-based or related projects.[8-10] The goal of the iHMP has been to define the genetic and functional diversity of the organ specific microbiomes and their relationship to disease(s).[9] The NMP and iNMP research projects demonstrated that each individual has their unique composition of microbiota strains. Though current studies in cancer have focused on bacteria, other microorganisms including the commensal viruses, fungi, and archaea cannot be neglected because they most certainly also have a role in cancer and immuno-oncology (for an in-depth review, see The Integrative HMP Research Netword Consortium,[8] Voth and Khanna,[9] and the NIH Human Microbiome Portfolio Analysis Team[10]).

Studies of the gut microbiome, for example, demonstrated the importance of maternal colonization and a period during newborn development with flora of low diversity, referred to as the period of "founder species." The gut microbiome is seeded in utero and evolves early in life to a mature colonization. Composition of the gut microbiota is influenced by geography, ethnicity, diet, mode of delivery (vaginal vs cesarean section), illness, and use of antibiotics during the host's early development.[11] The intestinal microbiome is estimated to contain over 100 trillion microorganism cells that encode more than 3 million genes.[12-14] The gut microbiota with its complex organization of microbes exists in symbiosis with the host and provides a remarkable array of protein products that play a critical role in host physiology.[15]

During the past decade as a result of the NIH investments in the NMP, research has found increasing evidence for a strong relationship between the gut microbiome and cancer, including colon and rectum, esophageal, gastric, pancreatic, lung, melanoma, breast cancer, as well as hematologic malignancies.[16] In this chapter, we will review what is known regarding the role the gut microbiome plays in the initiation and progression of cancer as well as its effect on cancer treatment especially immunotherapy.

The Microbiome and Immune System Development

The bacterial component of the human microbiota is by far the most researched of the microbiota communities. These microbiota communities consist of bacteria, archaea, bacteriophages, viruses, fungi, and protozoa. The colonies of the microbiota can be found on the surfaces of digestive tract, respiratory system, urogenital tracts, and skin.[13,14] It is demonstrated that the host immune system, both innate and adaptive, evolved along with the colonization of the host microbiota to establish a healthy coexistence between the organisms of the microbiota and the responding capability of the host immune system.[4,17] This evolving relationship actually begins in utero and reaches a mature status somewhere between the ages of 3 and 5 years.[18] This commensal relationship and the integrity of the immune system, however, are ongoing throughout life. The integrity and cellular makeup of the immune system is subject to alteration or impairment throughout life as a result of changes in the microbiota. Gut microbiota forces impacting the integrity of the immune system may be as simple as host dietary changes and as complex as may occur with the onset of certain chronic diseases and the administration of antibiotics[19,20] (for an in-depth review, see Maynard et al.[17]).

In the gastrointestinal (GI) tract, the Bacteroidetes and Firmicutes phyla account for an estimated 90% of the bacterial colonies. The remaining 10% is made up of colonies of the phyla Actinobacteria, Cyanobacteria, Fusobacteria, Proteobacteria, and Verrucomicrobia.[21] The greatest bacterial density in the GI tract occurs in the colon. Research using advanced genomic techniques has demonstrated that the GI microbiome actively affects a number of host functions including metabolism, immunity, the development and progression of cancer, and the host responses to pharmacogenomic interventions.[4,21-25]

The actual development of the immune system begins in utero, as does the growing relationship of the immune system with the developing fetal microbiota. Because the initial microbiota of the neonate is acquired by vertical transmission from the mother, there exists an inherited tolerogenic immunity to the colonizing microbiota.[18] It has been demonstrated that transvaginal delivery is also an important source of seeding the newborn microbiome with the mother's native and tolerated vaginal microbiota.[11] Breast milk is also an important source of immune regulating factors involved in the early education and formation of the newborn immune system. Breast milk contains a number of immune stimulating factors such as actual live bacteria, protein metabolites, immunoglobulin (Ig) A antibodies, certain immune cytokines, and even cells of the immune system.[26-28] Accumulating evidence has confirmed the critical role the early seeding and maturation of the newborn microbiota has to the postnatal imprinting and maturation of the immune system. In a sense, the constant priming of the host immune system by an intact microbiome is critical for an immune system ready to optimize the host's ability to effect efficient antitumor therapies. Any effect on the normal development of the newborn microbiota can affect host immunity throughout life.[4,15,18,26-28]

Conditions that occur in the host required for the host to eliminate an invading pathogen can become a risk to the host if these immune responses become chronic in nature. Such chronic inflammatory responses have the potential to cause dysbiosis within the microbiota and as a result alter host immunity. Host efforts to curb inflammation can be detrimental to the host's antitumor response.[29] The host's efforts to curb inflammation can be thought of as being competitive to the host's capacity to adequately mount a robust antitumor response during the early stages of tumor initiation[30] (for an in-depth review, see Belkaid and Harrison[20]).

The Microbiome and Cancer Initiation and Progression

Over the past two decades, there has been increasing evidence that the intestinal microbiota has a critical relationship with the human peripheral immune system. As noted previously, more than 1000 different microbial species and an estimated 3.8×10^{13} microorganisms can be found in the human gut, mostly in the lower colon.[31] This varied microbiota expresses more than 3 million genes, the products of which have significant metabolic activity affecting normal host physiology and health. When there is a shift or dysbiosis in the gut microbiota composition causing disruption of the normal host microbiota homeostasis, the host is at risk for a broad array of altered physiology and even the onset of chronic diseases including cancer.[32,33] A dysbiosis within the GI tract may also significantly affect the immune system's normal ability to eliminate cancer at its earliest stages of formation by suppressing innate immune surveillance and the adaptive antitumor immune response.[34]

In addition to a dysbiosis that may impair normal immune surveillance and an anticancer immune response, there is accumulating evidence that certain gut microbes and their metabolites have the ability to alter DNA in somatic cells of the host. Alterations of somatic cell DNA may interfere with the host's genes responsible for controlling the cell cycle, causing increased cell proliferation, and also generate metabolites that disrupt normal cell death programs. Alterations in the GI tract microbiota and the resultant induced events in DNA coding and in gene transcription increase the risk for the development of somatic cells with malignant potential.

Perhaps the best-known pathogens directly involved in the inflammation–cancer pathway are *Helicobacter pylori* in gastric cancer, human papillomavirus in cervical and head and neck cancer, and hepatitis B and C viruses in hepatocellular cancers (Table 11.1).[17,19,20,30-34]

In addition, certain pathogens can promote inflammation and bacterial metabolites that directly trigger tumor initiation. An estimated 15% to 20% of human cancers have been connected either directly or indirectly to having microbial origins.[30,31] *Enterococcus faecalis*, for example, produces reactive oxygen species responsible for the formation of a DNA-damaging compound. Important to the relationship between the microbiome and the antitumor immune response is the observation that bacterial microbes originating in the gut can be found in both the tumor and the tumor microenvironment, where they secret factors that promote tumor cell growth and suppress antitumor immunity (Table 11.2).[19,33,35-39]

Alterations in the gut microbiota have been shown to promote inflammation in the intestinal tract and epithelial cell proliferation through the activation of the interleukin (IL)-6 signaling pathway.[40] Epithelial inflammation results in microbial-generated products such as lipopolysaccharides (LPS) causing immune cell proliferation and migration along with an upregulation of Toll-like receptors (TLRs). Bacterial products produced in excess as a result of gut dysbiosis and inflammation can activate nuclear factor kappa B (NF-κB), c-Jun N-terminal Kinase (c-Jun/JNK), and Janus Kinase/signal transducer and activator of transcription (JAK/STAT3) pathways,

TABLE 11.1 ■ **A List of Microbes Designated by the International Agency for Research on Cancer as Class I Carcinogens**

Class I Microbes	
Carcinogenic Microbe	**Site of Cancer**
Helicobacter pylori	Stomach
Hepatis B	Liver
Hepatis C	
Opisthorchis viverrini	
Clonorchis sinensis	
Human papilloma virus	Cervix, vagina, vulva, anus, penis, oropharynx
Epstein-Barr virus	Nasopharynx, non-Hodgkin lymphoma, Hodgkin lymphoma
Kaposi sarcoma–associated herpes virus	Kaposi sarcoma
	Primary effusion lymphoma
Human T-cell lymphotropic virus type I	Adult T-cell lymphoma
Schistosoma haematobium	Bladder
Bacteroides fragilis, *Clostridium* cluster 1	

Adapted from Bhatt et al.,[33] table I.

TABLE 11.2 ■ **Gut Bacteria Metabolic Proteins Associated With Carcinogenesis**

Bacterial Metabolites	**Potential Cancer-Causing Action**
Sulfate-reducing bacteria (H_2S)	H_2S has cytotoxic and genotoxic actions.
Nitrate reduction to nitrite; N-nitroso compounds	Multiple gut bacteria involved, can form DNA adducts
Polyamine production such as ornithine	Multiple gut bacteria are capable; associated with increased inflammatory tumor microenvironment
Secondary bile acids, deoxycholic acid, lithocholic acid	Multiple *Clostridium* sp., tumor-promoting activity

Adapted in part from Hullar et al.,[31] table 1.

all of which have well-demonstrated actions causing abnormal cell proliferation and suppression of the antitumor immune response (Fig. 11.1).[41-44]

The Microbiome and Cancer Immunotherapy

Spontaneously arising cancers in humans are well recognized for the development of their capacity to avoid immune surveillance and to withstand tumor cell destruction by the adaptive immune response. Immunotherapy first became an option for treatment of malignant diseases with the introduction of monoclonal antibodies and the use of stem cell transplantation.[45,46] The ability to reverse tumor cell resistance to the host antitumor immune response has been demonstrated with the blocking of immune checkpoints responsible for down regulation of the antitumor T-cell response (ICI). ICI immunotherapy involves using monoclonal antibodies against the cytotoxic T lymphocyte–associated protein 4 (CTLA-4) and against the programmed cell death protein 1 (PD-1) or its programmed cell death ligand 1 (PD-1L) immune checkpoints. These monoclonal antibody inhibitors have had rather impressive responses and represent the first real breakthrough in immunotherapy. As a result, ICI has become the standard of therapy for a number of solid tumors and hematologic malignancies.[47]

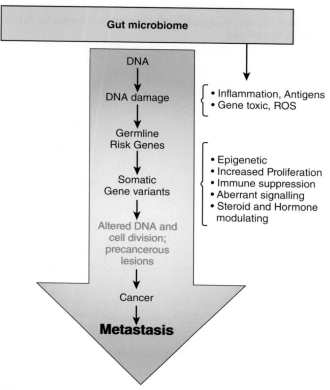

Gut microbiome

DNA

DNA damage

- Inflammation, Antigens
- Gene toxic, ROS

Germline
Risk Genes

Somatic
Gene variants

- Epigenetic
- Increased Proliferation
- Immune suppression
- Aberrant signalling
- Steroid and Hormone
  modulating

Altered DNA and
cell division;
precancerous
lesions

Cancer

Metastasis

Fig. 11.1 The gut microbiota may influence cancer risk by colonization of pathogenic organisms (e.g., specific cancer-causing bacteria or viruses), by the production of carcinogenic metabolites toxic to DNA, by producing endogenous host compounds such as hormones and steroids, and by inflammation causing microbial antigens that stimulate the host immune response. Adapted in part from Hullar et al.,[31] fig. 1.

In addition to the revolutionary success with ICI, a variety of cell-based therapies including adaptive T-cell therapy (ATC), in vitro expansion of tumor-infiltrating lymphocytes (TILs), T-cell receptor–engineered T cells (TCR), and chimeric antigen receptor gene–transduced T cells (CAR T cells) have demonstrated promising cell-based antitumor efficacy and are currently the subject of intense investigation.[30,46-50]

The Intestinal Microbiome and ICI Immunotherapy

Two observations have suggested that the response to ICI may be more complex than the simple antibody blocking of the cellular checkpoint. The first observation suggested that patients with cancer with a high body mass index (BMI) have a significantly higher ICI response rate than that observed for patients with a normal or low BMI.[51,52] The second observation found that patients with cancer who had received courses of antibiotics immediately before or early in their ICI treatment had much lower ICI response rates than those without an antibiotic use history.[53] This accumulating evidence therefore began to support the conclusion that ICI nonresponders may have an imbalance in gut flora composition that correlates with impaired immune cell activity[54-56] (for an in-depth review, see Frankel et al.[56]).

Routy and colleagues reported their studies of fecal samples from patients with lung cancer and kidney cancer being treated with checkpoint inhibitors. They discovered that those patients having a poor response to PD-1 blockade had low levels of the bacterium *Akkermansia muciniphila*.[57] In 2018, Matson and colleagues reported similar studies of patients with progressive metastatic melanoma undergoing anti-PD-1 blockade.[58] In these studies, they analyzed baseline stool samples before ICI therapy using integrated analysis of 16S ribosomal RNA gene sequencing, metagenomic shotgun sequencing, and quantitative polymerase chain reaction (qPCR) of selected bacteria. They found that responders to ICI had more abundant bacterial species of *Bifidobacterium longum*, *Collinsella aerofaciens*, and *Enterococcus faecium* than nonresponders. They also used germ-free mice whose GI tracts were reconstituted with fecal material obtained from ICI-responding patients with melanoma. The mice demonstrated improved tumor ICI response and tumor control and greater T-cell immune responses.[58]

In another report examining the oral and gut microbiome of patients with metastatic melanoma being treated with anti-PD-1 immunotherapy, analysis of 30 ICI responders and 13 nonresponders found that responders had significantly greater alpha diversity ($p < 0.01$) and a relative abundance of bacteria of the Ruminococcaceae family ($p < 0.01$).[59] In the nonresponders the *Bacteroidales* order was found to be enriched. Metagenomic WGS also showed enrichment of *Faecalibacterium* species in responders and nonresponders were enriched for *Bacteroides thetaiotaomicron*, *Escherichia coli*, and *Aaerotruncus colihominis*. The investigators supplemented these initial clinical studies by using fecal microbiota transplantation (FMT) from patients to germ-free mice. They concluded that nonresponders had an unfavorable gut microbiome with low diversity and an abundance of Bacteroidales leading to an impaired systemic antitumor immune response. They showed that the impaired immune response resulted from impaired lymphoid and myeloid cell tumor infiltration and a suppressed capacity for antigen presentation.[59] There have been a number of studies directed at characterizing the ICI responder gut taxa and how these species relate to the antitumor immune response (Table 11.3).

A number of preclinical studies in mouse tumor models and these early clinical studies have clearly documented the critical relationship between the gut microbiota and the ability to generate a response to ICI interventions in patients with advanced cancer. Documentation of the existing microbial deficiencies in the ICI nonresponders compared with responders spurred an intense interest in attempts to correct the nonresponder taxa deficiencies and to generate a responder gut microbial environment. Though there are a number of therapeutic approaches one might undertake in manipulating the gut microbiome, clinical experience using fecal microbiota transplantation (FMT) has currently generated the most clinical interest. The experience gained using FMT to treat recurrent *Clostridium difficile* infection, for example, has made FMT a proven and readily available tool for correcting ICI nonresponder microbiome deficiencies.[71,72] As a result, several clinical studies using FMT to enhance ICI outcomes have been successfully undertaken[73] (for an in-depth review, see Zerdan et al.[73]).

In a single-arm clinical study (NCT03341143), investigators treated a group of patients with advanced melanoma resistant to anti-PD-1 therapy with a treatment combination of fecal microbiota harvested from long-term anti-PD-1 responders with melanoma.[74] The trial was designed to evaluate the safety and efficacy of using long-term responder FMT in combination with anti-PD-1 (pembrolizumab) therapy. Sixteen patients with advanced melanoma who had no prior history of a response to anti-PD-1 either as single agent treatment or in combination with anticytotoxic T lymphocyte–associated protein-4 or other investigational agents were accrued to the study. All patients were confirmed to have progressive disease at the time of accrual and all had pretreatment native microbiota depletion using vancomycin and neomycin.

The investigators found the treatment combination to be well tolerated, with responders demonstrating an increased abundance of taxa previously documented to be associated with a response to anti-PD-1 checkpoint therapy. Fifteen patients received the planned experimental regimen and

TABLE 11.3 ■ **Effect of Microbiome Species on ICI Immunotherapy**

ICI Immunotherapy	Involved Microbes	Mechanisms of Effect on Outcome
Anti-CTLA-4 mAbs	Bacteroides fragilis, Bacteroides thetaiotaomicron, and Burkholderia cepacia	Stimulation of CD1b+ DCs increased IL-12-dependent Th1 antitumor response.[60]
	Bifidobacterium	Enhanced suppressive activity of Tregs decreasing immunopathology caused by ICI.[61,62]
	Bifidobacterium pseudolongum and Akkermansia muciniphila	Inosine from bacteria acted on adenosine 2A receptors, stimulating Th1 in the presence of costimulators from DCs, enhancing antitumor response.[63] A. muciniphila produced butyrate can cause proinflammatory immune response suppressing Tregs present in the TME and activate IL-12-mediated ICI responses.[47,49]
Anti-PD-1 and PD-L1	Bifidobacterium breve and Bifidobacterium longum	Activates DCs for CD8+ T-cell priming and for infiltration into the tumor microenvironment to enhance antitumor immune response induced by ICI.[64] Overrepresentation in responders.[58,65] Possible secretion of Hippurate, decreasing PD-1 molecule expression to activate NK cells, causing antitumor activity.[66]
	Akkermansia muciniphila	Increasing TCM, CD4/Foxp3 ratio in tumor and TME, increases IL-12 and IFN-γ production, resulting in synergistic effect with PD-1 blockade.[57,67]
	Lactobacillus rhamnosus GG	Activates DCs via cGAS-STING-TBK1-IRF7-IFN-β cascade to enhance CD8+ T-cell activity against cancer cells.[68]
	Bifidobacterium breve	Molecular mimicry between SVY antigen of B. breve and SIY neoantigen of mouse melanoma stimulated cross-reactive T-cell response against melanoma cancer cells.[69]
	Bacteriophage-infecting Enterococcus hirae	TMP of bacteriophage stimulated memory CD8+ T-cell cross-reactivity with cancer antigen PSMB4 protein.[70]

CTLA-4, cytotoxic T lymphocyte-associated antigen-4; *CD1b*, a transmembrane glycoprotein; *cGAS*, cyclic GMP-AMP synthase; *GMP*, guanosine monophosphate; *AMP*, adenosine monophosphate; *DCs*, dendritic cells; *FoxP3*, Fork head box P3 DNA binding protein; *ICI*, immune checkpoint inhibition; *IFN-γ*, interferons; *IRF7*, interferon regulatory factor 7; *IL*, interleukin; *PD-1*, programmed cell death protein-1; *PD-L1*, programmed death-ligand1; *PSMB4*, proteasome subunit beta type-4; *STING*, stimulator of interferon genes; *Th*, T helper cells; *Tregs*, T regulatory cells; *TME*, tumor microenvironment.
Adapted in part from Ting et al.,[50] table 2.

were evaluable for response. A complete response (CR) was observed in one patient and two patients demonstrated partial response (PR) (20%). Three additional patients had stable disease (SD) for more than 12 months (20%). One patient reportedly has had an ongoing PR for greater than 2 years. In this study, responders were found to have increased CD8+ T-cell activation and a lower abundance of interleukin-8-expresssing myeloid cells. The authors concluded that FMT can change the gut microbiome to a more favorable responder taxa and reprogram the tumor microenvironment to have a more favorable antitumor immune cellularity.[74]

A similar trial involved 10 patients with progressive melanoma treated at the Ella Lemelbaum Institute for Immuno-Oncology at the Sheba Medical Center in Tel-HaShomer, Israel. In this small Israeli trial, there were two advanced melanoma FMT donors and both had documented complete responses to anti-PD-1 (nivolumab) therapy. The authors reported two patients experiencing a PR and one patient experiencing a CR.[75]

In a systematically conducted review of publications of adult patients with solid tumors undergoing ICI treatment, the authors reported identifying 22 publications focused on the effect of antibiotic usage on ICI outcomes and 6 studies that reported the effect of FMT on ICI response.[76] Though these early, somewhat limited, clinical studies of FMT have certainly been promising and have not reported serious immune-Related Adverse Events (irAEs) or adverse FMT events, one must keep in mind the existence of certain risks using FMT. The added risks of FMT occur in the context of patients with hematologic and solid tumor malignancies undergoing targeted immunotherapy. The most concerning risk, of course, remains the potential FMT introduction of an infectious complication. This is especially true in a patient with cancer with neutropenia who is immunocompromised. The risk of special concern, in even the heavily screened donor FMT, is the incidence of bacterial species containing extended-spectrum beta-lactamases (ESBLs). ESBLs cause bacteria to be resistant to commonly used antibiotics.[77] To date, this has been a rare event based on the use of intense donor specimen screening.

Larger clinical trials will be required to answer key questions regarding ICI and the microbiota. Focusing on the gut microbiome, for example, several questions come to mind. Will the favorable ICI responder taxa of the gut be specific to the anti-PD-1 antibody (ICI) immunotherapy in general? Or will the responder taxa vary depending on the cancer, specific to each organ site as in pancreatic cancer, lung cancer, or melanoma, for example? It is hoped that all of this knowledge will lead to optimally designed approaches to establishing a patient's responder gut taxa using approaches such as FMT. In melanoma, for example, evidence supports the importance of an abundance of the phyla Actinobacteria with Bifidobacteriaceae species and Coriobacteriacear species, along with the phyla Firmicutes with Ruminococcacea species and Lachospiraceae species as being the most favorable for a successful response to ICI.[56-59] How stable will the FMT taxa be in the ongoing treatment of the patient? Will oral FMT capsules equate to direct colonic implantation?

These observations in humans are also supported by experimental work using germ-free mice and specific pathogen-depleted mouse cancer models generated with antibiotics. These microbiome-depleted mouse models demonstrated ablated antitumor immune responses, suppressed myeloid cell proliferation, and decreased cytokine production.[78] Specific microbiome-depleted mice gavaged with bacterial strains *Alistipes shahii* or *Ruminococci* reversed this condition, but gavage using *Lactobacillus fermentum* failed to provide immunotherapy benefit.[72]

Chen and colleagues, using a Lewis lung cancer mouse model treated with cisplatin, found that the addition of broad-spectrum antibiotics disrupted the balance of gut microflora in the antibiotic-treated group resulting in a poor antitumor response compared with controls.[79] In the group of cisplatin-treated mice to which an oral gavage of *Akkermansia muciniphila* (AKK) was administered daily, the growth of the tumor was significantly slowed. The tumors in these mice had decreased levels of Ki-67, p53, and FasL proteins and upregulated Fas proteins, interferon gamma (IFN-γ), interleukin (IL)-6, and tumor necrosis factor alpha (TNF-α). There was also evidence for suppression of regulatory T (Treg) cells, suggesting that AKK may be a beneficial microbe in treatment of lung cancer.[79] Others have found similar suppressed or ablated immune responses, decreased myeloid cell proliferation, and cytokine production in germ-free murine tumor models or when subjecting mouse models to specific antibiotic regimens. Studies showed that oral gavage to restore response only occurred when using selected bacterial species.[65,70]

Frankel and colleagues reviewed reports in the literature of a number of mouse tumor ICI models confirming the importance of the gut microbiome in terms of response and survival.[56] In their review, the authors also cited several human studies that associated gut microbiome profiles and pathways with the host antitumor response to ICI immunotherapy. Several of the clinical studies included the collection of patient stool specimens for fecal transplantation into ICI-treated murine tumor models. In each of these FMT experiments using human responder fecal samples, the experimental model showed improved antitumor response and tumor infiltration with CD8+ T cells and myeloid DCs.[56]

The Intestinal Microbiome and Cell-Based Immunotherapy

As indicated in the previous section, the majority of research regarding the role of the gut microbiome and the effect of specific microbes on immunotherapy in cancer has primarily centered on ICI therapies.[49,50] Only limited efforts have been undertaken to understand the role the gut microbiome plays in cell-based immunotherapy.[46,47,80] The introduction into cancer treatment of tumor-infiltrating lymphocytes (TILs), T-cell receptor (TCR)-engineered T cells, and chimeric antigen receptor gene–transduced T cells (CAR-Ts) have all shown promise in producing improved patient outcomes.[47,49] The responses to these cell-based therapies, however, are heterogeneous across patient populations, and when a response is observed, its duration is also quite varied. Biomarkers to provide therapy guidance are currently lacking.[47,49,80-83]

Evidence regarding the role the gut microbiome plays in ICI responses has certainly spurred a similar interest in determining the importance of the gut microbiome in adoptive T-cell transfer immunotherapies. The importance of conducting studies designed to define the commensal relationship between the patient's microbiome, their malignancy, and the application of cell-based immunotherapy is further supported by the fact that adoptive T-cell transfers generally involve preconditioning of the patient by lymphodepletion using either chemotherapy or irradiation. Pretreatment lymphodepletion has a dysbiosis effect on the gut microbiome and induces microbial translocation that amplifies the function of effector T cells.[80,84] Preconditioning, however, places the patient at increased risk of infectious complications. Infectious complications are a significant morbidity associated with all forms of adoptive T-cell transfer treatment and, as such, require the use of broad-spectrum antibiotics.[85] As a result, antibiotics are often used as a prophylactic measure prior to initiation of cell-based therapy.

One of the earliest studies of the gut microbiome in patients undergoing anti-CD19 CAR T-cell therapy was reported in an abstract presented at the annual American Society of Hematology (ASH) meeting by M. Smith and the laboratory of Marcel van den Brink at Memorial Sloan Kettering Cancer Center.[86] This retrospective study involved 137 patients with non-Hodgkin's lymphoma (NHL) and 91 patients with acute lymphocytic leukemia (ALL) treated with CD19-CAR-T cell immunotherapy. Sixty percent of the patients received some amount of varied broad-spectrum antibiotics. Of this 60%, 47% were treated with an obligate anaerobe-targeting broad-spectrum regimen consisting of piperacillin/tazobactam, imipenem/cilastatin, and meropenem (P-I-M). Patients treated with P-I-M antibiotic regimen were more likely to experience cytokine release toxicity and neurotoxicity during CAR-T therapy.[86]

The investigators prospectively collected stool samples before CAR T-cell therapy in 48 patients. They observed that responders had a very unique baseline microbiota compared with nonresponders. Patients with a greater relative abundance of *Ruminococcus*, *Bacteroides*, and *Faecalibacterium* bacterial species in their gut microbiome were more likely to respond. The distinctive microbiome structure between responders and nonresponders interestingly belonged to the same Firmicutes phylum. They observed in prospectively collected stool samples that day 100 CAR T-cell responses were associated with species within the class Clostridia. Patients who achieved complete remission had more abundance of *Lachnospiraceae* and *Ruminococcaceae*, whereas those who did not respond well had a greater abundance of *Peptostreptococcaceae* and *Clostridiales*. Microbiome diversity, however, was not observed to differ when comparing responders with nonresponders.[87]

From these early, somewhat limited, studies, it appears appropriate to conclude that one cannot simply extract the microbiota knowledge gained from studies of ICI immunotherapy and apply such to adoptive T-cell (ATC) therapies including engineered CAR T-cell responses and toxicities. Nevertheless, avoiding dysbiosis of the gut microbiome and the risk that such dysbiosis would result in the production of metabolites and excess microbiota antigens having negative effects on the antitumor immune response seems to be appropriate when possible. The existing patient variability in loss of initial CAR T-cell response, the existence of nonresponders, and similarities in ATC therapies to ICI in terms of therapeutic augmentation of the antitumor immune response provides strong evidence that manipulations of the gut microbiome will also benefit engineered T-cell therapies. As with ICI, the immunosuppressive action of Tregs is a factor in success of ATC therapies including CAR T-cell treatment. Interestingly, CAR T-cell therapy has been observed to increase PD-1 expression (Fig. 11.2)[46,88] (for an in-depth review, see Schubert et al.[46]).

Novel oral therapies directed at protecting the gut microbiota integrity during pretreatment lymphodepletion are already in preclinical and early clinical study. The goal of these agents is to prevent gut dysbiosis and promote the growth of response favorable microbial species. Other efforts are being made to therapeutically eliminate gut inflammatory mediators. Further clinical studies are needed to validate the role of probiotics and for the use of fecal transplantation including pretreatment auto transplantation. As noted in the discussion of ICI, FMT has been gaining considerable interest as an approach to alter the gut microbiota to generate an ICI responder intestinal taxa.

For the oncologist, the common use of broad-spectrum antibiotics, proton-pump inhibitors, aggressive multidrug chemotherapy, radiation, and immunosuppression are all common to cancer

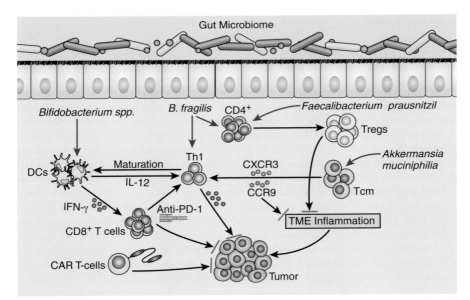

Fig. 11.2 There is an evolving fund of knowledge regarding the multiple mechanisms by which individual microorganisms of the intestinal microbiota are critical to the antitumor activity of immunotherapies. This figure provides a schematic designed to illustrate some of these interactions. *Bifidobacterium* activates DCs causing secretion of IFN-γ, enhancing tumor antigen presentation, initiating proliferation of CD8+ T cells, and stimulating their antitumor effectiveness. *Bacteroides fragilis* activates Th1 cells to cross-react with bacterial antigens and tumor antigens, enhancing the anticheckpoint response. *B. fragilis* also promotes the differentiation of CD4+ T cells into Tregs, which act to promote an enhanced antitumor inflammatory response. *Faecalibacterium prausnitzii* activates DCs and the proliferation of CD4+ T cells. *Akkermansia muciniphila* stimulates activation of the CCXR3/CCR9 chemokine receptor axes expressed by CD4+ central memory T cells (Tcms) further enhancing the antitumor immunotherapy response. The antitumor adaptive immune response in this schematic depicts newer approaches that are combining checkpoint blockade and engineered T cells such as CAR T cells in immunotherapy.

treatment and all are recognized causes of refractory *Clostridioides difficile* (CDI) in patients with cancer. As a result, oncologists have developed a familiarity with the use of FMT to address the complication of refractory CDI. In addition, as more has been learned regarding the commensal immune regulatory functions resident in the intestinal microbiota, clinical trials have been initiated to evaluate the use of FMT as a host immune–modulating intervention in patients with allogeneic HSCT experiencing corticosteroid-refractory acute graft-vs-host disease (GVHD). In a review published in 2022, the authors summarized eight clinical reports of 72 such patients treated with FMT. Responses to FMT treatment were observed in more than 50% of the patients with GVHD.[73,89,90]

Based on these preliminary observations, it will be critical to institute the clinical studies needed to define the beneficial from the harmful microbial species in the use of CAR T-cell therapy and with other forms of adoptive T-cell transfer immunotherapies. Future adoptive T-cell transfer therapies will undoubtedly involve methods to maintain desirable taxa necessary to optimize cancer treatment. Using specific antibiotics to deplete harmful species and even the development of probiotics and FMT seems certain to become critical additions to the application of cell-based therapies. As each new generation of CAR T cells is designed and taken into clinical trials, it will be necessary to understand the possible variations that each brings to its relationship with the various species of the gut microbiome. It is possible, because each new generation of CAR T cells (now into the third generation) attacks the tumor using somewhat different approaches to enhance antitumor immunity, that the involvement of the patient's microbiome will also need to be appropriately aligned[47,76,91] (for an in-depth review, see Angrish and Pezo[76]).

Pharmacomicrobiomics

The concept of an important relationship between the processing of medications and the microbiota of the gastrointestinal tract began to be significantly discussed in 2010.[92,93] *Pharmacomicrobiomics* is defined as the effect of variations or dysbiosis of the microbiome on drug metabolism, action, and toxicity. It reflects the observation that in reality the human microbiota functions as an organ system with significant metabolic capacity. In terms of the gut microbiota role as defined by pharmacokinetics (modifications of drug absorption, distribution, and metabolism) and pharmacodynamics (alterations of drug sensitivity) of administered oral medications, very little has been well defined. The frequent administration of antibiotics today further complicates this issue.

Pharmacomicrobiomics is a subfield of the sciences of genomics, microbiology, nutrition, and pharmacology. As has been noted, the majority of our knowledge today concerns the gut microbiota and, for the purposes of this chapter, its relationship to the new applications of anticancer immunotherapy. The characterization of the gut microbiome has the potential to serve as a biomarker for predicting patient response to all antitumor therapies, including surgery, radiotherapy, chemotherapy, and immunotherapy. Characterization of the gut microbiota may also prove to be a valuable part of anticancer therapy considering the potential to monitor the microbiota pretreatment and during treatment. Opportunities will exist for manipulating the microbiome of the patient with cancer to optimize treatment response, to decrease therapy morbidities, and to maintain a durable long-term response.

Some Thoughts in Conclusion

There is certainly significant accumulating evidence that the microbiome of the patient with cancer is intimately involved with the antitumor immune response and therefore plays a critical role in the host response to currently available immunotherapies. Most of our evidence for the important role of the gut microbiome has been accumulated in patients receiving ICI therapy, and studies are only beginning to be initiated to better understand the role that the microbiota plays in cell-based interventions. The important role the gut microbiota plays as a biomarker for patient selection and in the management of pretreatment lymphodepletion should perhaps not come as a surprise. Long before the availability of next-generation sequencing, oncologists were well aware that the use of chemotherapies such as 5-FU, irinotecan, and others altered the oral and fecal microbiota of tumor-bearing mice with an expansion of gram-negative anaerobes.[94-96] Clinically, there is plenty of evidence for an altered microbiota in patients with cancer receiving intense chemotherapy. GI toxicities in patients undergoing multidrug chemotherapy are common.

Enabling technologies of 16S and shotgun WGS, along with the computational power available today to provide the required in-depth analysis, provides for a new era of microbiota study in cancer. Early results of such studies are providing strong evidence that analysis of the microbiota of patients with cancer and especially the microbiome of the gut will become an integral part of cancer treatment management in the future. Such information will be essential in the use of immunotherapies targeted to optimize the anticancer immune response.

How this new knowledge will be used in patient selection for immunotherapy and how such information of microbiota alterations that occur during treatment will inform patient management remains to be carefully studied. Will supporting therapies such as probiotics be developed specific to the use of immunotherapies and individualized to the patient? Will pretreatment assessment of the gut microbiome become routine? Will the selection of antibiotics be based on pretreatment gut microbiome information? Will FMT, including autologous FMT, become an important tool? These are all questions that preliminary findings suggest will become critical to know in optimizing future immunotherapy. It appears at this early stage of clinical studies that such integrated management of the gut flora may need to be quite patient specific.

In this chapter, the focus has been to provide the early clinical evidence that is accumulating regarding the role the microbiota has with the rapid introduction of very promising immunotherapies, recognizing that there is still much to learn. One could also easily discuss at great length the very critical role that the microbiota plays in the actual risk of cancer. Many have stated that our estimation of 20% of cancers having an infectious origin is a vast underestimate. Undoubtedly, analysis and research regarding the microbiota will also point us in the direction of the microbiota as a knowledge-based cancer prevention strategy of the future.

Our understanding of the relationships between the microbiota, with the gut being only part of the puzzle, and the antitumor immune response (complex as it is) will be further complicated by the introduction of immune modulating therapies. Defining the intricacies of these complicated relationships will certainly be challenging, but the challenge is critical to advancing the progress in treating cancer. The excitement in addressing this challenge comes in the tremendous power of today's available tools, supported by the ability to apply high-powered computation and the ability to generate very large, searchable data sets to empower the science. These advances, I believe, will be revolutionary to the future management of health and disease, especially the prevention and treatment of cancer.

Key References

17. Maynard CL, Elson CO, Hatton RD, Weaver CT. Reciprocal interactions of the intestinal microbiota and immune system. *Nature*. 2012;489:231-241.
20. Belkaid Y, Harrison OJ. Homeostatic immunity and the microbiota. *Immunity*. 2017;46:562-576.
31. Hullar MA, Burnett-Hartman AN, Lampe JW. Gut microbes, diet, and cancer. *Cancer Treat Res*. 2014;159:377-399. doi:10.1007/978-3-642-38007-5-22.
33. Bhatt AP, Redinbo MR, Bultman SJ. The role of the microbiome in cancer development and therapy. *CA Cancer J Clin*. 2017;67(4):326-344. doi:10.3322/caac.21398.

46. Schubert M-L, Rohrbach R, Schmitt M, Stein-Thoeringer CK. The potential role of the intestinal mi- cromilieu and individual microbes in the immunobiology of chimeric antigen receptor T-cell therapy. *Front Immunol.* 2021;12:670286. doi:10.3389/fimmu.2021.670286.

50. Ting NL-N, Lau HC-H, Yu J. Cancer pharmacomicrobiomics: targeting microbiota to optimize cancer therapy outcomes. *Gut.* 2022;71:1412-1425. doi:10.1136/gutjnl-2021-326264.

56. Frankel AE, Deshmukh S, Reddy A, et al. Cancer immune checkpoint inhibitor therapy and the gut microbiota. *Integr Cancer Ther.* 2019;18:1-10. doi: 10.1177/1534735419846379.

57. Routy B, Chatelier E, Delrosa L, et al. Gut microbiome influences efficacy of PD-1-based immuno- therapy against epithelial tumors. *Science.* 2017;359(6371):91-97. doi:10.1126/science.aan3706.

58. Matson V, Fessler J, Bao R, et al. The commensal microbiome is associated with anti-PD-1 efficacy in metastatic melanoma patients. *Science.* 2018;359:104-108.

73. Zerdan MB, Niforatos S, Nasr S, et al. Fecal microbiota transplant for hematologic and oncologic dis- eases: principles and practice. *Cancers.* 2022;14:691. doi:10.3390/cancers14030691.

74. Davar D, Dzutsev A, McCulloch JA, et al. Fecal microbiota transplant overcomes resistance to anti- PD-1 therapy in melanoma patients. *Science.* 2021;371(6529):595-602. doi:10.1126/science.abf3363.

75. Baruch EN, Youngster I, Ben-Betzalel G, et al. Fecal microbiota transplant promotes response in immu- notherapy-refractory melanoma patients. *Science.* 2021;371(6529):602-609.

76. Angrish MD, Pezo RC. Impact of gut-microbiome altering drugs and fecal microbiota transplant on the efficacy and toxicity of immune checkpoint inhibitors: a systematic review. *Adv Cancer Biol Metastasis.* 2021;4:100020. doi:10.1016/j.adcanc.2021.100020.

79. Chen Z, Quian X, Chen S, Fu X, Ma G, Zhang A. Akkermansia muciniphila enhances the antitumor effect of cisplatin in Lewis lung cancer mice. *J Immunol Res.* 2020;2020:2969287. doi:10.1155/2020/2969287.

80. Paulos CM, Wrzesinski C, Kaiser A, et al. Microbial translocation augments the function of adoptively transferred self/tumor-specific CD8+ T cells via TLR4 signaling. *J Clin Invest.* 2007;117(8):2197-2204.

86. Smith M, Littmann ER, Slingerland JB, et al. Intestinal microbiota composition prior to CAR T cell infusion correlates with efficacy and toxicity. *Blood.* 2018;132(suppl 1):3492. doi:10.1182/blood-2018- 99-118628.

87. Smith M, Dai A, Ghilardi G, et al. Gut microbiome correlates of response and toxicity following anti- CD19 CAR T cell therapy. *Nat Med.* 2022;28(4):713-723. doi:10.1038/s41591-022-01702-9.

89. Kakihana K, Fujioka Y, Suda W, et al. Fecal microbiota transplantation for patients with steroid-resistant acute graft-versus-host disease of the gut. *Blood.* 2016;128:2083-2088.

90. Zhao Y, Li X, Zhou Y, et al. Safety and efficacy of fetal microbiota transplantation for Grade IV steroid refractory GI-GVHD patients: interim results from FMT2017002 trial. *Front Immunol.* 2021;12:678476.

Visit Elsevier eBooks + (eBooks.Health.Elsevier.com) for complete set of references.

CHAPTER 12

The Clinical Application of Immuno-Therapeutics

Sophia Y. Chen ■ Thatcher R. Heumann ■ Parul Agarwal ■ Lei Zheng

SUMMARY OF KEY FACTS

- Immuno-oncology (IO) is one of the fastest-growing therapeutic areas within oncology.
- IO agents work indirectly via the host's adaptive and innate immune systems to recognize and eradicate tumor cells.
- Current FDA-approved classes of IO agents include immune checkpoint inhibitors (ICIs), chimeric antigen receptor (CAR) T-cell therapy, bispecific T-cell engager (BiTE) antibody therapy, cancer vaccine therapy, and oncolytic virus therapy.
- Cancer immunotherapy has made progress in several cancer types including melanoma, non-small cell lung cancer (NSCLC), renal cell carcinoma (RCC), and urothelial carcinoma; however, several cancers remain refractory to immunotherapy.
- CAR T-cell therapies have a promising role for the treatment of many liquid malignancies.
- Immune-related adverse events (irAEs) associated with ICIs may present immediately or delayed and can affect any tissue or organ. Early recognition, diagnosis, and prompt treatment are needed. Severe toxicities will generally require permanent discontinuation of the offending agent.
- Future directions of IO include exploration in the neoadjuvant setting, combination strategies, and optimizing patient selection through improved biomarkers.

Introduction

Conventional chemotherapy has been the cornerstone of systemic treatment for oncologic malignancies. However, advances in medicine in the late 1990s and early 21st century have led to breakthroughs in the field of immuno-oncology (IO) therapy, an oncologic subspecialty widely regarded as one of the fastest growing areas within oncology. Whereas conventional chemotherapy mounts an indiscriminate, toxic, and direct attack on both malignant and normal cells, immunotherapy agents work indirectly via the host's adaptive and innate immune system to recognize and eradicate tumor cells. Such an approach makes cancer immunotherapy extraordinarily promising given its potential for specificity, breadth of response, memory, and durability.

Historical Background

The historical origins of the clinical application of immunotherapy in the treatment of cancer dates as far back as the late 19th century. In 1863, Rudolf Virchow noted infiltration of immune cells in human tumors.[1] Approximately 30 years later, William Coley, an American surgical oncologist, observed cancer remission in some patients who had sustained bacterial infections. Coley hypothesized that the link between the potential positive effect of infection on malignant tumors may be due to the body's provoked immune response. This led to an experiment where a bacterial broth containing streptococcus, now known as "Coley's toxins," was injected into patients' unresectable soft tissue tumors with the hope of inducing immune responses that would attack tumor cells.[2] Though Coley was met with skepticism during his lifetime, his scientific contributions have since been appropriately acknowledged. Advances in science and in medicine from the 1970s onward have spurred the development of engineered antibodies, cytokine treatments, and vaccines. It was not until the 1990s to 2000s, however, that a major breakthrough would transform the field of IO. A crucial discovery was that T-cell immune responses are controlled through immune checkpoints that function like on/off switches via the cytotoxic T lymphocyte–associated protein 4 (CTLA-4) pathway or the programmed cell death protein 1 (PD-1)/programmed cell death protein 1 ligand (PD-L1) pathway.[3] The characterization of immune checkpoints and their mechanisms of action would ultimately revolutionize the field and lead to the development of promising immunotherapies for previously refractory cancers.

General Classes of Cancer Immunotherapy Agents

There are five classes of U.S. Food and Drug Administration (FDA)-approved cancer immunotherapy agents that target various stages of the antitumor response and can be used for treatment: immune checkpoint inhibitors (ICIs), chimeric antigen receptor T-cell therapy (CAR-T), bispecific T-cell engager (BiTE) antibody therapy, cancer vaccine therapy, and oncolytic virus therapy.

ICIs use monoclonal antibodies to target immune checkpoints, which ultimately leads to enhanced T-cell effector function. Targets of currently approved ICIs include the CTLA-4 pathway and the PD-1/PD-L1 pathway. CTLA-4 is an immune checkpoint molecule that competes with CD28 to bind to CD80 and CD86, thereby downregulating T-cell activation.[4] PD-1 is also a negative regulator of T-cell activity and is induced by T-cells at the time of an inflammatory response.[5] PD-1 is expressed on a variety of immune cell types and limits immune response and T-cell activity in peripheral tissues. PD-L1 and PD-L2 are important mediators of the PD-1 pathway.[6,7]

CAR T-cell therapy is a class of immunotherapy that combines the antigen-binding site of a monoclonal antibody with the signal-activated machinery of a T-cell, thereby circumventing the more restrictive process of antigen recognition by major histocompatibility complex (MHC). In CAR T-cell therapy, a patient's own T-cells are genetically engineered to express a synthetic receptor to bind to a tumor antigen; these cells are then infused into the patient's body to attack chemotherapy-resistant cancer (Fig. 12.1).

BiTE antibodies are designed to engage and enhance T-cell activation by directing cytotoxic T-cells to CD19-expressing B cells. BiTE antibodies can recruit antigen-experienced T-cells without pre- or costimulation to directly kill tumor-associated antigen cells.

Cancer vaccines have been tested for the treatment of cancers, with the aim to elicit immune response against antigens expressed by tumor cells such as tumor-associated antigens or mutation-derived antigens (neoantigens). Finally, oncolytic virus therapy is another class of cancer immunotherapy that uses viruses to infect and kill tumor cells.

Skin Cancer

MELANOMA

Melanoma is the malignant transformation and proliferation of melanocytes, found predominantly in the skin but also present elsewhere in the gastrointestinal and genitourinary mucosa, the uvea, and the meninges/central nervous system.[8] Though localized melanoma is highly curable

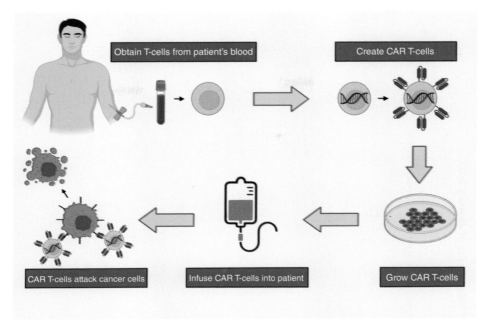

Fig. 12.1 **Overview of chimeric antigen receptor (CAR) T-cell therapy.** Normal T-cells are obtained from the patient's peripheral blood. CAR T-cells are created in the laboratory and grown in vitro. Expanded CAR T-cells are reinfused into the patient to attack tumor cells bearing the specific antigen the CARs are directed against. Created with BioRender.com.

with surgery, those with unresectable, metastatic disease have poor survival outcomes, with a 5-year overall survival (OS) of 29.8%.[9] The development of ICIs has revolutionized the treatment of advanced/metastatic melanoma.[10] In 2011, the FDA approved ipilimumab as a first-line therapy for unresectable stage III/IV melanoma after it demonstrated an improved OS of 11.2 months compared with 9.1 months in the placebo group.[11] This marked the beginning of the use of ICIs to treat cancers and transformed the oncologic therapeutic landscape. Since then, numerous clinical trials have been conducted with various ICIs approved for specific melanoma indications, as detailed in Table 12.1.

The approvals of ipilimumab, pembrolizumab, and nivolumab as monotherapy agents paved way for subsequent trials assessing the role of combination therapies. Results from the Check-Mate 069 trial led to the accelerated approval of the first immunotherapy combination immune checkpoint blockade of PD-1 (nivolumab) and CTLA-4 (ipilimumab) for patients with BRAFV600 wild-type unresectable/metastatic melanoma. Patients receiving combination CTLA-4 and PD-1 blockade demonstrated an improved 2-year OS of 63.8%, compared with a 2-year OS of 53.6% for patients receiving ipilimumab monotherapy.[12] This combination was also approved for patients with unresectable BRAFV600 mutation-positive melanoma after the CheckMate 067 trial demonstrated improved median progression-free survival (PFS) of 11.5 months in the combination group compared with 2.9 months in the ipilimumab mono-therapy group.[13] For patients with disease progression despite prior systemic therapies, ICIs are also approved as second-line monotherapy, with several trials demonstrating improved response rates, median OS, and PFS compared with standard chemotherapy regimens.[14-16]

Though ICIs have dominated the IO landscape for advanced/metastatic melanoma, the FDA has also approved talimogene laherparepvec (T-VEC), a genetically modified herpes simplex

TABLE 12.1 ■ Key Clinical Trials Leading to FDA Approval of Immuno-oncology Agents for Melanoma *(as of January 2022)*

Melanoma

Clinical Trial	FDA Agent	Phase	N	Study Population	Treatment Arm	Control Arm	Primary Endpoint	Results	Grade 3+ AE
First-Line Monotherapy									
NCT00324155	Ipilimumab (Yervoy)	3	502	Unresectable stage III/IV melanoma	Ipilimumab + Dacarbazine	Placebo + Dacarbazine	OS	OS: 11.2 vs 9.1 months	56.3% vs 27.5%
KEYNOTE-006 (NCT01866319)	Pembrolizumab (Keytruda)	3	834	Unresectable stage III/IV melanoma with no more than one prior systemic therapy	Pembrolizumab every 2 weeks; Pembrolizumab every 3 weeks	Ipilimumab	PFS, OS	ORR: 33.7%; 32.9% vs 11.9%; 1-year OS: 74.1%; 68.4% vs 58.2%; 6-month PFS: 47.3%; 46.6% vs 26.5%	13.3%; 10.1% vs 19.9%
CheckMate 066 (NCT01721772)	Nivolumab (Opdivo)	3	418	Unresectable stage III/IV melanoma without *BRAF* mutation	Nivolumab	Dacarbazine	OS	ORR: 40.0% vs 13.9%; 1-year OS: 72.9% vs 42.1%; median PFS: 5.1 vs 2.2 months	11.7% vs 17.6%
Second-Line Monotherapy									
NCT00094653	Ipilimumab (Yervoy)	3	676	Unresectable stage III/IV melanoma previously treated with dacarbazine, temozolomide, fotemustine, carboplatin, or IL-2	Ipilimumab + GP100; Ipilimumab alone	GP100	OS	Median OS: 10.0; 10.1 vs 6.4 months	10%–15% vs 3%
CheckMate 037 (NCT01721746)	Nivolumab (Opdivo)	3	631	Unresectable stage IIIC/IV metastatic melanoma BRAFV600+ pts with progression on anti-CTLA-4 and BRAF inhibitor BRAF wild-type pts with progression after anti-CTLA-4	Nivolumab	Chemotherapy	ORR, OS	ORR: 31.7% vs 10.6%	5% vs 9%

Trial (NCT)	Drug	Phase	Population	Treatment	Comparator	Endpoint	Results	
KEYNOTE-002 (NCT01704287)	Pembrolizumab (Keytruda)	2	Unresectable stage III/IV melanoma with progression after ipilimumab, BRAF, and/or MEK inhibitor	Pembrolizumab 2 mg/kg; Pembrolizumab 10 mg/kg	Chemotherapy	PFS	6-Month PFS: 34%; 38% vs 16%	11%; 14% vs 26%
First-Line Combination Therapy								
CheckMate 069 (NCT01927419)	Nivolumab (Opdivo) + Ipilimumab (Yervoy)	2	Unresectable stage III/IV melanoma	Nivolumab + Ipilimumab	Placebo + Ipilimumab	ORR	2-Year OS: 63.8% vs 53.6%; median OS: not reached	Tx arm: grade 3: 44%; grade 4: 11% Control arm: grade 3: 17%; grade 4: 2%
CheckMate 067 (NCT01844505)	Nivolumab (Opdivo) + Ipilimumab (Yervoy)	3	Unresectable stage III/IV melanoma	Nivolumab + Ipilimumab Nivolumab alone	Ipilimumab	PFS, OS	Median PFS: 11.5; 6.9 vs 2.9 months; PD-L1 positive: median PFS: 14.0 vs 5.3 months PD-L1 negative: median PFS 11.2 vs 5.3 months	55.0%; 16.3% vs 27.3%
IMspire150 (NCT02908672)	Atezolizumab (Tecentriq)	3	Unresectable stage IIIC/IV BRAFV600+ melanoma	Atezolizumab + Vemurafenib + Cobimetinib	Placebo + Vemurafenib + Cobimetinib	PFS	Median PFS: 15.1 vs 10.6 months	79% vs 73%
Adjuvant Therapy								
CheckMate 238 (NCT02388906)	Nivolumab (Opdivo)	3	Resected stage IIIB/IIIC/IV melanoma	Nivolumab	Ipilimumab	RFS	1-Year RFS: 70.5% vs 60.8%	14.4% vs 45.9%

Continued on following page

TABLE 12.1 ■ Key Clinical Trials Leading to FDA Approval of Immuno-oncology Agents for Melanoma *(as of January 2022)* (Continued)

								Melanoma	
Clinical Trial	FDA Agent	Phase	N	Study Population	Treatment Arm	Control Arm	Primary Endpoint	Results	Grade 3+ AE
EORTC 18071 (NCT00636168)	Ipilimumab (Yervoy)	3	951	Resected stage IIIA/IV melanoma metastatic to LN only	Ipilimumab	Placebo	RFS	5-Year RFS: 40.8% vs 30.3%; 5-year OS: 65.4% vs 54.4%; 5-year distant metastasis–free survival: 48.3% vs 38.9%	TRAE: 54.1% vs 26.2% irAE: 41.6% vs 2.7%
KEYNOTE-054 (NCT02362594)	Pembroli-zumab (Keytruda)	3	1019	Resected stage III melanoma	Pembrolizumab	Placebo	RFS	1-Year RFS: 75.4% vs 61.0% PD-L1 positive: 1-year RFS 77.1% vs 62.6%	14.7% vs 3.4%
Oncolytic Virus									
OPTIM (NCT00769704)	Talimogene laher-parepvec [T-VEC] (IMLYGIC)	3	436	Unresectable stage IIIB/IV melanoma	T-VEC	GM-CSF	DRR	ORR: 26.4% vs 5.7%; median OS: 23.3 vs 18.9 months; DRR: 16.3% vs 2.1%	≥2%

AE, adverse event; *DRR,* durable response rate; *FDA,* Food & Drug Administration; *irAE,* immune-related adverse event; *ORR,* objective response rate; *OS,* overall survival; *PFS,* progression-free survival; *RFS,* recurrence-free survival; *TRAE,* treatment-related adverse event; *Tx,* treatment.

virus (HSV) type 1 oncolytic virus therapy, for unresectable stage III/IV melanoma, based on a phase 3 trial that demonstrated a significant overall response rate (ORR) of 26.4% in the T-VEC group compared with 5.7% in the subcutaneous granulocyte-macrophage colony-stimulating factor (GM-CSF) group.[17] Although T-VEC is currently indicated for only melanoma treatment, it is the hope that oncolytic viruses, which are designed to selectively replicate within the tumor cell, eradicate the cells and, in doing so, induce tumor-directed immune responses, may eventually also demonstrate benefit for other cancer types.[18]

NONMELANOMA SKIN CANCERS

ICIs have received FDA approval for the treatment of advanced/metastatic nonmelanoma skin cancers including Merkel cell carcinoma (MCC), cutaneous squamous cell carcinoma (cSCC), and basal cell carcinoma (BCC), based on several phase 2 clinical trials (Table 12.2).

Two ICIs are currently FDA-approved for MCC. Avelumab was the first ICI approved in 2017 in the second-line setting for metastatic MCC, following results from the JAVELIN Merkel 200 trial that demonstrated an ORR of 31.8% at a median follow-up of 10.4 months.[19] One year later, pembrolizumab was approved for patients with recurrent locally advanced/metastatic MCC who had not received prior systemic therapy, based on results from the KEYNOTE-017 trial that demonstrated an ORR of 56% at median follow-up of 14.9 months, a 2-year PFS of 48.3% with median PFS of 16.8 months, and a 2-year OS of 68.7%.[20]

For cSCC, cemiplimab and pembrolizumab can be used as first-line agents for locally advanced/metastatic cSCC. Cemiplimab was FDA-approved in 2018 for locally advanced/metastatic cSCC, based on results from Study 1423 (phase 1)[21] and Study 1540 (phase 2).[22] In 2020, pembrolizumab was approved for recurrent/metastatic cSCC not amenable to surgery and radiation after the KEYNOTE-629 trial demonstrated an ORR of 34.3% at median follow-up of 11.4 months, a disease control rate of 52.4%, and a median PFS of 6.9 months.[23] For BCC, cemiplimab was approved in 2021 as a second-line therapy for patients with locally advanced/metastatic disease.[24]

Lung Cancer
NON-SMALL CELL LUNG CANCER

Lung cancer is the leading cause of all cancer mortality. Although lung cancer traditionally was characterized by late-stage disease at diagnosis with limited treatment options, immunotherapy breakthroughs over the early 21st century have provided encouraging results (Table 12.3).[25] Prior to ICIs, platinum-based chemotherapy was the cornerstone of treatment for early stage and advanced non-small cell lung cancer (NSCLC).

ICIs were initially evaluated in the second-line setting for patients with advanced NSCLC. Several clinical trials demonstrated significant improved OS with either nivolumab (CheckMate 017,[26] CheckMate 057[27]), pembrolizumab (KEYNOTE-010[28]), or atezolizumab (POPLAR,[29] OAK[30]) as monotherapy compared with standard, second-line chemotherapy control groups, ultimately leading to FDA approvals.

The promising results from the use of ICIs in the second-line setting led to further evaluation of these drugs as potential first-line therapies. KEYNOTE-001 was a phase 1 study that assessed the efficacy and safety of pembrolizumab in advanced NSCLC and showed that previously untreated patients with PD-L1 expression (determined by Tumor Proportion Score [TPS]) ≥ 50% had a response rate of 50%.[31] KEYNOTE-024 subsequently compared pembrolizumab with platinum-based chemotherapy in patients with untreated advanced NSCLC with TPS expression ≥50%; results from this study found higher response rates (44.8% vs 27.8%), PFS (10.3 vs

TABLE 12.2 ■ Key Clinical Trials Leading to FDA Approval of Immuno-oncology Agents for Non-Melanoma Skin Cancers *(as of January 2022)*

Merkel Cell Carcinoma (MCC)

Clinical Trial	FDA Agent	Phase	N	Study Population	Treatment	Primary Endpoint	Results	Grade 3+ AE
First-Line Therapy								
KEYNOTE-017 (NCT02267603)	Pembroli-zumab (Keytruda)	2	50	Metastatic/recurrent MCC refractory to chemo, un-amenable to surgery and radiation	Pembrolizumab	ORR	ORR: 56%; 2-year PFS: 48.3%, median PFS: 16.8 months; 2-year OS: 68.7%, median OS: not reached	28%
Second-Line Therapy								
JAVELIN Merkel 200 (NCT02155647)	Avelumab (Bavencio)	2	88	Stage IV MCC refractory to chemo	Avelumab	ORR	ORR: 31.8%	5%

Cutaneous Squamous Cell Carcinoma (cSCC)

Clinical Trial	FDA Agent	Phase	N	Study Population	Treatment	Primary Endpoint	Results	Grade 3+ AE
First-Line Therapy								
Study 1423 (NCT02383212)	Cemiplimab (LIBTAYO)	1	Phase 1: 26; Phase 2: 59	Locally advanced/metastatic cSCC unamenable to surgery and radiation	Cemiplimab	ORR	ORR phase 1: 50%; ORR phase 2: 47%	42%

Clinical Trial	FDA Agent	Phase	N	Study Population	Treatment	Primary Endpoint	Results	Grade 3+ AE
Study 1540 (NCT02760498)	Cemiplimab (Libtayo)	2	115	Locally advanced/metastatic cSCC unamenable to surgery and radiation	Cemiplimab 250 mg q3w; Cemiplimab 3 mg/kg q2w	ORR	ORR: 41.1%; 49.2%	39.3%; 50.8%
KEYNOTE-629 (NCT03283324)	Pembrolizumab (Keytruda)	2	105	Recurrent/metastatic cSCC unamenable to surgery and radiation	Pembrolizumab	ORR	ORR: 34.3%; disease control rate: 52.4%; median PFS: 6.9 months; median OS: not reached	5.7%

Basal Cell Carcinoma (BCC)

Clinical Trial	FDA Agent	Phase	N	Study Population	Treatment	Primary Endpoint	Results	Grade 3+ AE

Second-Line Therapy

Study 1620 (NCT03132636)	Cemiplimab (Libtayo)	2	84	Locally advanced/metastatic BCC after first-line HHI therapy or if not candidates for HHI	Cemiplimab	ORR	ORR: 31%	48%

AE, adverse event; BCC, basal cell carcinoma; cSCC, cutaneous squamous cell carcinoma; FDA, Food & Drug Administration; HHI, hedgehog inhibitor; MCC, Merkel cell carcinoma; ORR, objective response rate.

TABLE 12.3 ■ Key Clinical Trials Leading to FDA Approval of Immuno-oncology Agents for Non-Small Cell Lung Cancer (as of January 2022)

Non-Small Cell Lung Cancer (NSCLC)

Clinical Trial	FDA Agent	Phase	N	Study Population	Treatment Arm	Control Arm	Primary Endpoint	Results	Grade 3+ AE
First-Line Monotherapy									
KEYNOTE-024 (NCT02142738)	Pembrolizumab (Keytruda)	3	305	Stage IV NSCLC with no EGFR/ALK mutations with PD-L1 TPS ≥ 50%	Pembrolizumab	Platinum-based chemo	PFS	ORR: 44.8% vs 27.8%; median PFS: 10.3 vs 6.0 months; 6-month OS: 80.2% vs 72.4%	26.6% vs 53.3%
KEYNOTE-042 (NCT02220894)	Pembrolizumab (Keytruda)	3	1274	Stage III/IV NSCLC with no EGFR/ALK mutations unamenable to surgery or CRT with PD-L1 TPS ≥ 1%	Pembrolizumab	Platinum-based chemo	OS	Median OS: TPS ≥ 1% 16.7 vs 12.1 months; TPS ≥ 20% 17.7 vs 13.0 months; TPS ≥ 50% 20 vs 12.2 months	8% vs 41%
IMPower 110 (NCT02409342)	Atezolizumab (Tecentriq)	3	572	Stage IV NSCLC with PD-L1 TPS ≥ 1%	Atezolizumab	Platinum-based chemo	OS	Median OS: 20.2 vs 13.1 months; median PFS: 8.1 vs 5.0 months; ORR 38% vs 29%	30.1% vs 52.5%
EMPOWER-Lung 1 (NCT03088540)	Cemiplimab (Libtayo)	3	710	Stage IIIB-C/IV NSCLC with PD-L1 TPS ≥ 50%	Cemiplimab	Platinum-based chemo	PFS, OS	PD-L1 ≥ 50%: median OS not reached vs 14.2 months; median PFS: 8.2 vs 5.7 months	28% vs 39%

First-Line Combination Therapy

Trial (NCT)	Drug	Phase	N	Population	Treatment Arm	Control Arm	Endpoint	Results	
KEYNOTE-021 (NCT02039674)	Pembrolizumab (Keytruda)	2	123	Stage IIIB/IV NSCLC with no EGFR/ALK mutations	Pembrolizumab + Platinum-based chemo	Platinum-based chemo	ORR	ORR: 55% vs 29%	39% vs 26%
KEYNOTE-189 (NCT02578680)	Pembrolizumab (Keytruda)	3	616	Stage IV non-squamous NSCLC with no EGFR/ALK mutations	Pembrolizumab + Platinum-based chemo	Placebo + Platinum-based chemo	PFS, OS	1-Year OS: 69.2% vs 49.4%; median PFS: 8.8 vs 4.9 months	67.2% vs 65.8%
KEYNOTE-407 (NCT02775435)	Pembrolizumab (Keytruda)	3	559	Stage IV squamous NSCLC	Pembrolizumab + Platinum-based chemo	Placebo + Platinum-based chemo	PFS, OS, ORR	Median OS: 15.9 vs 11.3 months; median PFS: 6.4 vs 4.8 months; ORR: 58% vs 35%	69.8% vs 68.2%
IMPower 150 (NCT02366143)	Atezolizumab (Tecentriq)	3	692	Stage IV non-squamous NSCLC with wild-type or high effector T-cell gene (T_{eff}) signature	ABCP: Atezolizumab + Bevacizumab + Carboplatin + Paclitaxel	BCP: Bevacizumab + Carboplatin + Paclitaxel	PFS, OS	Wild-type pts: median PFS 8.3 (ABCP) vs 6.8 (BCP) months, median OS 19.2 vs 14.7 months T_{eff} pts: median PFS: 11.3 (ABCP) vs 6.8 (BCP)	ABCP: grade 3–4: 55.7%; grade 5: 2.8% BCP: grade 3–4: 47.7%; grade 5: 2.3%
IMPower 130 (NCT02367781)	Atezolizumab (Tecentriq)	3	724	stage IV NSCLC	Atezolizumab + Platinum-based chemo	Platinum-based chemo	PFS, OS	Median OS: 18.6 vs 13.9; median PFS: 7.0 vs 5.5 months	Tx arm: grade 3: 50%; grade 4: 23%; grade 5: 2% Control arm: grade 3: 47%; grade 4: 13%; grade 5: <1%

Continued on following page

TABLE 12.3 ■ Key Clinical Trials Leading to FDA Approval of Immuno-oncology Agents for Non-Small Cell Lung Cancer (as of January 2022) (Continued)

Non-Small Cell Lung Cancer (NSCLC)

Clinical Trial	FDA Agent	Phase	N	Study Population	Treatment Arm	Control Arm	Primary Endpoint	Results	Grade 3+ AE
CheckMate 227 (NCT02477826)	Nivolumab (Opdivo)	3	Part 1a: 793	Recurrent/stage IV NSCLC with no EGFR/ALK mutations with PD-L1 ≥ 1%	Nivolumab + Ipilimumab	Platinum-based chemo	OS	Median OS: 17.1 vs 14.9 months; median PFS 5.1 vs 5.6 months; ORR 36% vs 30%; median DoR 23.2 vs 6.2 months	32.8% vs 36.0%
CheckMate 9LA (NCT03215706)	Nivolumab (Opdivo) + Ipilimumab (Yervoy)	3	1150	Recurrent/stage IV NSCLC	Nivolumab + Ipilimumab + Platinum-based chemo	Platinum-based chemo	OS	Median OS: 15.6 vs 10.9 months	Tx arm: grade 3: 35%; grade 4: 12% Control arm: grade 3: 32%; grade 4: 6%
Second-Line Therapy									
CheckMate 017 (NCT01642004)	Nivolumab (Opdivo)	3	272	Previously treated, recurrent stage IIIB/IV squamous NSCLC	Nivolumab	Docetaxel	OS	Median OS: 9.2 vs 6.0 months; 1-year OS: 42% vs 24%; ORR: 20% vs 9%; median PFS: 3.5 vs 2.8 months	7% vs 55%

Continued on following page

Trial	Drug	Phase	Population	N	Treatment arm	Control arm	Endpoint	Results	Toxicity
CheckMate 057 (NCT01673867)	Nivolumab (Opdivo)	3	Previously treated, recurrent stage IIIB/IV nonsquamous NSCLC	582	Nivolumab	Docetaxel	OS	Median OS: 12.2 vs 9.4 months; 1-year OS: 51% vs 39%; 1.5-year OS: 39% vs 23%; ORR: 19% vs 12%	10% vs 54%
KEYNOTE-010 (NCT01905657)	Pembrolizumab (Keytruda)	2 + 3	Previously treated, stage IV NSCLC with PD-L1 TPS ≥ 1%	1034	Pembrolizumab 2 mg/kg; Pembrolizumab 10 mg/kg	Docetaxel	PFS, OS	Median OS: 10.4; 12.7 vs 8.5 months; median PFS: 3.9; 4.0; vs 4.0 months PD-L1 positive: OS 14.9; 17.3 vs 8.2 months; PFS: 5.0; 5.2 vs 4.1 months	13%; 16% vs 35%
POPLAR (NCT01903993)	Atezolizumab (Tecentriq)	2	Previously treated, stage III/IV NSCLC	287	Atezolizumab	Docetaxel	OS	OS: 12.6 vs 9.7 months	Tx arm: grade 3–4: 11%; grade 5: 1% Control arm: grade 3–4: 39%; grade 5: 2%
OAK (NCT02008227)	Atezolizumab (Tecentriq)	3	Previously treated stage IIIB/IV NSCLC with PD-L1 TPS ≥ 1%	1225	Atezolizumab	Docetaxel	OS	OS: 13.8 vs 9.6 months; OS PD-L1 ≥ 1%: 15.7 vs 10.3 months	15% vs 43%
Maintenance Therapy									
PACIFIC (NCT02125461)	Durvalumab (IMFINZI)	3	Unresectable stage III NSCLC after platinum-based CRT	709	Durvalumab	Placebo	PFS, OS	Median PFS: 17.2 vs 5.6 months; 2-year OS: 66.3% vs 55.6%	30.5% vs 26.1%

TABLE 12.3 ■ Key Clinical Trials Leading to FDA Approval of Immuno-oncology Agents for Non-Small Cell Lung Cancer (as of January 2022) (Continued)

Non-Small Cell Lung Cancer (NSCLC)

Clinical Trial	FDA Agent	Phase	N	Study Population	Treatment Arm	Control Arm	Primary Endpoint	Results	Grade 3+ AE
Adjuvant Therapy									
IMPower 010 (NCT02486718)	Atezolizumab (Tecentriq)	3	990	Resected stage II/IIIA NSCLC with PD-L1 TPS ≥ 1%	Atezolizumab	Platinum-based chemo	DFS	DFS: HR 0.79 (P = .020) DFS ITT: HR 0.81 (P = .040) DFS PD-L1 ≥ 1%: HR 0.66 (P = .039)	Tx arm: grade 3–4: 22%; grade 5; 2% Control arm: grade 3–4: 12%; grade 5: 1%
Neoadjuvant Therapy[a]									
CheckMate 816 (NCT02998528)	Nivolumab (OP-DIVO)	3	358	Resectable stage IB-IIIA NSCLC	Nivolumab + Platinum-based chemo followed by surgery	Platinum-based chemo followed by surgery	pCR, EFS	pCR: 24.0% vs 2.2%; improved EFS in tx arm compared with control; MPR: 36.9% vs 8.9%; ORR: 53.6% vs 37.4%; radiographic down-staging rates: 30.7% vs 23.5%	Grade 3: 33.5% vs 36.9% Grade 4: 11.4% vs 14.8%

[a]NOTE: As of January 2022, no immunotherapy drugs have been approved by the FDA as neoadjuvant therapy for NSCLC. However, this is currently evolving with continual changes in clinical practice. Results from the CheckMate 816 trial have shown promising results for the possible role of immunotherapy as neoadjuvant for NSCLC.

AE, adverse event; ALK, anaplastic lymphoma kinase; DFS, disease-free survival; DoR, duration of response; EFS, event-free survival; EGFR, epidermal growth factor receptor; ES-SCLC, extensive-stage small cell lung cancer; FDA, Food & Drug Administration; ITT, intention-to-treat; MPR, major pathologic response (defined as ≤ 10% of residual viable tumor in posttherapy specimen); NSCLC, non-small cell lung cancer; ORR, objective response rate; OS, overall survival; pCR, pathologic complete response (defined as 0% viable tumor cells in resected lung and lymph nodes); PFS, progression-free survival; TPS, tumor proportion score; tx, treatment.

6.0 months), and 6-month OS (80.2% vs 72.4%) compared with chemotherapy, leading to its FDA approval as a first-line therapy.[32] To investigate whether pembrolizumab could also be used for patients with lower PD-L1 expression, the investigators of KEYNOTE-042 compared patients with untreated locally advanced/metastatic NSCLC with PD-L1 expression ≥1% to those on standard platinum-based chemotherapy and found a significant survival advantage of 16.7 months in the treatment arm compared with 12.1 months in the control arm.[33] This paved the way for approval of pembrolizumab as a first-line agent for patients with untreated advanced/metastatic NSCLC with PD-L1 expression ≥1%. Atezolizumab (IMPower 110[34]) and cemiplimab (EMPOWER-Lung1[35]) were approved in 2020 and 2021, respectively, as first-line monotherapy agents for patients with advanced NSCLC with PD-L1 expression on tumors demonstrating improvement in OS compared with platinum-based chemotherapy.

Combinational therapy has also been an active area of investigation for treatment of this disease. Several clinical trials have led to the first-line approval of pembrolizumab in combination with chemotherapy (KEYNOTE-021,[36] KEYNOTE-189,[37] KEYNOTE-407[38]). Similarly, atezolizumab with chemotherapy was approved for metastatic NSCLC based on the IMPower 130 trial.[39] The IMPower 150 study, which randomized patients to receive atezolizumab + carboplatin + paclitaxel (ACP), bevacizumab + carboplatin + paclitaxel (BCP), or atezolizumab + BCP (ABCP), demonstrated improved PFS (8.3 vs 6.8 months) and median OS (19.2 vs 14.7 months) in the ABCP group compared with the BCP group, resulting in the approval of this combination regimen.[40] Regarding the combination of multiple ICIs, nivolumab plus ipilimumab is currently approved for advanced NSCLC after results from the CheckMate 227 trial showed improved median OS (17.1 vs 14.9 months), PFS (5.1 vs 5.6 months), and duration of response (DoR; 23.2 vs 6.2 months) compared with chemotherapy for patients with PD-L1 TPS ≥1%.[41] In 2020, nivolumab with ipilimumab and platinum-doublet chemotherapy was approved as first-line treatment for patients with recurrent/metastatic NSCLC after demonstrating improved median survival of 15.6 months compared with 10.9 months in the standard chemotherapy arm.[42]

For locally advanced NSCLC, durvalumab has been approved as a maintenance therapy for patients with unresectable, stage III NSCLC after platinum-based chemoradiation therapy as a result of the PACIFIC trial.[43,44]

One of the breakthroughs in the clinical application of immunotherapy in the 2020s is the use of ICIs in treating early-stage NSCLCs. As a result of the IMPower010 study, atezolizumab is indicated as a single-agent adjuvant therapy after resection and platinum-based chemotherapy for adult patients with stage II–IIIA NSCLC whose tumors have PD-L1 expression on ≥1% of tumor cells.[45] Although the application of immunotherapy as neoadjuvant therapy for NSCLC has yet to be FDA-approved, several trials have demonstrated findings that may lead to changes in clinical practice. The CheckMate 816 trial is a phase 3 study that compares nivolumab plus platinum-based chemotherapy as neoadjuvant with platinum-based chemotherapy alone for patients with resectable stage IB-IIIA NSCLC. An interim analysis of this trial showed improved pathologic complete response (pCR; 24.0% vs 2.2%), major pathologic response (MPR; 36.9% vs 8.9%), ORR (53.6% vs 37.4%), and event-free survival (EFS) in the neoadjuvant nivolumab plus chemotherapy treatment arm compared with the control arm, with no effect on surgical outcomes.[46-48] Together with the results from the IMPower010 trial, the findings from CheckMate 816 trial have changed the treatment paradigm of early-stage NSCLCs. Determining the role of neoadjuvant versus adjuvant ICI therapy for patients with stage IB–IIIA NSCLCs, however, remains to be addressed.

SMALL CELL LUNG CANCER

The positive results of PD-1/L1 inhibitors for the treatment of NSCLC ignited interest in evaluating these agents for the treatment of SCLC (Table 12.4). Although SCLC is initially

TABLE 12.4 ■ **Key Clinical Trials Leading to FDA Approval of Immuno-oncology Agents for Small Cell Lung Cancer (as of January 2022)**

Small Cell Lung Cancer (SCLC)

Clinical Trial	FDA Agent	Phase	N	Study Population	Treatment Arm	Control Arm	Primary Endpoint	Results	Grade 3+ AE
First-Line Therapy									
IMpower133 (NCT02763579)	Atezolizumab (Tecentriq)	3	403	ES-SCLC	Atezolizumab + Etoposide + Carboplatin	Placebo + Etoposide + Carboplatin	PFS, OS	Median OS: 12.3 vs 10.3 months; median PFS: 5.2 vs 4.3 months	Tx arm: grade 3–4: 56.6%; grade 5: 1.5% Control arm: grade 3–4: 56.1%; grade 5: 1.5%
CASPIAN (NCT03043872)	Durvalumab (Imfinzi)	3	537	ES-SCLC	Durvalumab + Etoposide + Platinum-based chemo	Platinum-based chemo	OS	Median OS: 13.0 vs 10.3 months; ORR 68% vs 58%	62% vs 62%
Third-Line Therapy									
KEYNOTE-028 (NCT02054806), KEYNOTE-158 (NCT02628067)	Pembrolizumab (Keytruda)	1 + 2	83	Stage IV SCLC with progression after platinum-based chemotherapy and 1+ prior line of therapy	Pembrolizumab	N/A	ORR, DRR	ORR: 19%; 6-month DRR 94%; 1-year DRR 63%; 18-month DRR: 56%	9.6%–9.9%

AE, adverse event; *DRR*, durable response rate; *ES-SCLC*, extensive-stage small cell lung cancer; *FDA*, Food & Drug Administration; *ORR*, objective response rate; *OS*, overall survival; *PFS*, progression-free survival; *tx*, treatment.

sensitive to chemoradiation, many patients may relapse within 6 months, with 5-year survival rates as low as 5% for patients with extensive-stage disease (ES-SCLC).[49] In 2018, nivolumab was the first ICI to be granted accelerated approval by the FDA as a third-line option for stage IV SCLC. That same year, pembrolizumab was approved as third-line therapy for the same indication based on the KEYNOTE-028 and KEYNOTE-158 studies.[50]

Though standard, first-line treatment for ES-SCLC is platinum-based chemotherapy with etoposide, outcomes continued to remain poor with median OS of approximately 10 months.[51] Two ICIs, atezolizumab (Impower133[52]) and durvalumab (CASPIAN[53]), approved as first-line therapies for untreated ES-SCLC in combination with etoposide and a platinum-based chemotherapy regimen, have shown improvements in median OS to 12 to 13 months.

MALIGNANT PLEURAL MESOTHELIOMA

Malignant pleural mesothelioma (MPM) is an aggressive cancer often unresectable at the time of diagnosis. Though platinum agents with folate antimetabolites such as pemetrexed have been approved as standard first-line therapies, prognosis remains poor, with a median 5-year OS of <10%.[54] Currently, nivolumab in combination with ipilimumab is the available immunotherapy for first-line treatment of unresectable MPM, based on the CheckMate 743 trial that demonstrated an OS of 18.1 months in the treatment arm compared with 14.1 months in the standard chemotherapy (platinum + pemetrexed chemotherapy) arm and a 2-year OS of 41% vs 27%, respectively (Table 12.5).[55]

Triple-Negative Breast Cancer

Triple-negative breast cancer (TNBC) is an aggressive subtype that is difficult to treat, owing to the lack of targeted agents. Though chemotherapy including taxanes or platinum-based agents remains the standard of care for systemic treatment, these tumors can become rapidly resistant to chemotherapy. In 2021, pembrolizumab in combination with chemotherapy was approved in the first-line setting for metastatic disease, as well as in the neoadjuvant and adjuvant setting (Table 12.6). The approval of pembrolizumab as first-line therapy for metastatic TNBC stemmed from the KEYNOTE-355 study, which demonstrated significant PFS (9.6 vs 5.6 months) in the pembrolizumab plus chemotherapy arm compared with the placebo plus chemotherapy arm for patients with PD-L1 expression with combined positive score (CPS) ≥10.[56] Pembrolizumab's approval as neoadjuvant therapy in combination with chemotherapy for high-risk stage II/III TNBC followed by adjuvant treatment after surgery was based on findings from KEYNOTE-522 that showed a pCR rate of 63% in the pembrolizumab arm compared with 56% in the chemotherapy arm.[57]

Gastrointestinal Malignancies

GASTRIC/GASTROESOPHAGEAL JUNCTION CANCERS

Gastric cancer, including gastroesophageal junction (GEJ) cancer, is the fourth leading cause of cancer-related deaths worldwide. Outcomes remain poor with standard-of-care fluoropyrimidine and platinum-based chemotherapy in unresectable disease.[58,59] Current ICIs approved as first-line agents for advanced or metastatic gastric/GEJ include nivolumab in conjunction with chemotherapy (CheckMate 649)[60] and pembrolizumab in conjunction with chemotherapy and trastuzumab for human epidermal growth factor receptor 2 positive (HER2+) tumors (KEYNOTE-811).[61] Nivolumab and pembrolizumab have also been approved as second-line indications for advanced or metastatic esophageal/GEJ cancers that have progressed after prior lines of therapy, based on findings from the KEYNOTE-180,[62] KEYNOTE-181,[63] and ATTRACTION-3[64]

TABLE 12.5 ■ **Key Clinical Trial Leading to FDA Approval of Immuno-oncology Agent for Malignant Pleural Mesothelioma (as of January 2022)**

Clinical Trial	FDA Agent	Phase	N	Study Population	Treatment Arm	Control Arm	Primary Endpoint	Results	Grade 3+ AE
Mesothelioma									
First-Line Therapy									
CheckMate 743 (NCT02899299)	Nivolumab (Opdivo) + Ipilimumab (Yervoy)	3	605	Unresectable malignant pleural mesothelioma	Nivolumab + Ipilimumab	Platinum + Pemetrexed chemo	OS	OS: 18.1 vs 14.1 months; 2-year OS: 41% vs 27%	30% vs 32%

AE, adverse event; *FDA*, Food & Drug Administration; *OS*, overall survival.

TABLE 12.6 ■ Key Clinical Trials Leading to FDA Approval of Immuno-oncology Agents for Triple-Negative Breast Cancer (as of January 2022)

Triple-Negative Breast Cancer (TNBC)

Clinical Trial	FDA Agent	Phase	N	Study Population	Treatment Arm	Control Arm	Primary Endpoint	Results	Grade 3+ AE
First-Line Therapy									
KEYNOTE-355 (NCT02819518)	Pembrolizumab (Keytruda)	3	847	Unresectable, recurrent/stage IV TNBC with PD-L1 (CPS ≥ 10)	Pembrolizumab + Chemo	Placebo + Chemo	PFS, OS	Median PFS: 9.6 vs 5.6 months	68% vs 67%
Neoadjuvant/Adjuvant Therapy									
KEYNOTE-522 (NCT03036488)	Pembrolizumab (Keytruda)	3	1174	Untreated high-risk stage II/III TNBC	Pembrolizumab + Chemo	Placebo + Chemo	Pathologic complete response rate, event free survival	Pathologic complete response: 63% vs 56%; event-free survival: 16% vs 24%	76.8% vs 72.2%

AE, adverse event; CPS, combined positive score; FDA, Food & Drug Administration; OS, overall survival; PFS, progression-free survival.

trials, as detailed in Tables 12.7 to 12.9. In addition, nivolumab is approved in the adjuvant setting for patients with stage II/III disease after definitive treatment with chemoradiation and surgical resection with residual disease.[65]

COLORECTAL CANCER

Patients with metastatic colorectal cancer (mCRC) have a median 5-year OS of 14.7%.[66] Currently, all IO agents approved for the treatment of colorectal cancers have been limited to MSI-H/dMMR metastatic colorectal cancers (mCRC) (Table 12.10).[67] In 2017, the FDA granted approval for nivolumab as a single agent for patients with microsatellite instability-high (MSI-H) and mismatch repair protein–deficient (dMMR) mCRC that progressed after treatment with a fluoropyrimidine, oxaliplatin, and irinotecan. Ipilimumab for use in combination with nivolumab was subsequently approved for the same indication. Both approvals were based on findings from CheckMate 142.[68] Pembrolizumab was approved in 2020 as first-line therapy for unresectable/metastatic MSI-H/dMMR mCRC after the KEYNOTE-177 study showed superior median PFS (16.5 vs 8.2 months) and 2-year OS (13.7 vs 10.8 months) in the pembrolizumab treatment arm compared with the standard chemotherapy (5-fluorouracil-based therapy +/− bevacizumab or cetuximab) arm. The durable response of these ICI for patients with mCRC with MSI-H/dMMR subtype highlights the promising role of immunotherapy.

HEPATOCELLULAR CARCINOMA

ICIs were first approved in the second-line setting for patients with advanced hepatocellular carcinoma (HCC) previously treated with sorafenib (Table 12.11). The approval of nivolumab plus ipilimumab was based on a phase 1/2 trial that demonstrated a durable ORR of 20%.[69] Similarly, another phase 1/2 trial demonstrated a durable ORR of 17% for patients treated with pembrolizumab monotherapy.[70] For patients with unresectable, metastatic HCC, atezolizumab in combination with bevacizumab was approved as first-line therapy in 2020 after results from IMbrave150 showed superior OS and PFS in the atezolizumab + bevacizumab group compared with sorafenib (1-year OS: 67.2% vs 54.6%; median PFS: 6.8 vs 4.3 months).[71]

Gynecologic Malignancies

CERVICAL CANCER

Although the incidence of cervical cancer has declined since the early 2000s owing to cancer screening programs and vaccination against the human papillomavirus (HPV), cervical cancer remains a significant cause of deaths, particularly in less developed nations. Patients with recurrent/metastatic cervical cancer continue to have poor prognoses with limited second-line or later treatment options because it it is relatively chemotherapy resistant. Cisplatin with radiation therapy is the primary therapy used for treating patients with advanced cervical cancer; however, ORRs range from 13% to 23% with generally low DoR.[72] Several studies have reported relatively high PD-1/PD-L1 expression in cervical tumors, providing potential targets for ICI.[73,74] Currently, immunotherapy for gynecologic malignancies has been limited to the use of pembrolizumab as monotherapy or combination therapy for recurrent/metastatic cervical cancer expressing PD-L1 (CPS ≥ 1) (Table 12.12). Pembrolizumab was first approved in 2018 as monotherapy for patients with PD-L1-positive (CPS ≥ 1), recurrent/metastatic cervical cancer after first-line standard chemotherapy; this was based on results from KEYNOTE-158 that showed that treatment with pembrolizumab in patients with PD-L1-positive tumors resulted in an ORR of 12.2% and a DCR of 30.6%.[75] Later in 2021, pembrolizumab in combination with platinum-based

TABLE 12.7 ■ Key Clinical Trials Leading to FDA Approval of Immuno-oncology Agents for Gastric Cancer (as of January 2022)

Gastric Cancer

Clinical Trial	FDA Agent	Phase	N	Study Population	Treatment Arm	Control Arm	Primary Endpoint	Results	Grade 3+ AE
First-Line Therapy									
CheckMate 649 (NCT02872116)	Nivolumab (Opdivo)	3	1581	Unresectable, locally advanced, stage IV gastric/GEJ/esophageal adenocarcinoma	Nivolumab + Chemo	Chemo	PFS, OS	Median OS: 13.8 vs 11.5 months CPS ≥ 5: PFS 7.7 vs 6.0 months, median OS 14.4 vs 11.1 months	59% vs 44%
KEYNOTE-811 (NCT03615326)	Pembrolizumab (Keytruda)	3	264	Unresectable/stage IV HER2+ gastric/GEJ cancer	Pembrolizumab + Trastuzumab + Chemo	Placebo + Trastuzumab + Chemo	PFS	ORR: 74.4% vs 51.9%	57.1% vs 57.4%

AE, adverse event; *CPS*, combined positive score; *FDA*, Food & Drug Administration; *GEJ*, gastroesophageal junction; *OS*, overall survival; *PFS*, progression-free survival.

TABLE 12.8 ■ **Key Clinical Trials Leading to FDA Approval of Immuno-oncology Agents for Esophageal/Gastroesophageal Junction Adenocarcinoma (as of January 2022)**

				Esophageal/Gastroesophageal Junction (GEJ) Adenocarcinoma					
Clinical Trial	FDA Agent	Phase	N	Study Population	Treatment Arm	Control Arm	Primary Endpoint	Results	Grade 3+ AE
First-Line Therapy									
CheckMate 649 (NCT02872116)	Nivolumab (Opdivo)	3	1581	Locally advanced, unresectable/stage IV gastric/GEJ/esophageal adenocarcinoma	Nivolumab + Chemo	Chemo	PFS, OS	Median OS: 13.8 vs 11.5 months CPS ≥ 5: PFS 7.7 vs 6.0 months; OS 14.4 vs 11.1 months	59% vs 44%
KEYNOTE-590 (NCT03189719)	Pembrolizumab (Keytruda)	3	749	Locally advanced, unresectable/stage IV esophageal adenocarcinoma or SCC, GEJ adenocarcinoma	Pembrolizumab + 5-FU + Cisplatin	Placebo + 5-FU + Cisplatin	PFS, OS	Median OS: 12.4 vs 9.8 months, PFS 6.3 vs 5.8 months SCC group: median OS 12.6 vs 9.8 months, PFS 6.3 vs 5.8 months PD-L1 w/CPS ≥ 10: median OS 13.5 vs 9.4 months, PFS 7.5 vs 5.5 months SCC and PD-L1 CPS ≥ 10: median OS 13.9 vs 8.8 months	72% vs 68%
Second-Line Therapy									
KEYNOTE-180 (NCT02559687)	Pembrolizumab (Keytruda)	2	121	Locally advanced, unresectable/stage IV esophageal adenocarcinoma or SCC, GEJ adenocarcinoma that progressed after 2+ lines of therapy	Pembrolizumab	N/A	ORR	ORR: 9.9%	12.4%

Trial	Drug	Phase	N	Population	Intervention	Comparator	Endpoint	Result	
KEYNOTE-181 (NCT02564263)	Pembrolizumab (Keytruda)	3	628	Locally advanced, unresectable/stage IV esophageal adenocarcinoma or SCC, GEJ adenocarcinoma that progressed after first-line chemo	Pembrolizumab	Chemo	OS	1-Year OS: 43% vs 20% CPS ≥ 10: median OS 9.3 vs 6.7 months SCC group: median OS: 8.2 vs 7.1 months	18.2% vs 40.9%
ATTRACTION-3 (NCT02569242)	Nivolumab (Opdivo)	3	419	Locally advanced, unresectable/recurrent esophageal SCC that progressed after one line of therapy	Nivolumab	Chemo	OS	OS: 10.9 vs 8.4 months	18% vs 63%
Adjuvant Therapy									
CheckMate 577 (NCT02743494)	Nivolumab (Opdivo)	3	794	Resected stage II/III esophageal adenocarcinoma or SCC, GEJ cancer after neoadjuvant CRT, surgery with residual pathologic disease	Nivolumab	Placebo	DFS	Median DFS: 22.4 vs 11.0 months	13% vs 6%

AE, adverse event; CPS, combined positive score; CRT, chemoradiation therapy; DFS, disease-free survival; FDA, Food & Drug Administration; GEJ, gastroesophageal junction; ORR, objective response rate; OS, overall survival; PFS, progression-free survival; SCC, squamous cell carcinoma.

TABLE 12.9 ■ Key Clinical Trials Leading to FDA Approval of Immuno-oncology Agents for Esophageal Squamous Cell Carcinoma (as of January 2022)

	Esophageal Squamous Cell Carcinoma (SCC)								
Clinical Trial	FDA Agent	Phase	N	Study Population	Treatment Arm	Control Arm	Primary Endpoint	Results	Grade 3+ AE
First-Line Therapy									
KEYNOTE-590 (NCT03189719)	Pembrolizumab (Keytruda)	3	749	Locally advanced, unresectable/stage IV esophageal adenocarcinoma or SCC, GEJ adenocarcinoma	Pembrolizumab + 5-FU + Cisplatin	Placebo + 5-FU + Cisplatin	PFS, OS	Median OS: 12.4 vs 9.8 months, PFS 6.3 vs 5.8 months SCC group: median OS 12.6 vs 9.8 months, PFS 6.3 vs 5.8 months PD-L1 w/CPS ≥ 10: median OS 13.5 vs 9.4 months, PFS 7.5 vs 5.5 months SCC and PD-L1 CPS ≥ 10: median OS 13.9 vs 8.8 months	72% vs 68%
Second-Line Therapy									
KEYNOTE-180 (NCT02559687)	Pembrolizumab (Keytruda)	2	121	Locally advanced, unresectable/stage IV esophageal adenocarcinoma or SCC, GEJ adenocarcinoma that progressed after 2+ lines of therapy	Pembrolizumab	N/A	ORR	ORR: 9.9%	12.4%

Trial	Drug	Phase	N	Population	Intervention	Comparator	Endpoint	Results	AE
KEYNOTE-181 (NCT02564263)	Pembrolizumab (Keytruda)	3	628	Locally advanced, unresectable/stage IV esophageal adenocarcinoma or SCC, GEJ adenocarcinoma that progressed after first-line chemo	Pembrolizumab	Chemo	OS	1-Year OS: 43% vs 20% CPS ≥ 10: median OS 9.3 vs 6.7 months SCC group: median OS: 8.2 vs 7.1 months	18.2% vs 40.9%
ATTRACTION-3 (NCT02569242)	Nivolumab (Opdivo)	3	419	Locally advanced, unresectable/recurrent esophageal SCC that progressed after one line of therapy	Nivolumab	Chemo	OS	OS: 10.9 vs 8.4 months	18% vs 63%
Adjuvant Therapy									
CheckMate 577 (NCT02743494)	Nivolumab (Opdivo)	3	794	Resected stage II/III esophageal adenocarcinoma or SCC, GEJ cancer after neoadjuvant CRT, surgery with residual pathologic disease	Nivolumab	Placebo	DFS	Median DFS: 22.4 vs 11.0 months	13% vs 6%

AE, adverse event; *CPS*, combined positive score; *CRT*, chemoradiation therapy; *DFS*, disease-free survival; *FDA*, Food & Drug Administration; *GEJ*, gastroesophageal junction; *ORR*, objective response rate; *OS*, overall survival; *PFS*, progression-free survival; *SCC*, squamous cell carcinoma.

TABLE 12.10 ■ Key Clinical Trials Leading to FDA Approval of Immuno-oncology Agents for MSI-H/dMMR or TMB-H Solid Tumors *(as of January 2022)*

Clinical Trial	FDA Agent	Phase	N	Study Population	Treatment Arm	Control Arm	Primary Endpoint	Results	Grade 3+ AE
Microsatellite Instability–High or Mismatch Repair–Deficient (MSI-H/dMMR) Solid Tumors									
First-Line Therapy									
KEYNOTE-177 (NCT02563002)	Pembrolizumab (Keytruda)	3	307	MSI-H/dMMR unresectable/ mCRC	Pembrolizumab	5-FU based therapy +/– Bevacizumab/ Cetuximab	PFS, OS	Median PFS: 16.5 vs 8.2 months; 2-year OS: 13.7 vs 10.8 months; ORR: 43.8% vs 33.1%	22% vs 66%
Second-Line Therapy									
CheckMate 142 (NCT02060188)	Nivolumab (Opdivo)	2	74	MSI-H/dMMR recurrent/ mCRC who progressed on or after fluoropyrimidine and oxaliplatin or irinotecan	Nivolumab	N/A	ORR	ORR: 31%	Grade 3: 18% Grade 4: 3%
KEYNOTE-016 (NCT01876511)	Pembrolizumab (Keytruda)	2	41	Unresectable/stage IV MSI-H/dMMR solid tumors progressed from prior treatment with no alternative options; colorectal cancer progressed after fluoropyrimidine, oxaliplatin, and irinotecan.	Pembrolizumab	N/A	ORR, PFS	dMMR: ORR 40% vs 78%: median PFS and OS not reached Non-dMMR: median PFS 2.2 months, OS 5.0 months	41%

Clinical Trial	FDA Agent	Phase	N	Study Population	Treatment Arm	Control Arm	Primary Endpoint	Results	Grade 3+ AE
GARNET (NCT02715284)	Dostarlimab (Jemperli)	1	209	dMMR recurrent/advanced solid tumors progressed after systemic therapy	Dostarlimab	N/A	ORR, DoR	ORR: 41.6%, DoR: 34.7 months	8.3%
Third-Line Therapy									
CheckMate 142 (NCT02060188)	Nivolumab (Opdivo) + ipilimumab (Yervoy)	2	119	MSI-H/dMMR recurrent/mCRC who progressed on or after fluoropyrimidine and oxaliplatin or irinotecan	Nivolumab + Ipilimumab	N/A	ORR	ORR: 55%; PFS: 76% vs 71%; OS: 87% vs 85%	32%

Tumor Mutational Burden-High (TMB-H) Solid Tumors

Clinical Trial	FDA Agent	Phase	N	Study Population	Treatment Arm	Control Arm	Primary Endpoint	Results	Grade 3+ AE
Second-Line Therapy									
KEYNOTE-158	Pembrolizumab (Keytruda)	2	1066	Unresectable/metastatic TMB-H solid tumors progressed from prior treatment with no alternative options	Pembrolizumab	N/A	ORR	ORR: 29%	15%

AE, adverse event; *dMMR*, mismatch repair deficient; *DoR*, duration of response; *FDA*, Food & Drug Administration; *MSI-H*, microsatellite instability-high; *ORR*, objective response rate; *OS*, overall survival; *PFS*, progression-free survival; *TMB-H*, tumor mutational burden-high.

TABLE 12.11 ■ Key Clinical Trials Leading to FDA Approval of Immuno-oncology Agents for Hepatocellular Carcinoma (as of January 2022)

Hepatocellular Carcinoma (HCC)

Clinical Trial	FDA Agent	Phase	N	Study Population	Treatment Arm	Control Arm	Primary Endpoint	Results	Grade 3+ AE
First-Line Therapy									
IMbrave150 (NCT03434379)	Atezolizumab (Tecentriq)	3	336	Unresectable metastatic HCC	Atezolizumab + Bevacizumab	Sorafenib	PFS, OS	Median PFS: 6.8 vs 4.3 months; OS: 67.2% vs 54.6%	56.5% vs 55.1%
Second-Line Therapy									
CheckMate 040 (NCT01658878)	Nivolumab (Opdivo)	1 + 2	262	Advanced HCC previously tx w/ sorafenib	Nivolumab	N/A	ORR	ORR: 20% in dose-expansion phase; 15% in dose escalation phase	25%
CheckMate 040 (NCT01658878)	Nivolumab (Opdivo)	1 + 2	148	Advanced HCC previously tx w/ sorafenib	Arm A: Nivolumab 1 mg/kg + Ipilimumab 3 mg/kg q3w, followed by Nivolumab 240 mg q2w Arm B: Nivolumab 3 mg/kg + Ipilimumab 1 mg/kg q3w, followed by Nivolumab 240 mg q2w Arm C: Nivolumab 3 mg/kg q2w plus Ipilimumab 1 mg/kg q6w	N/A	ORR	Arm A: ORR 32%, median DoR: not reached Arm B: ORR 27%, median DoR: 15.2 months Arm C: ORR 29%, median DoR: 21.7 months	Arm A: 53% Arm B: 29% Arm C: 31%
KEYNOTE-240 (NCT02702401)	Pembrolizumab (Keytruda)	3	413	Advanced HCC previously tx w/ sorafenib	Pembrolizumab	Placebo	PFS, OS	Median PFS: 3.0 vs 2.8 months; median OS: 13.9 vs 10.6 months	52.7% vs 46.3%

AE, adverse event; DoR, duration of response; FDA, Food & Drug Administration; HCC, hepatocellular carcinoma; ORR, objective response rate; OS, overall survival; PFS, progression-free survival; tx, treated.

TABLE 12.12 ■ Key Clinical Trials Leading to FDA Approval of Immuno-oncology Agents for Cervical Cancer *(as of January 2022)*

Cervical Cancer

Clinical Trial	FDA Agent	Phase	N	Study Population	Treatment Arm	Control Arm	Primary Endpoint	Results	Grade 3+ AE
Second-Line Therapy									
KEYNOTE-158 (NCT02628067)	Pembrolizumab (Keytruda)	2	98	Recurrent/stage IV cervical cancer with progression on or after chemo with PD-L1 (CPS ≥ 1)	Pembrolizumab	N/A	ORR	ORR: 12.2%; median DoR: not reached PD-L1 positive: ORR 14.6%	12.2%
KEYNOTE-826 (NCT03635567)	Pembrolizumab (Keytruda)	3	617	Persistent/recurrent/ stage IV cervical cancer with PD-L1 (CPS ≥ 1)	Pembrolizumab + Platinum-based chemo +/− Bevacizumab	Placebo + Platinum-based chemo +/− Bevacizumab	PFS, OS	ITT: PFS 10.4 vs 8.2; 2-year OS: 50.4% vs 40.4% PD-L1 CPS ≥ 1: PFS 10.4 vs 8.2; 2-year OS: 53.0% vs 41.7% PD-L1 CPS ≥ 10: 10.4 vs 8.1; 2-year OS: 54.4% vs 44.6%	81.8% vs 75.1%

AE, adverse event; *CPS*, combined positive score; *DoR*, duration of response; *FDA*, Food & Drug Administration; *ORR*, objective response rate; *OS*, overall survival; *PFS*, progression-free survival; *ITT*, intention-to-treat.

chemotherapy +/− bevacizumab was approved in the first-line setting for metastatic cervical cancer expressing PD-L1 (CPS ≥ 1). KEYNOTE-826 demonstrated a significant survival benefit from adding checkpoint blockade to standard chemotherapy compared with standard chemotherapy alone in 2-year OS (50.4% vs 40.4%) and median PFS (10.4 vs 8.2 months).[76]

ENDOMETRIAL CANCER

Thus far, there have been two notable IO advances specific to the treatment of endometrial carcinoma (Table 12.13). In 2021 the FDA granted accelerated approval for dostarlimab (anti-PD-1) in the second-line setting, after standard platinum-based chemotherapy, for patients with dMMR/MSI-H endometrial cancers. This approval was based on an interim analysis of the early-phase GARNET study that showed an ORR of 42.3% (including a 12.7% complete response [CR] rate) and 6-month DoR of 93.3% (median DOR not reached) in 71 patients with dMMR recurrent or advanced endometrial cancer.[77] In the same year, the oral tyrosine kinase inhibitor lenvatinib in combination with pembrolizumab was approved in the second-line setting for patients with proficient mismatch repair (pMMR) and microsatellite instability-low (MSI-L) endometrial cancer, based on KEYNOTE-775. This trial demonstrated that the combination lenvatinib plus pembrolizumab led to superior disease responses compared with physician's choice treatment (ORR 30% vs 15%; DOR 9.2 months vs 5.7 months) in patients with advanced pMMR endometrial cancers after at least one prior platinum-based regimen.[78]

Genitourinary Malignancies

RENAL CELL CARCINOMA

Renal cell carcinoma (RCC) comprises 90% of all kidney cancers, with clear cell being the most common subtype. Approximately 33% of patients have advanced or metastatic disease at diagnosis. Although RCC is notably resistant to chemotherapy, it is relatively sensitive to immunotherapy and antiangiogenic treatment compared with other tumor types.[79] Prior to IO agents, agents such as sunitinib that target the vascular endothelial growth factor (VEGF) pathway have been standard-of-care first-line therapy for advanced disease; however, many patients may have either resistance to antiangiogenic drugs or progressive disease. Though nivolumab was the first IO agent approved by the FDA as a second-line agent for previously treated advanced/metastatic clear cell RCC based on findings from the CheckMate 025 trial,[80] there are now three ICIs approved as first-line agents for advanced clear cell RCC, in combination with either another ICI or with antiangiogenic inhibitors. CheckMate 214 was a phase 1 study that investigated the combination of nivolumab + ipilimumab compared with sunitinib in advanced clear cell RCC.[81] Results from this study showed that the nivolumab + ipilimumab combination group had significantly higher ORR (39% vs 32%) and OS (not reached vs 32.9 months) compared with the control (sunitinib) arm. Nivolumab plus ipilimumab is currently the combination of ICI approved as first-line therapy for advanced clear cell RCC. Other combination therapies that have been found to improve ORR, PFS, and OS compared with sunitinib are multiple combinatorial regimens of single-agent PD-1/PD-L1 inhibitors with antiangiogenic tyrosine kinase inhibitors (TKIs), such as pembrolizumab + axitinib (KEYNOTE-426),[82] avelumab + axitinib (JAVELIN Renal 101),[83] nivolumab + cabozantinib (CheckMate 9ER),[84] and pembrolizumab + lenvatinib (KEYNOTE-581).[85] Key findings from these trials are summarized in Table 12.14. Because there has yet to be a direct head-to-head trial comparing dual checkpoint inhibition and checkpoint blockade plus antiangiogenic TKI regimens, first-line therapy selection remains a topic of active debate.

TABLE 12.13 ■ Key Clinical Trials Leading to FDA Approval of Immuno-oncology Agents for Endometrial Cancer (*as of January 2022*)

Endometrial Cancer

Clinical Trial	FDA Agent	Phase	N	Study Population	Treatment Arm	Control Arm	Primary Endpoint	Results	Grade 3+ AE
Second-Line Therapy									
GARNET (NCT02715284)	Dostarlimab (Jemperli)	1	104	dMMR recurrent/advanced endometrial cancer with progression on or after platinum-doublet chemo w/no more than yeo prior lines of therapy	Dostarlimab	N/A	ORR, DoR	ORR: 42.3%; median DoR: not reached	46.2%
KEYNOTE-775 (NCT03517449)	Pembrolizumab (Keytruda)	3	827	Advanced endometrial cancer that is not MSI-H/ dMMR with progression on or after platinum-based chemo, unamenable to surgery or radiation	Pembrolizumab + Lenvatinib	Doxorubicin or Paclitaxel	PFS; OS	Median PFS: 6.6 vs 3.8 months; median OS: 17.4 vs 12.0 months; ORR: 30% and 15%; median DoR: 9.2 vs 5.7 months	88.9% vs 72.7%

AE, adverse event; *dMMR*, mismatch repair deficient; *DoR*, duration of response; *FDA*, Food & Drug Administration; *MSI-H*, microsatellite instability-high; *ORR*, objective response rate; *OS*, overall survival; *PFS*, progression-free survival.

TABLE 12.14 ■ Key Clinical Trials Leading to FDA Approval of Immuno-oncology Agents for Renal Cell Carcinoma *(as of January 2022)*

Renal Cell Carcinoma (RCC)								
Clinical Trial	FDA Agent	Phase	N	Study Population	Treatment Arm	Control Arm	Primary Endpoint	Results	Grade 3+ AE
First-Line Therapy								
CheckMate 214 (NCT02231749)	Nivolumab (Opdivo) + ipilimumab (Yervoy)	3	1096	Untreated advanced clear cell RCC	Nivolumab + Ipilimumab	Sunitinib	OS, ORR, PFS	18-Month OS: 75% vs 60%; median OS: not reached vs 26.0 months; ORR 42% vs 27%; median PFS: 11.6 vs 8.4 months	46% vs 63%
KEYNOTE-426 (NCT02853331)	Pembrolizumab (Keytruda)	3	861	Advanced/recurrent/stage IV clear cell RCC	Pembrolizumab + Axitinib	Sunitinib	OS, PFS	1-Year OS: 89.9% vs 78.3%; median PFS: 15.1 vs 11.1 months; ORR: 59.3% vs 35.7%	75.8% vs 70.6%
JAVELIN Renal 101 (NCT02684006)	Avelumab (Bavencio)	3	886	Advanced clear cell RCC	Avelumab + Axitinib	Sunitinib	OS, PFS	Median PFS 13.8 vs 8.4 months PD-L1 positive: median PFS 13.8 vs 7.2 months; ORR 55.2% vs 25.5%	71.2% vs 71.5%

Trial (NCT)	Drug	Phase	n	Population	Treatment	Comparator	Endpoint	Results	
CheckMate 9ER (NCT03141177)	Nivolumab (Opdivo)	3	651	Advanced clear cell RCC	Nivolumab + Cabozantinib	Sunitinib	PFS	Median PFS: 16.6 vs 8.3 months; 1-year OS: 85.7% vs 75.6%; ORR: 55.7% vs 27.1%	75.3% vs 70.6%
KEYNOTE-581 (NCT02811861)	Pembrolizumab (Keytruda)	3	1069	Advanced clear cell RCC	Arm 1: Pembrolizumab + Lenvatinib; Arm 2: Everolimus + Lenvatinib	Sunitinib	PFS	Arm 1: median PFS 23.9 vs 9.2 months; OS HR 0.66, p = 0.005; Arm 2: median PFS 14.7 vs 9.2 months	82.4%; 83.1% vs 71.8%
Second-Line Therapy									
CheckMate 025 (NCT01668784)	Nivolumab (Opdivo)	3	821	Advanced/metastatic clear cell RCC previously treated with 1+ antiangiogenic therapy	Nivolumab	Everolimus	OS	Median OS: 25.0 vs 19.6 months; ORR: 25% vs 5%; median PFS: 4.6 vs 4.4 months	19% vs 37%
Adjuvant Therapy									
KEYNOTE-564 (NCT03142334)	Pembrolizumab (Keytruda)	3	984	Clear cell RCC with high risk for recurrence after nephrectomy +/− metastasectomy	Pembrolizumab	Placebo	DFS	2-Year DFS: 77.3% vs 68.1%	32.4% vs 17.7%

AE, adverse event; *DFS*, disease-free survival; *FDA*, Food & Drug Administration; *ORR*, objective response rate; *OS*, overall survival; *PFS*, progression-free survival; *RCC*, renal cell carcinoma.

UROTHELIAL CARCINOMA

Urothelial carcinoma (UC) is the most common subtype of bladder cancer in the United States and Europe. Current standard, first-line therapy for advanced UC is platinum-based chemotherapy; however, due to renal dysfunction, poor performance status, and other comorbidities, some patients are ineligible for this treatment, whereas others do not respond to this treatment and have short response durations and/or disease progression. The advent of immunotherapy has introduced more therapeutic options for patients who are either ineligible for or have progressed despite platinum-containing chemotherapy (Table 12.15).[86]

The two current immunotherapy classes approved for the treatment of UC include the Bacillus Calmette-Guerin (BCG) vaccine and ICIs. The BCG vaccine was first demonstrated in 1980 to show a reduction in tumor recurrence for patients with high-grade non-muscle-invasive bladder cancer (NMIBC) compared with observation alone or intravesicular chemotherapy, leading to its approval in 1990.[87] For advanced-stage disease, pembrolizumab has been approved as first-line therapy for platinum-ineligible advanced/metastatic UC. This approval was based on results from KEYNOTE-052, which demonstrated an ORR of 24% in all comers, with a notably higher ORR of 38% in patients with CPS ≥10%.[88] However, pembrolizumab did not show additive clinical benefit when combined with first-line platinum-based chemotherapy for advanced/metastatic UC (KEYNOTE-361).[89] Avelumab has been approved as maintenance therapy in patients with advanced/metastatic UC previously treated with platinum-based chemotherapy with no disease progression, following the results of JAVELIN Bladder 100, which showed that maintenance avelumab increased OS by 7 months and nearly doubled PFS compared with best supportive care alone in all comers.[90] For patients with advanced/metastatic UC who were previously treated with first-line platinum-based chemotherapy but who developed disease progression or recurrence, nivolumab (CheckMate 275[91]), pembrolizumab (KEYNOTE-045,[92] KEYNOTE-057[93]), and avelumab (JAVELIN Solid Tumor[94]) are available as second-line therapies after first-line chemotherapy. For adjuvant therapy, nivolumab has become the first immunotherapy agent approved in 2021 for patients with muscle-invasive bladder cancer (MIBC) after radical cystectomy who are deemed high-risk for recurrence, based on results from CheckMate 274 that showed that it nearly doubled time to recurrence/death compared with placebo (20.8 months vs 10.8 months).[95]

Prostate Cancer

Despite prostate cancer cells having been reported to express tumor-associated antigens such as prostate-specific antigen, prostatic acid phosphatase, and prostate-specific membrane antigen, thereby providing potential targets for immunotherapies, Sipuleucel-T, a personalized, cell-based ex vivo processed dendritic cell vaccine, is the first FDA-approved cancer-specific vaccine (Table 12.16). The D9901 study, a placebo-controlled phase 3 study of patients with metastatic castration-resistant prostate cancer, demonstrated survival advantage of 4.5 months in the vaccine-treated group.[96] D9902B, or the Immunotherapy for Prostate Adenocarcinoma Treatment (IMPACT) study, demonstrated improved median OS (25.8 vs 21.7 months) in the sipuleucel-T group vs placebo.[97] This therapy is recommended in patients with castrate-resistant prostate cancer who are minimally symptomatic from their disease. Due to the complexity of its manufacturing, sipuleucel-T is currently not marketed in the United States. ICIs have yet to take an approved role in the treatment of prostate cancer, but studies are ongoing.

Head and Neck Squamous Cell Carcinoma

Head and neck squamous cell carcinoma (HNSCC) includes cancers of the oral cavity, oropharynx, hypopharynx, and larynx. Although locoregional HNSCC is treated with curative intent,

TABLE 12.15 ■ Key Clinical Trials Leading to FDA Approval of Immuno-oncology Agents for Urothelial Carcinoma *(as of January 2022)*

Urothelial Carcinoma (UC)

Clinical Trial	FDA Agent	Phase	N	Study Population	Treatment Arm	Control Arm	Primary Endpoint	Results	Grade 3+ AE
Vaccine Therapy									
BCG vaccine	BCG vaccine	N/A	37	Superficial bladder cancer	BCG + Surgery	Surgery	Recurrence	Reduction in tumor recurrence in treatment vs control (P = .029)	N/A
First-Line Therapy									
KEYNOTE-052 (NCT02335424)	Pembrolizumab (Keytruda)	2	370	Cisplatin-ineligible locally advanced/unresectable/metastatic UC	Pembrolizumab	N/A	ORR	PD-L1 > 10%: ORR 38%	Grade 3: 14% Grade 4: 1% Grade 5: <1%
JAVELIN Bladder 100 (NCT02603432)	Avelumab (Bavencio)	3	700	Locally advanced/metastatic UC w/ no disease progression with first-line platinum-containing chemo	Avelumab + Best supportive care	Best supportive care	OS	1-Year OS: 71.3% vs 58.4%; median PFS: 3.7 vs 2.0 months PD-L1 positive: 79.1% vs 60.4%; median PFS: 5.7 vs 2.1 months	47.4% vs 25.2%
KEYNOTE-361 (NCT02853305)	Pembrolizumab (Keytruda)	3	1010	Unresectable/locally advanced/metastatic UC	Arm 1: Pembrolizumab Arm 2: Pembrolizumab + Platinum-based chemo	Platinum-based chemo	PFS, OS	Arm 1: median OS 15.6 vs 14.3 months Arm 2: median PFS 8.3 vs 7.1 months, median OS 17.0 vs 14.3 months	Arm 1: grade 3: 12%; grade 4: 1%; grade 5: 1% Arm 2: grade 3: 14%; grade 4: 2% Control arm: grade 3: 6%; grade 4: <1%

Continued on following page

TABLE 12.15 ■ Key Clinical Trials Leading to FDA Approval of Immuno-oncology Agents for Urothelial Carcinoma (as of January 2022) (Continued)

Urothelial Carcinoma (UC)

Clinical Trial	FDA Agent	Phase	N	Study Population	Treatment Arm	Control Arm	Primary Endpoint	Results	Grade 3+ AE
Second-Line Therapy									
CheckMate 275 (NCT02387996)	Nivolumab (Opdivo)	2	270	Unresectable, locally advanced/metastatic UC with progression/recurrence on or after platinum-based chemo	Nivolumab	N/A	ORR	ORR 19.6% PD-L1 < 1%: ORR 16.1% PD-L1 ≥ 5%: ORR 28.4%	18%
KEYNOTE-045 (NCT02256436)	Pembrolizumab (Keytruda)	3	542	Second-line: locally advanced/metastatic UC w/disease progression/recurrence after platinum-based chemo	Pembrolizumab	Chemo	OS, PFS	Median OS: 10.3 vs 7.4 months PD-L1 ≥ 10%: median OS 8.0 vs 5.2 months	15.0% vs 49.4%
JAVELIN Solid Tumor (NCT01772004)	Avelumab (Bavencio)	1	249	Locally advanced/metastatic UC with progression/recurrence after platinum-based chemo	Avelumab	N/A	ORR	ORR: 17%	8%

Trial	Drug	Phase	N	Population	Treatment	Control	Endpoint	Results	
KEYNOTE-057 (NCT02625961)	Pembrolizumab (Keytruda)	2	101	BCG-unresponsive, high-risk, NMIBC w/CIS +/− papillary tumors who are ineligible for or have elected not to undergo cystectomy	Pembrolizumab	N/A	Complete response rate	Complete response rate: 41%	13%
Adjuvant Therapy									
CheckMate 274 (NCT02632409)	Nivolumab (Opdivo)	3	709	Adjuvant: MIBC who had undergone radical surgery	Nivolumab	Placebo	DFS	Median DFS 20.8 vs 10.8; 6-month DFS 74.9% vs 60.3%; recurrence-free survival 22.9 vs 13.7 months; 6-month RFS 77.0% vs 62.7% PD-L1 ≥ 1%: 74.5% vs 55.7%	17.9% vs 7.2%

AE, adverse event; CIS, carcinoma in situ; DFS, disease-free survival; FDA, Food & Drug Administration; NMIBC, nonmuscle invasive bladder cancer; ORR, objective response rate; OS, overall survival; PFS, progression-free survival; UC, urothelial carcinoma.

TABLE 12.16 ■ **Key Clinical Trials Leading to FDA Approval of Immuno-oncology Agents for Prostate Cancer (as of January 2022)**

| | | | | | **Prostate Cancer** | | | |
Clinical Trial	FDA Agent	Phase	N	Study Population	Treatment Arm	Control Arm	Primary Endpoint	Results	Grade 3+ AE
D9901 (NCT00005947)	Sipuleucel-T (Provenge)	3	127	Metastatic hormone refractory prostate cancer	Sipuleucel-T	Placebo	TTP	Median TTP: 11.7 vs 10.0 weeks; median OS: 25.9 vs 21.4 months	N/A
D9902B (IMPACT; NCT00849290)	Sipuleucel-T (Provenge)	3	512	Metastatic castration-resistant prostate cancer	Sipuleucel-T	Placebo	OS	3-Year OS: 31.7% vs 23.0%; median OS: 25.8 vs 21.7 months	31.7% vs 35.1%

AE, adverse event; *FDA*, Food & Drug Administration; *OS*, overall survival; *TTP*, time to progression.

patients who develop recurrent/metastatic HNSCC were traditionally treated with chemotherapy (platinum plus 5-fluorouracil) and cetuximab as first-line therapy with a historic median overall survival of approximately 10 months.[98] ICIs have not only demonstrated manageable safety in HNSCC but have also been shown to improve OS compared with previous standard of care (Table 12.17). Pembrolizumab is currently approved as first-line therapy for unresectable recurrent/metastatic HNSCC in combination with chemotherapy, based on results from KEYNOTE-048 that showed an improvement in median OS for the pembrolizumab plus chemotherapy arm compared with 10.7 months for the cetuximab plus chemotherapy arm (13.0 months vs 10.7 months; hazard ratio [HR] = 0.77; 95% confidence interval [CI], 0.63, 0.93; $P = 0.0067$).[99] Additionally, first-line single-agent pembrolizumab was approved based on results from the same trial that showed a similar OS benefit for the subgroups of patients with PDL1-positive (CPS $\geq$1) HNSCC randomized to pembrolizumab monotherapy compared with cetuximab plus chemotherapy.[99]

For patients with recurrent/metastatic HNSCC with disease progression on or after first-line platinum-containing chemotherapy without prior checkpoint inhibitor treatment, pembrolizumab (KEYNOTE-012[100]) and nivolumab (CheckMate 141[101]) are the currently available agents that have been shown to have good response rates. In CheckMate 141, nivolumab demonstrated a median OS of 7.5 months compared with 5.1 months in the control arm of standard single-agent systemic therapy (methotrexate, docetaxel, or cetuximab).[101]

Tissue/Site-Agnostic Malignant Solid Tumors

In 2017, the FDA granted accelerated approval of pembrolizumab for the treatment of adult and pediatric patients with unresectable or metastatic MSI-H/dMMR solid tumors that progressed on prior treatment, based on several clinical trials (see Table 12.10).[102,103] This decision marked the FDA's first tissue/site-agnostic approval based on a tumor's genetic features regardless of primary site and suggests the potential role of MSI-H/dMMR status as a biomarker to guide patient selection for immunotherapy. More recently, dostarlimab was approved in 2021 as a second-line therapy for recurrent/advanced dMMR solid tumors with progression after systemic therapy, based on the GARNET trial, which demonstrated a pan-tumor collective ORR of 41.6% and median DoR of 34.7 months.[104]

Tumor mutational burden (TMB), defined as the total number of somatic mutations per coding area of a tumor genome, has also been considered a potential biomarker to help guide IO treatment. TMB varies among cancer types and can even vary among patients within the same tumor types. It is hypothesized that tumors with high TMB (TMB-H; defined as $\geq$10 mutations/megabase) may produce more neoantigens that may increase T-cell reactivity, thereby allowing for more improved response with IO agents. Approval for TMB-H solid cancers was based on KEYNOTE-158, a phase 2 trial that showed improved clinical responses with pembrolizumab monotherapy treatment in patients with previously treated unresectable/metastatic TMB-H solid tumors (ORR of 29% in the TMB-H group vs 6% in the TMB-low group).[105]

Hematologic Malignancies

LEUKEMIA

The 21st-century breakthrough of CAR T-cell therapy has transformed the therapeutic landscape of hematologic malignancies and shows the promise of personalized medicine (Table 12.18).[106] Although 5-year OS for pediatric acute lymphoblastic leukemia (ALL) now approaches 80% to 90%, patients with relapsed ALL have 5-year OS of 30% to 50% after the first relapse and <20% after subsequent relapses.[107] The FDA approval of tisagenlecleucel in 2017 for

TABLE 12.17 ■ Key Clinical Trials Leading to FDA Approval of Immuno-oncology Agents for Head and Neck Squamous Cell Carcinoma (as of January 2022)

| | | | | **Head and Neck Squamous Cell Carcinoma (HNSCC)** | | | | |
Clinical Trial	FDA Agent	Phase	N	Study Population	Treatment Arm	Control Arm	Primary Endpoint	Results	Grade 3+ AE
First-Line Therapy									
KEYNOTE-048 (NCT02358031)	Pembrolizumab (Keytruda)	3	992	Unresectable, recurrent/stage IV HNSCC	Arm 1: Pembrolizumab Arm 2: Pembrolizumab + Chemo	Cetuximab + Chemo	PFS, OS	Arm 1: CPS ≥ 20: OS 14.9 vs 10.7 months CPS ≥ 1: OS 12.4 vs 10.3 months Arm 2: OS 13.0 vs 10.7 months CPS ≥ 20: OS 14.7 vs 1.0 months CPS ≥ 1: OS 13.6 vs 10.4 months	55%; 85% vs 83%
Second-Line Therapy									
KEYNOTE-012 (Cohort B/B2) (NCT01848834)	Pembrolizumab (Keytruda)	1b	60	PD-L1 positive recurrent/stage IV HNSCC with progression on/after platinum-based chemo	Pembrolizumab	N/A	ORR	ORR: 18%	17%
CheckMate 141 (NCT02105636)	Nivolumab (Opdivo)	3	361	Recurrent/stage IV HNSCC with progression on/after platinum-based chemo	Nivolumab	Chemo	OS	Median OS: 7.5 vs 5.1 months; median PFS: 2.0 vs 2.3 months; ORR: 13.3% vs 5.8%	13.1% vs 35.1%

AE, adverse event; CPS, combined positive score; FDA, Food & Drug Administration; HNSCC, head and neck squamous cell carcinoma; ORR, objective response rate; OS, overall survival; PFS, progression-free survival.

TABLE 12.18 ■ Key Clinical Trials Leading to FDA Approval of Immuno-oncology Agents for Leukemia (as of January 2022)

Leukemia

Clinical Trial	FDA Agent	Phase	N	Study Population	Treatment Arm	Control Arm	Primary Endpoint	Results	Grade 3+ AE
CAR T-Cell Therapy									
ELIANA (NCT02435849)	Tisagenlecleucel (Kymriah)	2	75	Patients up to age 25 years with relapsed/refractory B-cell precursor ALL	Tisagenlecleucel	N/A	Remission rate	Remission rate: 81%; complete remission rate: 60%; 6-month event-free survival: 73%; 6-month OS: 90%; 1-year event-free survival: 50%; 1-year OS: 76%	73%
ZUMA-3 (NCT02614066)	Brexucabtagene autoleucel (Tecartus)	2	71	Relapsed/refractory B-cell precursor ALL	Brexucabtagene autoleucel	N/A	Complete remission	overall complete remission: 56%; median duration of remission: 12.8 months; median relapse-free survival: 11.6 months; median OS: 18.2 months	Grade 3: 15% Grade 4: 62% Grade 5: 18%
Bispecific Antibodies (BiTE)									
ALCANTARA (NCT02000427)	Blinatumomab (Blincyto)	2	45	Relapsed/refractory Ph+ ALL after one second-generation or later TKI (or were intolerant to TKIs and/or imatinib)	Blinatumomab	N/A	Complete remission	complete remission: 36%; median relapse-free survival: 6.7 months; median OS: 7.1 months	Grade 3: 73% Grade 4: 36%
BLAST (NCT01207388)	Blinatumomab (Blincyto)	2	116	B-cell precursor ALL in first or later complete remission with persistent/recurrent MRD ≥ 0.1% after minimum of three blocks of chemo	Blinatumomab	N/A	Complete response	complete MRD response: 78% Ph-negative ALL: 18-month relapse-free survival 54%; median OS: 36.5 months	Grade 3: 33% Grade 4: 27%

AE, adverse event; ALL, acute lymphoblastic leukemia; FDA, Food & Drug Administration; MRD, minimal residual disease; OS, overall survival; Ph+, Philadelphia chromosome-positive; TKI, tyrosine kinase inhibitor.

patients with relapsed/refractory ALL younger than 25 years old marked a significant milestone as the first CAR-T therapy, gene therapy, and cancer therapy approved for a pediatric population before an adult population. Tisangenlecleucel is currently approved for pediatric relapsed/refractory B-cell precursor ALL after the ELIANA trial demonstrated a CR of 60%, an ORR of 81%, a 6-month OS of 90%, and 1-year OS of 76%.[108] Most recently, in 2021, brexucabtagene autoleucel, another CAR T-cell therapy, was approved for adults with relapsed/refractory B-cell precursor ALL after the ZUMA-3 trial showed a CR of 56% with median remission duration of 12.8 months, relapse-free survival (RFS) of 11.6 months, and OS of 18.2 months.[109]

Another class of immunotherapy agents, bispecific T-cell engager (BiTE) antibodies, have demonstrated promising results for the treatment of ALL. This novel class of immunotherapy is designed to engage and enhance T-cell activation by directing cytotoxic T-cells to CD19-expressing B cells. BiTE antibodies can recruit antigen-experienced T-cells without pre- or costimulation to directly kill tumor-associated antigen cells. Blinatumomab is currently an FDA-approved BiTE antibody for treating ALL. In the ALCANTARA study, the use of blinatumomab for relapsed/refractory Philadelphia chromosome-positive ALL after prior TKI therapy demonstrated a CR of 36%, a median RFS of 6.7 months, and a median OS of 7.1 months.[110] In the BLAST study, blinatumomab led to a CR of 78% for all comers; patients with Philadelphia chromosome–negative ALL had an 18-month RFS of 54% and a median OS of 36.5 months.[111]

LYMPHOMA

Traditionally, patients with first relapse of classical Hodgkin lymphoma (cHL) are treated with chemotherapy followed by autologous hematopoietic stem cell transplantation (HSCT); however, the 3-year freedom from treatment failure rate in this population is around 55%.[112] For patients who relapse after autologous HSCT, the prognosis is worse. The approval of ICI nivolumab (CheckMate 205[113]) and pembrolizumab (KEYNOTE-087,[114] KEYNOTE-204[115]) as second-line therapies for relapsed/refractory cHL after autologous HSCT has provided some encouragement, with trials demonstrating good response rates and improved median PFS (Table 12.19). Pembrolizumab has also been approved as a third-line therapy for relapsed/refractory primary mediastinal B-cell lymphoma (PMBCL) after the KEYNOTE-170 phase 2 trial demonstrated an ORR of 45%.[116]

Though ICIs have found less success with other lymphoma subtypes such as large B-cell lymphomas (LBCL), follicular lymphoma, and mantle cell lymphoma, CAR T-cell therapy has shown promise for these lymphoma subtypes. Three CAR T-cell agents, axicabtagene ciloleucel (ZUMA-1[117]), tisangenlecleucel (JULIET[118]), and lisocabtagene maraleucel (TRANSCEND[119]), are approved for relapsed/refractory LBCL including diffuse large B-cell lymphoma (DLBCL), high-grade B-cell lymphoma, PMBCL, and DLBCL arising from follicular lymphoma after two or more lines of systemic therapy, with phase 1/2 trials demonstrating good overall response rates ranging from 52% to 82%. Axicabtagene ciloleucel was also approved in 2021 for relapsed/refractory follicular lymphoma after two or more prior lines of systemic therapy (ZUMA-5[120]), and brexucabtagene autoleucel was approved for relapsed/refractory mantle cell lymphoma after prior treatment with Bruton's tyrosine kinase (BTK) inhibitor (ZUMA-2[121]), with both agents demonstrating ORR >90% in their respective clinical trials.

MULTIPLE MYELOMA

Multiple myeloma (MM) is characterized by the clonal expansion of malignant plasma cells that can lead to lytic bone lesions, anemia, renal dysfunction, and an immunocompromised state. The abundance of malignant plasma cells suppresses normal B cells, leading to deficiencies in

TABLE 12.19 ■ Key Clinical Trials Leading to FDA Approval of Immuno-oncology Agents for Lymphomas (as of January 2022)

Classical Hodgkin Lymphoma (cHL)

Clinical Trial	FDA Agent	Phase	N	Study Population	Treatment Arm	Control Arm	Primary Endpoint	Results	Grade 3+ AE
Second-Line Therapy									
CheckMate 205 (NCT02181738)	Nivolumab (Opdivo)	2	80	Recurrent cHL who failed to respond to autologous HSCT, brentuximab vedotin	Nivolumab	N/A	ORR	ORR: 66.3%	Grade 3: 30% Grade 4: 3.75%
KEYNOTE-087 (NCT02453594)	Pembrolizumab (Keytruda)	2	210	Relapsed/refractory cHL after 3+ prior lines of therapy	Pembrolizumab	N/A	ORR	ORR: 69.0%	6.7%
KEYNOTE-204 (NCT02684292)	Pembrolizumab (Keytruda)	3	304	Relapsed/refractory cHL ineligible for or had relapsed after autologous HSCT	Pembrolizumab	Brentuximab vedotin	PFS, OS	Median PFS: 13.2 vs 8.3 months	Tx arm: grade 3: 16%; grade 4: 3%; grade 5: 1% Control arm: grade 3: 21%; grade 4: 4%

Primary Mediastinal B-Cell Lymphoma (PMBCL)

Clinical Trial	FDA Agent	Phase	N	Study Population	Treatment Arm	Control Arm	Primary Endpoint	Results	Grade 3+ AE
Third-Line Therapy									
KEYNOTE-170 (NCT02576990)	Pembrolizumab (Keytruda)	2	53	Relapsed/refractory PMBCL after 2+ lines of therapy	Pembrolizumab	N/A	ORR	ORR: 45%	23%

Continued on following page

TABLE 12.19 ■ Key Clinical Trials Leading to FDA Approval of Immuno-oncology Agents for Lymphomas (as of January 2022) (Continued)

Clinical Trial	**FDA Agent**	**Phase**	**N**	**Study Population**	**Treatment Arm**	**Control Arm**	**Primary Endpoint**	**Results**	**Grade 3+ AE**

Large B-Cell Lymphoma (LBCL)

Clinical Trial	FDA Agent	Phase	N	Study Population	Treatment Arm	Control Arm	Primary Endpoint	Results	Grade 3+ AE
CAR T-Cell Therapy									
ZUMA-1 (NCT02348216)	Axicabtagene ciloleucel (Yescarta)	2	111	Relapsed/refractory LBCL after 2+ lines of systemic therapy, including DLBCL, DLBCL arising from FL, high-grade B-cell lymphoma, PMBCL	Axicabtagene ciloleucel	N/A	ORR	ORR: 82%; 18-month OS: 52%	95%
JULIET (NCT02445248)	Tisagenlecleucel (Kymriah)	2	93	Relapsed/refractory LBCL after 2+ lines of systemic therapy including DLBCL, DLBCL arising from FL, high grade B-cell lymphoma	Tisagenlecleucel	N/A	ORR	ORR: 52%	AE ≤ 8 weeks: 58% AE > 8 weeks: 22%
TRANSCEND (NCT02631044)	Lisocabtagene maraleucel (Breyanzi)	1	344	Relapsed/refractory LBCL after 2+ lines of systemic therapy, including DLBCL, high-grade B-cell lymphoma, PMBCL, and FL grade 3B	Lisocabtagene maraleucel	N/A	ORR	ORR: 73%	79%

Follicular Lymphoma (FL)

Clinical Trial	FDA Agent	Phase	N	Study Population	Treatment Arm	Control Arm	Primary Endpoint	Results	Grade 3+ AE
CAR T-Cell Therapy									
ZUMA-5 (NCT03105336)	Axicabtagene ciloleucel (Yescarta)	2	151	Relapsed/refractory FL after 2+ lines of systemic therapy	Axicabtagene ciloleucel	N/A	ORR, DoR	ORR: 91%; median DoR: not reached; 1-year continued remission: 76.2%	86%

Mantle Cell Lymphoma (MCL)

Clinical Trial	FDA Agent	Phase	N	Study Population	Treatment Arm	Control Arm	Primary Endpoint	Results	Grade 3+ AE
CAR T-Cell Therapy									
ZUMA-2 (NCT02601313)	Brexucabtagene autoleucel (Tecartus)	2	74	Relapsed/refractory MCL previously treated with BTK inhibitor	Brexucabtagene autoleucel	N/A	ORR	ORR: 93%	grade 3: 12%; grade 4: 3%

AE, adverse event; *BTK*, Bruton's tyrosine kinase; *cHL*, classical Hodgkin lymphoma; *DLBCL*, diffuse large B-cell lymphoma; *DoR*, duration of response; *FDA*, Food & Drug Administration; *HSCT*, hematopoietic stem cell transplant; *LBCL*, large B-cell lymphoma; *MCL*, mantle cell lymphoma; *ORR*, objective response rate; *OS*, overall survival; *PFS*, progression-free survival; *PMBCL*, primary mediastinal B-cell lymphoma.

humoral immunity. Upregulation of the PD-1/PD-L1 pathway in patients with MM further disrupts immune activation and promotes immune tolerance. There is currently no standard of care established for patients with disease progression despite receiving three classes of therapy of immunomodulatory agents, proteasome inhibitors, and anti-CD38 antibodies. Even with these therapies, many patients continue to have incomplete responses, a median PFS of 3 to 4 months, and a median OS of 8 to 9 months.[122]

The introduction of CAR T-cell therapy has provided a promising therapy for patients with MM with refractory disease (Table 12.20). Idecabtagene vicleucel, a B-cell maturation antigen (BCMA)-directed genetically modified CAR T-cell therapy, is the first approved CAR T-cell therapy agent for patients with relapsed/refractory MM after at least four prior lines of therapy and was approved by the FDA in 2021 after the KarMMa study that showed an ORR of 73% at median follow-up of 13.3 months and a median PFS of 8.8 months.[123]

Immune-Related Toxicities Associated With Checkpoint Blockade

Because cancer immunotherapies manipulate the host immune system to recognize and attack cancer cells, they have the potential to induce durable responses for various cancer types. However, cancer immunotherapies also carry distinct toxicity profiles compared with more traditional cancer systemic therapies. Whereas traditional chemotherapy may have acute-onset emetic and myelosuppressive effects, immune-related toxicities associated with ICIs can have more delayed onset with autoimmune/inflammatory-like responses. As noted in clinical trials, the onset of immune-related adverse events (irAEs) can occur anytime as early as within the first few weeks of treatment or even after treatment discontinuation. The disinhibition of T-cell function by ICIs can lead to a spectrum of irAEs that may affect any organ or tissue. The most common organ-related toxicities associated with ICIs involve the skin, gastrointestinal, and endocrine systems; the pulmonary, ocular, cardiac, hematologic, and central nervous systems are less commonly affected.[124-126] A list of common irAEs is summarized in Table 12.21. Differences in side effect profiles and severity are found even between anti-CTLA-4 and anti-PD-1/PD-L1 inhibitors. Whereas anti-CTLA-4 is associated with increased incidences of colitis, hypophysitis, and rash, anti-PD-1/PD-L1 is associated with increased incidences of pneumonitis, arthralgias, and hypothyroidism; several studies have also shown that anti-CTLA-4-mediated side effects are generally more severe and that combination checkpoint blockade may also increase the frequency of irAEs.[127] Though reasons for these differences are still under investigation, it has been hypothesized that these distinct irAE profiles may be driven by different immune cell activation and tissue-related factors.

Given these findings, it is important for the health care provider to monitor patients who have received ICI treatment with routine lab monitoring, comparisons to baseline, and focused history-taking and physical exams. Prior to the initiation of immunotherapy as well as throughout treatment and survivorship, health care providers should educate patients and their caregivers on the potential clinical profiles of irAEs. Main symptoms that may cause clinical suspicion of an irAE include changes in bowel pattern (e.g., diarrhea, colitis), cough, headaches, nausea, rashes, fatigue, muscle/joint pain, muscle weakness, and weight loss. However, a high level of suspicion should still be maintained for any new symptoms that may arise during and after ICI treatment. Dermatologic adverse events are usually the first to present.

Based on the 2021 American Society of Clinical Oncology (ASCO) Guidelines,[128] ICIs can generally be continued with close monitoring for patients with grade 1 toxicities, unless patients experience neurologic, hematologic, and cardiac toxicities. Clinicians should consider holding immunotherapies for patients experiencing grade 2 toxicities and resume when symptoms and/or labs revert to less than grade 1; corticosteroid administration can also be considered. For patients

TABLE 12.20 ■ Key Clinical Trial Leading to FDA Approval of Immuno-oncology Agent for Multiple Myeloma (as of January 2022)

Clinical Trial	FDA Agent	Phase	N	Study Population	Treatment Arm	Control Arm	Primary Endpoint	Results	Grade 3+ AE
Multiple Myeloma									
Fifth-Line Therapy									
KarMMa (NCT03361748)	Idecabtagene vicleucel (Abecma)	2	140	Adult patients with multiple myeloma who have not responded to, or whose disease has returned after, at least 4+ lines (different types) of therapy	Idecabtagene vicleucel	N/A	ORR	ORR: 73%; median PFS: 8.8 months	99%

AE, adverse event; *FDA*, Food & Drug Administration; *ORR*, objective response rate; *PFS*, progression-free survival.

TABLE 12.21 ■ **Common Immune-Related Adverse Events (irAEs)**

Neurologic

All-Grade Incidence: 3%–12%
Autoimmune encephalitis
Myasthenia gravis
Guillain-Barre syndrome
Peripheral neuropathy
Posterior reversible encephalopathy syndrome
Aseptic meningitis
Transverse myelitis

Ocular

All-Grade Incidence: < 1%
Dry eye/uveitis
Peripheral ulcerative keratitis
Choroidal neovascularization
Retinopathies

Cardiovascular

All-Grade Incidence: < 1%
Pericarditis
Cardiac fibrosis
Arrhythmias
New onset heart failure

Pulmonary

Pneumonitis (1%–4.9%)

Gastrointestinal

Colitis (1%–14%)
Diarrhea (20%–40+%)
Hepatitis (6%–22%)
Pancreatitis (<1%)

Renal

Acute kidney injury (0.4%–7%)

Endocrinopathies

All-Grade Incidence: 4%–14%
Hyperthyroidism
Myxedema
Thyroid storm
Primary adrenal insufficiency (0.6%–2.6%)
Hypophysitis (<1%–7.7%)

Musculoskeletal/Rheumatologic

All-Grade Incidence: 1%–7%
Arthritis/myalgia (~8%)
Sicca syndrome (~5%)
Myositis
Polymyalgia rheumatica and giant cell arteritis

TABLE 12.21 ■ **Common Immune-Related Adverse Events (irAEs)** (Continued)

Dermatologic

Maculopapular rash (0.7%–34.2%)
Hypersensitivity reaction
Dermatomyositis
Pyoderma gangrenosum
Bullous dermatitis
Stevens-Johnson syndrome/toxic epidermal necrosis

Hematologic

All-Grade Incidence: 3%–4%
Anemia
Thrombocytopenia
Leukopenia
Neutropenia

Source of reported irAE incidences as combination of anti-PD1/PDL1 and anti-CTLA-4 therapy: National Comprehensive Cancer Network[125] and Ramos-Casals et al.[126]

with grade 3 and higher toxicities, clinicians should hold immunotherapy and treat patients with high-dose corticosteroids (prednisone 1–2 mg/kg/d or equivalent) tapered over at least 4 to 6 weeks. In cases of steroid-resistant irAEs, other biologic immunosuppressive medications such as infliximab may need to be used. Patients with severe-grade toxicities should generally discontinue immunotherapy permanently. An exception to this is with particular endocrinopathies that can be sufficiently treated and managed long term with hormone replacement. Fortunately, retrospective studies have shown that treating irAEs with steroids or immunomodulators has yet to show any detrimental effects on the efficacy of immune checkpoint therapy in terms of OS and PFS.[124,129] Detailed consensus guidelines for the monitoring, diagnosis, and treatment of irAEs from ICIs are available from ASCO[128,130] and the National Comprehensive Cancer Network (NCCN).[125]

Toxicities Associated With CAR T-Cell Therapy

Although CAR T-cell therapy has demonstrated durable and objective responses for hematologic malignancies, literature suggests that many patients treated with CAR T-cell therapy experience side effects, the most common being cytokine release syndrome (CRS) and neurotoxicity.[131] CAR T-cells are activated by antigen recognition, which can lead to subsequent cytokine release and a positive feedback loop of further immune cell activation. This inflammatory response can result in organ dysfunction with wide-ranging symptoms such as hypoxia, hypotension, fevers, arthralgias, myalgias, fatigue, and coagulopathy; in severe cases, cardiogenic/vasodilatory shock, fulminant liver/kidney failure, acute respiratory distress syndrome, and even death can occur. Neurotoxic side effects of CAR T-cell therapy can range from mild cognitive changes to aphasia, seizures, and coma. Early detection, management, and understanding of CAR T-cell toxicities are therefore paramount to ensure the safety and tolerability of this therapy. Management of CAR T-cell toxicities generally requires supportive care measures such as the use of antipyretics, fluids, vasopressors, and antibiotics. Patients with more severe side effects may receive additional interventions including corticosteroids and tocilizumab, a monoclonal antibody that inhibits the interleukin (IL)-6 receptor to exert anti-CRS effects. Various grading systems have been used to assess CAR

T-cell–mediated CRS; however, this not only made it difficult to compare the safety profiles of different CAR T-cell therapies but also led to differences in reported rates of adverse events in clinical trials. In 2019, consensus guidelines for the monitoring, diagnosis, and treatment of CAR T-cell–associated toxicities were established by the American Society for Transplantation and Cellular Therapy to help standardize care.[132]

Prospective Directions

Cancer immunotherapy has revolutionized the clinical landscape of oncology and brought renewed hope to the treatment of previously difficult-to-treat malignancies. Yet, more questions and challenges continue to lie ahead. Though beyond the scope of this chapter, future directions of cancer immunotherapy should include the investigation of IO agents earlier in the cancer disease progression, such as in the context of neoadjuvant therapy. IO combination therapy in combination with various classes of immunotherapy agents, targeted therapies, chemotherapies, and/or with radiation therapy is currently being investigated. In the context of immunotherapy drug development, developing preclinical models that can translate to human immunity, understanding organ-specific tumor immune contexts and developing strategies to transform immunologically "cold" tumors into "inflamed" tumors, defining appropriate endpoints for cancer immunotherapy treatment and duration, assessing efficacy and safety in special populations often excluded from these trials (e.g., patients with autoimmune disease, chronic viral infections, Eastern Cooperative Oncology Group (ECOG) grade $\geq$ 2, transplant recipients/patients who are immunocompromised),[133] and using a personalized approach via composite biomarkers (e.g., PD-L1 expression, MSI-H/dMMR, TMB, etc.)[134] to select for patients who may respond to immunotherapy are ongoing challenges awaiting discovery. As our knowledge and understanding of cancer pathogenesis and immunotherapies continue to grow, we remain optimistic regarding the hope that immunotherapy may provide to countless patients.

Glossary of Clinical Trial Terms & Definitions

Term	Abbreviation	Definition
Overall Survival	OS	The length of time from either the date of diagnosis or the start of treatment that patients diagnosed with the disease are still alive.
Progression-Free Survival	PFS	The length of time during and after treatment for a disease that a patient lives with the disease but it does not get worse.
Event-Free Survival	EFS	The length of time after primary treatment for a cancer ends that the patient remains free of certain complications or events that the treatment was intended to prevent or delay, such as cancer recurrence and the onset of certain symptoms.
Relapse-Free Survival	RFS	The length of time after primary treatment for a cancer ends that the patient survives without any signs or symptoms of that cancer.
Duration of Response	DoR	The length of time that a tumor continues to respond to treatment without the cancer growing or spreading
Disease Control Rate	DCR	The percentage of patients with advanced/metastatic cancer who have achieved complete response, partial response, and stable disease to a therapeutic intervention.
Overall Response Rate	ORR	The percentage of patients who have a partial or complete response to the treatment within a certain period of time.

Glossary of Clinical Trial Terms & Definitions (Continued)

Term	Abbreviation	Definition
Partial Response	PR	The decrease in the size of a tumor or the amount of cancer in the body.
Complete Response	CR	The disappearance of all signs of cancer in response to treatment. This does not always mean the cancer has been cured. Also called complete remission.
Pathologic Complete Response	pCR	The lack of all signs of cancer in tissue samples removed during surgery or biopsy after treatment with radiation or systemic therapy. Also called pathologic complete remission.
Major Pathologic Response	MPR	Defined as ≤ 10% of viable tumor remaining in primary tumor after neoadjuvant treatment.
Tumor Proportion Score	TPS	The ratio of PD-L1 stained tumor cells to the total number of viable tumor cells.
Combined Positive Score	CPS	The ratio of potential PD-L1 expression including tumor cells and immune cells to the total number of viable tumor cells.

Adapted from: National Cancer Institute (NCI) Dictionary of Cancer Terms: https://www.cancer.gov/publications/dictionaries/cancer-terms

Key References

3. Pardoll DM. The blockade of immune checkpoints in cancer immunotherapy. *Nat Rev Cancer.* 2012;12(4):252-264. doi:10.1038/nrc3239.

7. Han Y, Liu D, Li L. PD-1/PD-L1 pathway: current researches in cancer. *Am J Cancer Res.* 2020; 10(3):727-742.

10. Barrios DM, Do MH, Phillips GS, et al. Immune checkpoint inhibitors to treat cutaneous malignancies. *J Am Acad Dermatol.* 2020;83(5):1239-1253. doi:10.1016/j.jaad.2020.03.131.

18. Chiocca EA, Rabkin SD. Oncolytic viruses and their application to cancer immunotherapy. *Cancer Immunol Res.* 2014;2(4):295-300. doi:10.1158/2326-6066.Cir-14-0015.

25. Patel SA, Weiss J. Advances in the treatment of non-small cell lung cancer: immunotherapy. *Clin Chest Med.* 2020;41(2):237-247. doi:10.1016/j.ccm.2020.02.010.

67. Ganesh K, Stadler ZK, Cercek A, et al. Immunotherapy in colorectal cancer: rationale, challenges and potential. *Nat Rev Gastroenterol Hepatol.* 2019;16(6):361-375. doi:10.1038/s41575-019-0126-x.

79. Rini BI, Battle D, Figlin RA, et al. The Society for Immunotherapy of Cancer consensus statement on immunotherapy for the treatment of advanced renal cell carcinoma (RCC). *J Immunother Cancer.* 2019;7(1):354. doi:10.1186/s40425-019-0813-8.

86. Tripathi A, Plimack ER. Immunotherapy for urothelial carcinoma: current evidence and future directions. *Curr Urol Rep.* 2018;19(12):109. doi:10.1007/s11934-018-0851-7.

106. Pehlivan KC, Duncan BB, Lee DW. CAR-T-cell therapy for acute lymphoblastic leukemia: transforming the treatment of relapsed and refractory disease. *Curr Hematol Malig Rep.* 2018;13(5):396-406. doi:10.1007/s11899-018-0470-x.

125. National Comprehensive Cancer Network. *Management of Immunotherapy-Related Toxicities (Version 4.2021).* Available at: https://www.nccn.org/professionals/physician_gls/pdf/immunotherapy.pdf. Accessed November 22, 2021.

126. Ramos-Casals M, Brahmer JR, Callahan MK, et al. Immune-related adverse events of checkpoint inhibitors. *Nat Rev Dis Primers.* 2020;6(1):38. doi:10.1038/s41572-020-0160-6.

127. Khoja L, Day D, Wei-Wu Chen T, Siu LL, Hansen AR. Tumour- and class-specific patterns of immune-related adverse events of immune checkpoint inhibitors: a systematic review. *Ann Oncol.* 2017;28(10): 2377-2385. doi:10.1093/annonc/mdx286.

131. Schubert ML, Schmitt M, Wang L, et al. Side-effect management of chimeric antigen receptor (CAR) T-cell therapy. *Ann Oncol.* 2021;32(1):34-48. doi:10.1016/j.annonc.2020.10.478.
132. Lee DW, Santomasso BD, Locke FL, et al. ASTCT Consensus Grading for cytokine release syndrome and neurologic toxicity associated with immune effector cells. *Biol Blood Marrow Transplant.* 2019;25(4): 625-638. doi:10.1016/j.bbmt.2018.12.758.
133. Ramnaraign BH, Chatzkel JA, Al-Mansour ZA, et al. Immunotherapy management in special cancer patient populations. *JCO Oncol Pract.* 2021;17(5):240-245. doi:10.1200/op.20.00996.
134. Gibney GT, Weiner LM, Atkins MB. Predictive biomarkers for checkpoint inhibitor-based immunotherapy. *Lancet Oncol.* 2016;17(12):e542-e551. doi:10.1016/s1470-2045(16)30406-5.

Visit Elsevier eBooks + (eBooks.Health.Elsevier.com) for complete set of references.

CHAPTER 13

The Effect of COVID-19 on Cancer Immunotherapy and Cancer Care

John E. Niederhuber

SUMMARY OF KEY FACTS

- SARS-CoV-2 was initially detected in December 2019 and is an enveloped, single-stranded RNA virus causing an extremely contagious severe respiratory illness with a high rate of mortality.
- Whole genome sequencing confirmed COVID-19 to be 79.6% similar to SARS and MERS, which belong to β-CoV genera, one of four identified coronavirus genera.
- SARS-CoV-2 is a respiratory virus and spreads mainly through person-to-person contact and inhalation of microdroplets and aerosols containing viral particles.
- To establish infection, the COVID-19 virus must target and enter cells to undertake viral replication. It does so through the virus S1 subunit of the spike protein, which binds to the human angiotensin-converting enzyme-2 (ACE2) receptor on host cells.
- Τηε World Health Organization declared SARS-CoV-2 (COVID-19) a global pandemic on March 11, 2020.
- Health care systems were rapidly overwhelmed with critically ill patients with COVID-19, causing significant disruptions in delivery of active cancer therapy and cancer screening.
- mRNA expression of ACE2 is upregulated in renal cell cancer, gastrointestinal cancer, and lung adenocarcinoma. ACE2 upregulation also correlates with increased PD-L1 expression.
- The promotor of ACE2 expression is hypomethylated during COVID-19 infection.
- Initial COVID-19 innate immune response occurs by germ-line encoded pattern recognition receptors (PRRs) and their recognition of viral PAMPs and infected host cell DAMPs (cDAMPs and iDAMPs). PRRs involve the Toll-like receptors, especially TLR-7, in innate system immunity.
- A weakened innate immune system response may be observed in individuals of advanced age, with obesity, and with associated chronic diseases including cancer.
- Patients with cancer have been highly vulnerable to COVID-19 infection, especially patients with hematologic malignancies, lung cancer, and patients receiving B-cell targeted therapy.
- Excessive and prolonged innate immune system response with secretion of cytokines in response to COVID-19 infection may cause organ damage (especially lung) in patients already responding to cancer and cancer immune therapies. High levels of cytokines correlate with greater COVID-19 morbidity and mortality.
- Increasing evidence supports infection-induced genetic alterations generating a form of innate response immunity/memory to infecting agents.

Continued on following page

SUMMARY OF KEY FACTS—cont'd

- Innate immune response goals are to (1) eliminate COVID-19 virus replication, (2) establish a proinflammatory response to kill infected cells, and (3) rapidly prime the antigen-specific adaptive immune response.
- Adaptive system goals are (1) generation of antigen-specific B-cell neutralizing antibodies, (2) expansion of antigen-specific cytotoxic $CD8^+$ T cells to eliminate virus infected cells, and 3) expansion of activated $CD4^+$ subpopulations and robust lymphocyte-based immune memory.
- The response of T lymphocytes is critical to surviving the COVID-19 acute infection and generating a robust vaccination response.
- Frequent reverse transcription polymerase chain reaction (RT-PCR) testing and timing of the use of vaccination are key to safely managing the patient with cancer during the COVID-19 pandemic.
- Evidence is accumulating that immune checkpoint inhibitor therapy does not predict a worse course or outcome if such patients become COVID-19 positive. Combination immunotherapy appears safe with careful patient selection and monitoring for the vaccinated patient with cancer.
- Avoiding therapy-induced lymphopenia (anti-CD20 therapy and chemotherapy are examples of lymphopenia inducing anti-cancer therapies) should be the goal by carefully managing therapy to minimize infection risk.

Introduction

The world of cancer care continues to be significantly affected by the severe acute respiratory syndrome coronavirus-2 (SARS-CoV-2; coronavirus disease 2019 [COVID-19]) global pandemic. COVID-19 has demonstrated unprecedented transmissibility as a highly infectious RNA respiratory virus causing serious morbidity and mortality. On March 11, 2020, the World Health Organization declared COVID-19 a global pandemic.[1] Health care systems everywhere were quickly overwhelmed as they were called upon to provide hospitalization for a sudden tremendous surge in COVID-19-infected patients. Hospitalized patients with COVID-19 often required intensive care (ICU) beds and ventilator support for severe respiratory distress. As expected, it was quickly observed that individuals with malignant disease were at a higher risk for COVID-19 infection and for having greater disease severity and mortality.[2-5] The tremendous effect of the pandemic on health care systems and health care workers immediately caused disruptions to the delivery of normal cancer care, both anticancer therapy and cancer screening. Patients with cancer frequently delayed or abandoned active treatment out of fear of becoming infected if they were to actually go to their point of care.[6,7]

Stressed hospitals were forced to delay surgical procedures. Cancer clinical trials were severally limited or even placed on hold as staff had to be shifted to COVID-19 patient care and research support staff was transferred to remote work. At major academic centers, clinical investigators were called upon to urgently shift their focus to COVID-19 research. At Johns Hopkins, a special COVID-19 Institutional Review Board (IRB) was established and throughout the remainder of 2020 and 2021 met every day of the week to expedite proposed COVID-19 research protocol reviews. By the end of 2020, there was a glimmer of hope, as safety and efficacy data generated by large-scale clinical trials of several candidate vaccines received U.S. Food and Drug Administration (FDA) review and emergency use authorization (EUA) in the United States as well as review and similar approval in other countries.[8-12]

Over the months since the introduction of the vaccines and priority access to vaccination for patients with cancer, cancer care, cancer research, and cancer screening have gradually begun to return to prepandemic status. Even with the current much lower incidence of infections in the population, it will take some time to completely understand the true disruption that COVID-19 has had on the incidence and mortality caused by cancer. Though the vaccines have had a major effect, it is important to recognize that the pandemic continues. On March 10, 2022, the Johns Hopkins Coronavirus Resource Center website reported that the number of global COVID-19 documented cases for the previous 28 days was 48,132,252, with 242,345 deaths. In the United States the 28-day total cases were 2,107,247 and there were 49,440 deaths. The total number of individuals documented as dying from COVID-19 in the United States since the beginning of the outbreak had reached 965,069. Many believe this to be a significant underestimation.[13]

During the 2 years since January 2020, much has been learned about this specific coronavirus, and much knowledge has been gained regarding the public health management of a serious viral pandemic. Though there exists considerable knowledge regarding the innate and adaptive immune responses and the heterogeneity of those responses to tumors of different organ sites and histologies, there is still much to learn regarding the effect of COVID-19 infection on the existing anticancer immune response and on the timing of cancer therapies, especially immunotherapy. Such knowledge regarding COVID-19's effect on cancer immune therapies is aided to some degree by previous experience in many patients with cancer harboring other chronic infections such as human immunodeficiency virus (HIV), human papillomavirus (HPV), hepatitis B, and hepatitis C.[14] This chapter will attempt to summarize what we currently know regarding COVID-19 and to do so in the context of malignancy and anticancer immune therapy.

The Emergence and Global Effect of SARS-CoV-2

In early December 2019, there was increasing awareness regarding an outbreak of a serious and novel life-threating acute respiratory viral illness spreading in and around the city of Wuhan in the Hubei Province of China. The exact origin of this virus has been an ongoing debate, with considerable difficulty encountered by epidemiologists in exercising a full-force investigation. The early cases of the severe respiratory illness were said to be related to an open-air market located in Wuhan, China. By January 26, 2020, there were 2794 laboratory-confirmed cases resulting in 80 deaths and evidence documenting the beginnings of global spread to at least 33 individuals in 10 countries.[2]

A complete genome sequence of isolates from hospitalized patients documented the causative agent to be an RNA coronavirus virus. The complete sequence was initially obtained by scientists at the Wuhan Institute of Virology, Center for Biosafety Mega-Science, Chinese Academy of Sciences, Wuhan, China.[2] The initial sequence and subsequent analysis was based on specimens obtained from seven severely ill hospitalized patients in Wuhan and showed that the novel disease-causing virus was 96% identical to a bat coronavirus and shared 79.6% sequence identity with viruses known to cause SARS.[2,15] Coronaviruses have previously been determined to cause SARS and Middle East respiratory syndrome (MERS).[3-12,14-18]

Spread of the COVID-19 respiratory virus is mainly through person-to-person contact and the inhalation of microdroplets and aerosols containing viral particles. This occurs when an infected person coughs, sneezes, or simply talks during direct person-to-person contact.[19-21] Less common modes of spread include a fecal–oral route, leading to identification of the virus in site-specific sewage and in wastewater at municipal treatment plants.[22-25] There has been evidence in a small percentage of cases of vertical maternal transmission to the newborn especially occurring during late stages of pregnancy.[19]

SARS-CoV-2 causes nasopharyngeal and lower respiratory tract infections. Most infections appear to be mild, and though it is difficult to be certain, somewhere between 20% and 40% of those infected are asymptomatic or only mildly symptomatic.[26-30] However, for a great number of patients the disease is much more severe, leading to hospitalization and acute respiratory distress syndrome (ARDS). Patients requiring hospitalization can present with a severe interstitial pneumonia, sometimes further complicated by systemic inflammation, thromboembolic events, evidence of cardiac complications, and massive cytokine release.[2,20,26-32] Currently recognized risks for severe disease requiring hospitalization include lack of complete vaccination and medical comorbidities such as immunodeficiency, obesity, cardiopulmonary diseases, and cancer.[33] During the beginning of the pandemic, the risk of COVID-19 infection was estimated to be seven times greater for the patient with cancer and even greater for the non-White population of patients with cancer.[34,35]

COVID-19 rapidly became a pandemic, putting extreme pressure on health care workers and the infrastructure of health care systems. Despite well-proven public health measures required to manage a global pandemic caused by a rapidly spreading respiratory virus, the attempted implementation of these measures in the United States became a major political challenge. This unfortunate turn of events and the lack of our medical system's preparedness for such an occurrence will certainly be the subject of debate for many years to come. At the time of this writing, we are improving from the latest wave of COVID-19, Omicron BA.1, but by no means are we able to declare that the pandemic is behind us as Omicron BA.2 begins to spread in the United States (https://coronavirus.jhu.edu/map.html, accessed March 10, 2022).[13] We must continue to be vigilant, increase the rate of maximum vaccination, increase the ease and availability of testing, and, above all, significantly enhance our genetic surveillance searching for new viral variants. One important lesson to be learned from our experience attempting to manage this global pandemic is the tremendous need for public education regarding the very basics of infectious disease and the methodologies of sound public health to minimize the effect of future pandemics.

The vast global and extremely rapid spread of COVID-19 provides significant opportunities for the occurrence of viral mutations as the virus replicates within the host's cells, producing new variants of the virus. The world has already experienced the challenges of several of these new variants of the original COVID-19, namely, Delta and Omicron BA.1 and BA.2.[22,36] The U.S. government through the Centers for Disease Control and Prevention (CDC) has significantly increased its approach to population sampling and virus sequencing in an effort to stay ahead of the development of new COVID-19 variants circulating in the population. The CDC has established a classification process for new COVID-19 variants that places newly identified viral variants into one of three groups: variants of interest, variants of concern, and variants of high consequence[22] (for in-depth review, see Xu et al.[22]).

SARS-CoV-2 Structure and Biology

SARS-CoV-2 (COVID-19) is an enveloped, single-stranded RNA virus and has proved to cause an extremely infectious and severe respiratory illness with clinical features of fever, cough, dyspnea, malaise, severe rapidly progressing interstitial pneumonia, and acute respiratory distress syndrome (ARDS).[30] SARS-CoV, MERS-CoV, and COVID-19 all belong to the β-CoV genera, one of the four described *Coronaviridae* genera.[3,37] Currently the β-CoV subgroup is recognized as having the highest human mortality rates among the four coronavirus genera.[3,19,20]

Structurally, COVID-19 is composed of four major proteins: the spike protein (S); the nucleocapsid protein (N); the membrane protein (M), which has a short N-terminal ectodomain with a cytoplasmic tail; and the hydrophobic envelope protein (E).[22,37] The nucleocapsid protein (N) is complexed with the genomic RNA to form a helical capsid. The spike or S protein is a type 1 glycoprotein that forms peplomers on the virus surface. The RNA virus has several open reading frames (ORFs) encoding accessory proteins (Fig. 13.1).[37-39]

The respiratory tract is the primary site for viral particle entry in humans. The main transmission of the virus occurs in the form of COVID-19 encapsulated virus particle aerosols and

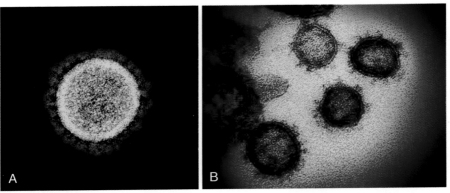

Fig. 13.1   (A) A microscopic image of a SARS-CoV-2 virion. Coronaviruses are named for the appearance of a halo or crown when viewed under a microscope. (B) An electron microscope photo of a cluster of SARS-CoV-2 virions. Courtesy the U.S. National Institute of Allergy and Infectious Diseases.

microdroplets released by infected hosts. For the virus to survive and replicate, it must enter into host cells.[40,41] This occurs via the S1 subunit of the spike protein on the virus surface that recognizes and binds to the human angiotensin-converting enzyme-2 (hACE-2) receptor expressed on respiratory tract cells, vascular endothelium, cardiovascular tissue, renal tissues, and intestinal epithelium.[19,22,42-44] The normal function of ACE2 is to convert angiotensin II to angiotensin-(1-7).[45] A serine protease, TMPRSS2, is also involved and acts to prime the S protein for ACE2 binding and host cell entry.[46]

The host cell entry process is assisted by other proteins including neurophilin-1, heparin sulfate proteoglycans, and C-type lectins.[47-50] In the infected cell cytoplasm, the viral RNA is translated into two polyproteins pp1a and pp1ab and 16 nonstructural proteins that function to form the viral replication–transcription complex generating an antisense negative-strand template of the viral RNA.[51] Double-membrane vesicles formed from membranes of the endoplasmic reticulum (ER) and the Golgi compartmentalize and isolate within the cytoplasm the process of viral replication.[52] The assembly of new viral particles within the ER–Golgi compartment generates virion-containing vesicles that fuse with the host cell plasma membrane for exocytosis and release of the virus into the extracellular space.[53,54] From these several steps in the pathologic process of viral infection and replication, there are numerous opportunities for the virus to be recognized as nonself, to initiate a host inflammatory response, and to first activate the innate immune response, followed quickly by the more critical adaptive immune system response (Fig. 13.2)[54] (for in-depth review, see Diamond and Kanneganti[54]).

The Angiotensin-Converting Enzyme 2, SARS-CoV-2 Infection, and Cancer

Angiotensin-converting enzyme 2 (ACE2) is the cell surface receptor required for SARS-CoV-2 entrance into the host cells.[46,55,56] As expected, studies quantitating the expression of ACE2 in various tissues correlate both the risk of becoming infected and the severity of the viral infection.[55,57,58] Ren and colleagues reported studies early in the pandemic (March 2020) focused on determining the level of ACE2 expression in normal patient tissues and in tissues of patients with cancer.[59] Their studies using primarily the Gene Expression Profiling Interactive Analysis (GEPIA) database and ONCOMINE to compare mRNA expression of ACE2 in tissues found that the kidneys, duodenum, intestine, gallbladder, and testis had the highest level of ACE2

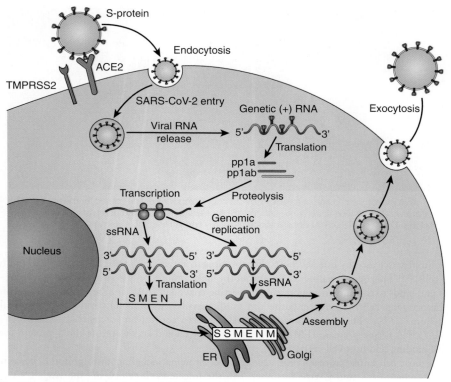

Fig. 13.2 A schematic depiction of SARS-CoV-2 viral entry into an epithelial cell to undergo virus replication. Depiction of the replication cycle illustrates COVID-19 virus spike (S) protein binding to ACE2 receptor on the cell surface. Entry is facilitated by a serine protease TMPRSS2 that cleaves the COVID-19 S protein. Viral entry involves fusion with the extracellular membrane and endocytosis. After entry, viral RNA is released and translated into viral polyproteins pp1a and pp1ab. Pp1a and pp1ab are further processed by virus-encoded proteases to produce full-length negative-strand viral RNA and viral subgenomic RNA. The latter is translated into structural and accessory proteins including spike (S), membrane (M), envelope (E), and nucleocapsid (N). S, E, M, and N proteins are inserted into the endoplasmic reticulum (ER) and Golgi membranes and transferred to an intermediate compartment where, along with newly synthesized COVID-19 single-stranded viral RNA (ssRNA), a new virion is formed and undergoes exocytosis as a new COVID-19 viral particle. Adapted from several sources including Diamond and Kanneganti.[54]

expression. The colon, rectum, and seminal vesicles displayed a moderate level of expression, with the lungs having the lowest expression.[59]

ACE2 is recognized to have a significant role in cancer prognosis, demonstrating a protective anticancer effect.[60] In these studies, ACE2 expression was upregulated in renal cancer, gastrointestinal tumors, and lung cancer.[59] Other studies of malignant tumors and cancer cell lines suggest that essentially all cancer tissues can express ACE2.[61] Studies indicated that ACE2 is overexpressed in colon adenocarcinoma, renal papillary cell carcinoma, pancreatic adenocarcinoma, rectal adenocarcinoma, gastric adenocarcinoma, and lung adenocarcinoma.[56,58,59,62]

In patients with cancer infected with COVID-19, there is evidence that the promotor for ACE2 expression is hypomethylated but not to the degree that it is in non-COVID-19-infected patients with cancer.[58,62] Studies documenting the importance of the level of ACE2 expression in patients with cancer demonstrate that upregulation of ACE2 in multiple cancer types is associated with suppression of multiple oncogenic pathways, including cell cycle proteins, vascular endothelial growth factor (VEGF), transforming growth factor beta (TGF-β), and the Wnt and Notch signaling pathways.[63] Increased levels of ACE2 in cancer are also directly correlated with enhancement of an antitumor immune response.[64-66] Taken together, ACE2 upregulation results in enhanced disease prognosis. More specific to the use of immunotherapies in cancer, ACE2 expression has been shown to directly correlate with expression of programmed death ligand 1 (PD-L1) in patients with cancer.[66] Tumors express PD-L1 to varying degrees, which binds to T cells, causing immunosuppression of the antitumor immune response and tumor progression.

SARS-CoV-2 Viral Infection and Innate Immunity

The infection and host inflammatory response is initiated by the binding of the COVID-19 S1 glycoprotein to the ACE2 receptor on the target cell membrane followed by entry of a viral RNA genome into the target cell cytoplasm. Studies show that the infected cells, shortly after viral entry, stimulate local inflammatory cells to secrete interleukin (IL)-8, which functions as a chemoattractant for monocytes and macrophages, dendritic cells, neutrophils, and T lymphocytes. These form the first stage of inflammation initiating the innate immune response to COVID-19 infection.[67]

Host cell–based sensors may detect the COVID-19 virion during this initial ACE2 binding process. This recognition occurs through pathogen-associated molecular patterns (PAMPs) and damage-associated molecular patterns (DAMPS) that occur within the inflammatory cells responding to the invading virus. PAMPs are evolutionarily highly conserved pathogen-specific structures on the invading COVID-19 virus. DAMPs (sometimes termed *alarmins*) are self molecules found in tissue macrophages and monocyte-derived macrophages under conditions of cell stress and cell damage as occurs with viral infection–induced inflammation. DAMPs are a heterogeneous group of host inflammatory cell–derived molecules and have been classed as continuous DAMPs (cDAMPs) and inducible DAMPs (iDAMPs).[68-71]

The host has a limited but quite effective number of germ line-encoded pattern recognition receptors (PRRs). In the case of COVID-19 infection, PPRs have been shown to involve the family of Toll-like receptors (TLRs), especially TLR-7. These PPR TLRs recognize PAMPs and DAMPs that are present in the infected cell's endosomes, resulting in secretion of a number of inflammatory cytokines. Other PRRs, such as retinoid acid–inducible gene I (RIG-I)-like receptors (RLRs), nucleotide-binding oligomerization domain (NOD)-like receptors (NLRs), C-type lectin receptors, and absent in melanoma 2 (AIM2)-like receptors also contribute to the initial virus-induced inflammatory response.[71-73]

There are a number of innate immune system cells that provide the source of PRRs capable of the early recognition of the COVID-19 array of PAMPs and DAMPs, including tissue resident macrophages, monocytes, antigen-presenting dendritic cells, neutrophils, cytotoxic natural killer (NK) cells, and gamma delta T lymphocytes (γδT cells). Many of these cell types are rapidly recruited by the initial PRR's, recognition of COVID-19 PAMPs and infected host cell DAMPs. The result is the initial release of interferon gamma (IFN-γ) and IL-8 followed by cytokines IL-1β, IL-6, TNF, IL-12, IL-18, and others along with a number of chemoattractants.[54]

The Toll-like receptor TLR-7 is expressed on monocytes–macrophages and dendritic cells. TLR-7 activates several key signaling pathways and transcription factors such as Janus kinase/signal transducer and activator of transcription (JAK/STAT), nuclear factor κB (NF-κB), activator protein 1 (AP-1), interferon response factor 3 (IRF3), and IRF7. In the next stage, the virus and the initial inflammatory response acts to trigger an adaptive immune response involving T and B lymphocytes. It should be noted that much of the knowledge regarding the immune system's response to SARS-CoV-2 comes from studies of prior coronaviruses SARS and MERS.[74,75] Neutrophils are rapidly recruited to sites of viral infection where extracellular traps (NETS) trap and eliminate virus and virus infected cells.[76]

For SARS-CoV-2 to be the cause of such a destructive global pandemic, it must have ways in which it can successfully evade immune attack. One therefore can conclude that COVID-19 is very capable of evading the initial innate recognition and innate system immune response. Failure to control the early stage of COVID-19 infection and a high risk of hospitalization, serious morbidity such as ARDS, and mortality has been associated with lack of early IFN I and IFN III responses leading to an ineffective or delayed innate immune response. Elevated C-X-C motif chemokine ligand 10 (CXCL 10), IL-6, and IL-8 in patients with COVID-19 appear to be indicators of a weak or delayed innate immune response. This provides the COVID-19 virus with a damaging head start and, most important, a significant delay in the innate immune system's priming of the adaptive anti-COVID-19 antigen-specific immune response.[77]

A weakened innate immune system response may be observed in individuals of advanced age, those with obesity, and those with other chronic diseases such as cancer, all known to affect the integrity of the host immune response. A concern in patients with COVID-19 with a compromised immune system must be the occurrence of a prolonged and overactive innate immune response that tries to overcome the lack of a good adaptive immune response. The excessive and prolonged secretion of cytokines and chemokines cause an increased inflammatory response with organ damage, especially damage to the lung. There is increasing evidence in patient studies that the cytokine profile of COVID-19 appears unique to the virus compared with other infections and inflammatory states. The presence of high levels of cytokines does correlate with a greater COVID-19 morbidity and mortality.[54,78-81]

In recent years (2010-2022) and perhaps relevant to individual susceptibility to SARS-CoV-2 infection, there has been experimental evidence supporting the presence of "innate immune memory" or "trained immunity."[71] This is a significant change in our understanding of the innate immune system. The concept of innate immune memory was first suggested in 2007 by experiments that observed histone modifications to be present in macrophages responding to bacterial-derived lipopolysaccharide (LPS).[82] These findings were supported by others demonstrating that there were other stimuli of the innate immune response that also produced specific persistent changes of histone acetylation and methylation resulting in a persistent alteration of the innate immune response to those stimuli. This form of innate immune system memory involves long-term changes in gene transcription.[71,83-87]

Recognizing that trained immunity in the innate immune system is a relatively new discovery raises a number of important questions regarding exactly when this memory response is positive for the host and when it might be detrimental. In addition, how does innate memory correlate with an early and/or enhanced adaptive immune response? Is there a role for trained immunity in the innate system with the initiation of cancer and cancer surveillance? These critical questions will be the subject of exciting future research.

One of the most worrisome effects of acute COVID-19 infection in the patient with cancer is an overly aggressive innate immune response to the virus inducing a massive release of a variety of cytokines, resulting in cytokine storm or, as it is more appropriately termed, cytokine release syndrome (CRS), causing added damage to the lung and other critical organ tissues.[88] Patients with cancer undergoing new immune-stimulating anticancer therapies such as immune checkpoint inhibitors (ICIs), chimeric antigen receptor (CAR) T-cell therapies, and bispecific T-cell engagers (BiTEs) have the potential, if infected with COVID-19, of experiencing an enhanced CRS, causing an even more aggressive COVID-19 attack and severe physiologic complications secondary to an immune attack on normal tissues.

Clearly, in the majority of COVID-19 cases the initial host innate immune response is sufficient to effectively clear the COVID-19 virus, as it does so often with the many viruses we regularly encounter. There are several goals of this initial host recognition of SARS-CoV-2 infection by the cells that comprise the innate immune response. The first goal is to eliminate replication of the virus. The second is to induce production of a number of cytokines and chemoattractants to establish a proinflammatory response to eliminate infected host cells and, third, to rapidly prime the process of adaptive antigen-specific immune activation, culminating in the production of neutralizing antibodies and cytotoxic T lymphocytes[89] (for an in-depth review, see Mogensen[89]).

Though this is just the early phase of research to carefully define the many aspects of the innate immune system's response to COVID-19, there are some important messages from these initial studies and from past efforts to clarify the protective role that the innate immune system plays regarding viral infections. For example, it has become clear that the innate immune system has a great deal of actual specificity through PRRs providing the host with the ability to quickly recognize nonself. Further, there exists a much greater connectivity between the innate response and the activation and imprinting of the adaptive immune response than was previously believed. In addition, there is now increasing evidence indicating the occurrence of genetic reprogramming of the cells involved in innate immunity to generate innate response memory. This latter observation holds significant promise regarding our resistance to cancer initiation as well.

The Adaptive Immune Response to SARS-CoV-2 Infection

The adaptive immune system comprises three major cell types, B lymphocytes, CD4+ T lymphocytes, and CD8+ T lymphocytes. B lymphocytes are the producers of the anti-COVID-19 neutralizing antibodies. CD4+ T lymphocytes are responsible for evolving a number of different T-cell subpopulations including T helper cells (Th1, Th2), T regulator cells, and other T cells with a variety of functional roles, including assisting the B-cell humoral response. The acute immune response to COVID-19 rapidly stimulates naïve CD8+ T lymphocytes to undergo antigen-specific vigorous proliferation to become antigen-specific cytotoxic cells (CTLs).[90,91] These three major cell populations of the immune system provide highly restricted antigen-specific recognition of the COVID-19 virus.

In response to the COVID-19 infection, the lymphocyte populations function in an integrated and complex fashion to generate SARS-CoV-2-specific neutralizing antibodies, to generate cytotoxic T lymphocytes to kill virus-infected cells, and, importantly, to create long-lasting host immunity through a successful response to the infection and, of course, through vaccination. The level of response and the balance of each of the involved lymphocyte subpopulations in the adaptive immune response is host dependent and influenced by comorbid diseases such as cancer. A healthy adaptive immune system capable of COVID-19 antigen-specific recognition and the generation of robust immune memory is key to a successful vaccination program and protection of patients with cancer against the risk of serious COVID-19 disease[89,91-94] (for an in-depth review, see Sette and Crotty[94]).

With the priming assistance of the front-line response by the innate immune system, viral COVID-19 antigen(s) are presented in the context of major histocompatibility complex (MHC) class I and MHC class II molecules to stimulate antigen-specific humoral and cellular immunity. COVID-19 antigen presentation and cellular response occurs approximately on days 7 to 14 from the onset of COVID-19 disease. Viral antigens are presented by antigen-presenting cells (APCs) to antigen-specific B cells, which produce specific antiviral neutralizing antibodies, and to antigen-specific CD4$^+$ and CD8$^+$ T cells. Antigen-specific CD8$^+$ cytotoxic T cells recognize and kill virus-infected cells.[67,95] The antigen triggering of the CD4$^+$ T lymphocytes results in an aggressive antiviral inflammatory response and the differentiation of additional T-cell subtypes with unique supporting functions.

The B-cell antibody response occurs with the assistance of antigen recognition by T cells and includes the production of immunoglobulin (Ig) M, IgG, and IgA neutralizing antibodies that have been confirmed to recognize antigenic determinants of the spike glycoprotein and of the nucleocapsid.[96,97] Studies demonstrate that seroconversion occurs within 5 to 15 days of initial infection with 90% conversion by day 10 of infection.[98] Observations in patients with COVID-19 indicate that the antibody response to the virus develops rapidly and primarily from naïve B cells and not from B cells with any memory to coronaviruses in general.[99] It has been suggested that the B-cell responses in infected patients appear to be lower than expected, especially in the severely ill. Further, the presence of a demonstrable Fc antibody-dependent cytotoxic component of the immune response to the virus is fairly negligible. Severity of COVID-19 disease has been strongly correlated with the level of neutralizing antibody.[100]

Alejo and colleagues, of the Department of Surgery, Johns Hopkins University School of Medicine, reported a study of healthy unvaccinated adults recruited between September 11, 2021, and October 8, 2021.[101] They divided the cohort into the following three groups: (1) 295 subjects laboratory confirmed to have experienced a COVID-19 infection, (2) 275 subjects unconfirmed but who believed they had been infected, and (3) 246 subjects who never tested positive and believed they were never infected. Antibodies to SARS-CoV-2 spike protein receptor-binding domain (RBD) were detected in 99% of individuals in group 1, in 55% of group 2, and in 11% of group 3. Anti-RBD antibodies were observed after a confirmed positive COVID-19 test for up to 20 months. Though these findings are encouraging, it remains to be demonstrated how serologic testing results may correlate with actual immunity.[101,102]

CD8[+] T cells are the T-lymphocyte cell population with the major responsibility for clearance of the COVID-19 disease. They do so through their ability to directly destroy infected cells. SARS-CoV-2-specific CD8[+] T cells have been detected very early in the disease and have been shown to recognize a range of COVID-19 antigens, primarily spike, nucleocapsid determinants, M-determinants, and ORF3a.[90,92,103] A demonstrated strong CD8[+] T-cell response correlates with a more favorable outcome to infection, which is also common for other severe viral infections such as SARS and MERS. Post-COVID-19 infection and after complete vaccination, protection from recurrent or breakthrough infection is strongly supported by the presence of memory SARS-CoV-2 CD8[+] T cells.[94]

CD4[+] T cells can be considered to be the more functionally critical lymphoid cells to achieving a successful overall adaptive immune response to COVID-19. Antigen-specific CD4[+] T cells, especially those specific to the spike antigenic determinants, are critically involved in supporting the generation of antigen-specific B-cell neutralizing antibodies. Antigen-specific CD4[+] T cells are detectable early in the infection, and the robustness of the CD4[+] T-cell response is more strongly associated with less severity of infection than the level of B-cell and CD8[+] T-cell responses.[90] In COVID-19, CD4[+] T cells differentiate into Th1 cells and T-follicular helper cells (Tfh) that directly support B-cell responses. Th1 cells produce antiviral IFN-γ and a variety of antiviral cytokines. CD4[+] T lymphocytes are also responsible for developing a critical memory element of the disease and from vaccination.[104-106] Observations in patients infected with SARS-CoV-2 also showed that the response of the T lymphocytes is critically important to ultimately surviving the disease. Importantly, the response in T cells is critical to the development of strong protection against the disease via vaccination[106] (for an in-depth review, see Shrotri et al.[106]).

COVID-19 Infection in Patients With Cancer

As with any viral infectious disease, a robust, healthy immune system is essential to fighting the infection and to mounting a strong protective antiviral vaccine response. There are striking similarities between the host's immune response to acute virus challenge and the response of the immune system to cancer initiation and progression. As we have seen, both challenges involve similar host cell populations and generate very similar inflammatory responses and humoral neutralizing antibody and antigen-specific T-cell immune responses.

Cancer, however, is a heterogeneous group of diseases with the resultant variability in the malignancy's interaction with the host immune system. The antitumor immune response can be further altered by active therapeutic interventions including surgery and the effect of tissue injury, radiation with tissue damage, chemotherapy, and, more recently, immunotherapy. As a consequence, one can assume that in the patient with cancer there is immune imbalance.[107-109] This immune imbalance in the patient with cancer creates a challenge to treating physicians in terms of managing the patient's response to the added burden of an active COVID-19 infection or simply to the ever-present risk of COVID-19 infection.

Evidence accumulated during the pandemic has confirmed that T-cell immunity, in contrast to humoral immunity, is the critical component of survival from SARS-CoV-2 infection and also for long-term vaccine protection against COVID-19. Studies have proposed the importance of the balance in the roles of Th1 versus Th2 cells in fighting the invading virus and in developing long-term immunity. The balance or differences between the roles of Th1 and Th2 and their functional integrity exist in the portfolio of cytokines unique to each subtype and the potential for cytolytic activities generated by each CD4[+] T-cell subtype. The balance between Th1 and Th2 response may, of course, be altered in cancer and therefore relevant to the development of a robust anti-COVID-19 immune response. A robustness in the integrity of Th1/Tc1 also appears particularly important to the development of vaccination-induced strong immunity. Perhaps in the future, being able to test for the Th1/Tc1 ratio and Th2 balance in functional T-cell integrity will be useful in optimizing the design of future antiviral vaccines.[109]

To further expand on the relevance of the Th1/Th2 CD4[+] subtypes, it is worth examining a recent extensive prospective cross-sectional analysis of several groups of healthy subjects and patients with cancer. In this study, investigators attempted to determine how the virus-specific T cell correlates of protection against COVID-19 infection are affected by the presence of cancer. They found that an imbalance between Th1/Th2 population recall responses conferred a greater susceptibility to COVID-19 in both cancer and noncancer populations. A more robust Th1/Tc1 level of immunity and their respective cytokines (IL-2/IL-5 ratio > 1) appeared to be significantly more protective against infection by COVID-19.[108] The results of these studies suggest that any defects/weaknesses in the performance of the Th1/Tc1 response affecting the recognition of the COVID-19 S1-RBD are associated with an increased susceptibility to infection by COVID-19. Importantly, the Th1/Tc1 defect was more prominent in patients with hematologic malignancies.[110]

As anticipated, COVID-19 infection can be especially challenging for the patient with cancer undergoing treatment, especially anticancer immunotherapies or therapies that are immunosuppressive. As it progresses, cancer generates a network of stromal cells and inflammatory immune cells. Early in the onset of the pandemic, it appeared that of COVID-19-infected patients, approximately 2% were being actively treated for cancer.[5,111] Multiple studies have reported that patients with cancer have a greater incidence of complications and mortality if they develop COVID-19 infection that is severe enough to require hospitalization. The hospitalized COVID-19-infected patient with cancer has a reported 30-day mortality rate of ~30% compared with 21% for noncancer patients.[5,112,113] As a result, there is consensus regarding the high priority for vaccination of patients with cancer, including those actively receiving therapy. Exceptions to this recommendation includes patients undergoing stem cell transplantation and adoptive cell-based therapy. Vaccination of these patients should be delayed appropriately until the immune system has had adequate time for recovery.

The cancer inflammatory process consists of antitumor immune responses and protumor inflammation blocking antitumor immunity as well as exerting tumor promoting signals.[114] The acute immune response to COVID-19 stimulates naïve CD8[+] T cells to undergo vigorous proliferation and differentiation to become effective killer cells like the natural killer (NK) cells of the first line of antiviral immune defense. The innate immune system response is directed against infected cells harboring the virus and expressing specific viral antigens. These viral antigens are presented in the context of MHC class I and class II molecules to the cells of the adaptive immune system. The resultant T-cell response is also associated with the release of a number of different inflammatory cytokines and chemokines.

Upon COVID-19 activation, CD8[+] T cells express increased numbers of inhibitory receptors (immune checkpoints) such as PD-1, Cytotoxic T-lymphocyte Antigen-4 (CTLA-4), and others that function to control for an excessive response to antigenic stimulation and, in doing so, avoid any damage to self tissues.[115] Once the CD8[+] T cells have accomplished clearance of the COVID-19-infected cells, the majority of these antigen-specific T cells undergo activation-induced cell death and are cleared, with a small percentage remaining as CD8[+] antigen-specific memory cells.[116,117]

For the patient with cancer infected with COVID-19, there exists the concern that their CD8[+] T cells, in responding to a progressing tumor, are already undergoing a chronic intense exposure to a variety of specific tumor antigens and are being pushed to their limits of potential immune response. This raises the possibility that if infected by the COVID-19 virus, the added CD4[+] and CD8[+] antigen stimulation could result in a phenomenon known as *T-cell exhaustion*. T-cell exhaustion results in a decreased production of effector cytokines such as IL-2, decreased T-cell proliferation, impaired cytotoxicity, and decreased production of antigen-specific memory cells.[115,118]

Patients with cancer undergoing chemotherapy and/or immunotherapy are recognized as having a weakened or altered immune response of both innate and adaptive immune systems. Cancer, more commonly a disease among those of older age (>65 years), is commonly associated with other diseases such as obesity, type 2 diabetes, and cardiopulmonary disease. These comorbidities may further compromise the integrity of the immune system. As a result, patients with cancer are at a greater risk for contracting infectious diseases, especially when faced with the severity of the current SARS-CoV-2 pandemic.[34,56,119] In a report by Lee and associates comparing cohorts of patients with cancer with and without COVID-19 infection in the United Kingdom, patients with hematologic malignancies experienced a more serious COVID-19 infection (odds ratio [OR] = 1.57; 95% confidence interval [CI], 1.15–2.15; $P < .0043$).[120] The in-hospital mortality for those patients recently receiving chemotherapy who became infected with COVID-19 was also increased (OR = 2.09; 95% CI, 1.09–4.08; $P = .028$).[56,120]

SARS-CoV-2 viral load has been reported to be an independent predictor for in-hospital mortality in patients with cancer contracting COVID-19. Patients with documented high, mid-range, or low viral load had mortality rates of 45.2%, 28%, and 12.1%, respectively ($P = .008$).[121] Jee and colleagues reported that both the severity of the hematologic malignancy in patients and the severity of the lung cancer stage in patients with lung cancer were predictive of an increase in the severity of a COVID-19 infection.[122] An interesting observation by Kong and colleagues suggests that patients with lung adenocarcinoma were actually more at risk of contracting COVID-19 infection than patients with squamous cell lung cancer.[123] Clearly, because the major feature of COVID-19 infection is pulmonary, patients with lung cancer are at higher risk of experiencing a more serious course of COVID-19 than patients with other solid tumor malignancies.

COVID-19 Vaccination and the Patient With Cancer

The protection of patients with cancer from the devastating morbidities and added mortality associated with infection by SARS-CoV-2 depends on the physical protective measures of masking and upon achieving long-term B- and T-cell immune memory protection by adequate vaccination.[8,124] As the year 2020 came to a close, the FDA had reviewed the results of clinical trials and granted emergency use authorization to two lipid nanoparticle-formulated, nucleoside-modified mRNA vaccines that encoded the S1 spike glycol of SARS-CoV-2 protein. The FDA also granted emergency use authorization to a replication-deficient adenovirus type 26 vaccine (Ad26.COV2.S).[125]

Initial clinical trials to confirm the efficacy and safety of COVID-19 vaccines, as expected, did not include patients with cancer with active disease.[9] Studies indicate that patients with cancer do not mount the same antibody response to mRNA platform vaccines as obtained in normal healthy subjects.[126] In Shroff et al.'s reported studies, the data indicated that most patients with cancer developed both CD4[+] and CD8[+] T-cell responses. Reports indicate a fairly rapid decline in the neutralizing capacity of vaccine induced antibodies against COVID-19 spike and nucleocapsid antigens, especially in the face of the development of variants of the original SARS-CoV-2 strain.[126] It appears that COVID-19 vaccination of patients with cancer even when they are undergoing active anticancer therapy will result in some degree of detectable neutralizing antibody and T-cell response, especially the latter.

A meta-analysis that included 621 patients with cancer and 256 control noncancer patients provides a useful look at the efficacy and safety of mRNA COVID-19 vaccines in patients with cancer. The meta-analysis identified and screened 39 citations of potential relevance that were subjected to inclusion/exclusion screening. The screening resulted in six manuscripts deemed suitable for meta-analysis inclusion. The meta-analysis confirmed that the majority of patients with cancer can be expected to have a good immunologic response to mRNA anti-COVID-19 vaccinations. The seropositive rates (anti-S IgG) in 281 patients with solid tumors after two doses of an mRNA vaccine were >90% in the group of patients with cancer and 100% in the control group. The cohort of 340 reported patients in the analysis with hematologic malignances consistently had a slightly lower (~85%) seroconversion. Recent chemotherapy (<15 days), patient frailty, patients with thoracic malignancies, and patients who received highly immunosuppressive cancer treatments showed significantly lower seroconversion rates. Obviously, the numbers available for analysis in these latter groups were small and heterogeneous, but the trends appeared as expected.[107,126-128] Patients with hematologic malignancies are certainly candidates for closer follow-up and specific testing to determine optimal timing of booster vaccination. More longitudinal clinical studies are needed to understand the duration of vaccine protection as well as the development of high-risk variants of the virus.

All accumulated data indicate that SARS-CoV-2 vaccination is safe when given to patients with cancer even for patients known to be immunocompromised.[129] Patients with hematologic malignancy and those patients with cancer receiving immunosuppressive systemic therapy should receive a third mRNA vaccine dose of the mRNA vaccine at least 28 days after receiving their second dose. This third dose has been shown to significantly improve the neutralizing antibody response, especially against the Omicron variants, in patients with cancer. The benefit is unfortunately less in patients with hematologic malignancy. In a prospective study, neutralizing antibodies were detected in only 19% of patients with hematologic malignancy after the second dose. The number of patients with detectable neutralizing antibodies was increased to 56% with the third dose.[130,131]

It is important to understand that the three-dose primary regimen is not equivalent to the common use of a "booster" dose for noncancer patients and nonimmunosuppressed patients.[132-134] Studies involving patients with cancer support the use of a three-dose primary regimen followed by the administration of a booster immunization (a fourth dose) 6 months after the three-dose primary regimen.[135] More studies will be needed to develop a more formal regimen for the administration of booster doses of the vaccines. The correlation between assays for B-cell immunity (enzyme-linked immunosorbent assay, ELISA) by determining levels of neutralizing antibody and by testing for T-cell function (enzyme-linked immune absorbent spot, ELISPOT) to determine the level of protection against COVID-19 remains to be demonstrated by cohort studies (Fig. 13.3).[136]

At the time of this writing, it can be anticipated that most newly diagnosed patients with cancer have had access to full COVID-19 vaccination. For those who have not been vaccinated, it may be best to consider holding the initiation of cancer treatment until the completion of the three-dose vaccination regimen. Timing decisions concerning vaccination and treatment initiation should, of course, take into account a patient history of COVID-19 infection balanced against the stage of cancer and degree of immunocompromise. Decisions need to be individualized based on

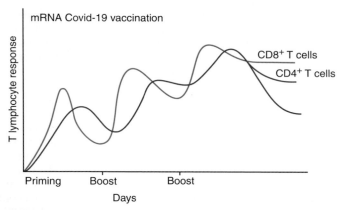

Fig. 13.3 **A conceptual graph depicting the CD8$^+$ and CD4$^+$ T-lymphocyte responses during administration of a three-dose course of mRNA COVID-19 vaccine.** In this response graph, boosting doses
occur at 28-day intervals. CD8$^+$ and CD4$^+$ S1 antigen-specific T cells undergo proliferation with each exposure to S1 antigen and develop long-lasting CD8$^+$ and CD4$^+$ memory cell populations. The subset of CD4$^+$
memory cells is depicted by the lower breakaway blue curve. Antigen-specific B-cell response has a similar
trajectory of cell expansion and neutralizing antibody production. The B-lymphocyte population also develops
an antigen-specific memory population for more rapid recall. The level of serum-detectable COVID-19 neutralizing antibody has not proven to be a good surrogate for the level of T-lymphocyte memory and antiviral
protection in the case of COVID-19.

BOX 13.1 ■ Optimizing COVID-19 Vaccination for the Patient With Cancer

- Optimal primary-course vaccination consists of three doses of mRNA vaccine administered 28 days
  apart (even for patients with a history of COVID-19).
- All existing evidence supports the conclusion that mRNA vaccines are safe.
- Booster vaccine doses continue to be important at ~4- to 6-month intervals.
- For newly diagnosed patients with cancer who are vaccinated, consider boosting immunity to
  COVID-19.
- Consider holding introduction of immunosuppressive anticancer treatment until vaccination is
  completed whenever possible.
- Administer any vaccine doses between therapy cycles to maximize immunity.
- At least 4 weeks post vaccine administration is required to achieve full benefit.
- Repeat primary vaccination regimen approximately 3 months after completion of hematopoietic cell
  transplant and CAR T-cell therapies.
- mRNA vaccination may cause temporary regional lymph adenopathy, which should be accounted for
  when using imaging in the patient with cancer.
- Participation in immunology-based clinical trials should be encouraged to examine long-term reciprocal interactions between COVID-19 vaccination and cancer immunotherapy.
- B-cell COVID-19 neutralizing antibody levels may be assayed by ELISA and plaque reduction
  neutralization test (PRNT).
- T-cell COVID-19 specific activity may be measured by ELISPOT.

---

general guidelines. For example, if initiation of immunosuppressive treatment is urgent,
COVID-19 vaccine may be given between therapy cycles (Box 13.1).

A special consideration exists for fully vaccinated patients who undergo stem cell transplantation or CAR T-cell therapy. For these patients, the CDC recommends repeating the full primary
three-dose series approximately 3 months after completion of these treatments.[137] If possible,

during the period of COVID-19 vaccination administration, it is ideal to avoid administering anticancer therapies that would be immunosuppressive to achieve some level of optimal vaccine protection. Should the patient with cancer receiving chemotherapy or immunotherapy become infected with COVID-19, the treatment course is interrupted (even in the asymptomatic patient) until recovery can be confirmed.

The mRNA-based COVID-19 vaccines (Pfizer BNT162b2 and Moderna mRNA-1273) may cause a degree of postvaccination axillary adenopathy that can interfere with imaging interpretation in the patient with cancer. Mammography, computed tomography (CT) and positron emission tomography (PET)-CT imaging should be scheduled prior to any COVID-19 vaccination or 4 to 6 weeks after completion of the three-dose primary vaccination or the administration of a COVID-19 booster dose.[138] It is important to know the history of vaccinations when obtaining imaging studies. Consideration should be given to administering the vaccine in the arm opposite to the site of the primary tumor. This is especially useful for imaging of patients with cancers of the breast and head and neck and cutaneous melanoma.[139,140]

Patients with cancer have the added risk of a tumor-compromised immune system and increased susceptibility to COVID-19 infection, secondary to the effect of progressing malignancy and/or anticancer therapy. Both the presence of malignancy and the anticancer therapy may cause an altered adaptive immune system with defects in Th1/Th2 and CTL recognition and binding of the COVID-19 spike protein. As discussed previously, studies indicate that defects in Th1, Th2, and CTL repertoires, especially the Th1/Tc1 response capacity, may affect the efficient recognition of the S1 receptor-binding domain on the spike protein as presented by current vaccines and result in a less-than-optimal sustained immunity. This potential defect appears to be more prominent in patients with hematologic malignancies compared with those with solid tumors.[110]

The burden on the immune system to generate an adaptive anticancer response and the significant potential for this process to produce alterations in the functions of the critical lymphocyte subpopulations have prompted increased attention on finding ways to optimize protective T-cell immunity and T-cell memory. Th1 cells and CD8$^+$ cytotoxic T lymphocytes (CTLs) have a similar profile of active cytokines including IL-2, IFN-γ, and TNF-α. These Th1 and CTL cytokines work together to drive the host response to COVID-19 vaccination.[126] During the response to vaccination, CD4$^+$ T cells and Th2 cells also provide antigen-specific memory and optimal help for both B-cell antiviral responses and protective mucosal immunity.

There have not been extensive clinical studies on the potential negative effect of COVID-19 vaccination of the patient with cancer on active immunotherapy. The severity of the viral disease in patients with cancer has led to a balancing of the risks of the viral illness with that of vaccination. A report by Waissengrin and colleagues, though limited by a small number of study participants, suggested that administration of BNT162b2 mRNA COVID-19 vaccine to patients with cancer being treated with checkpoint inhibitors (CPIs) showed an increase in all vaccination side effects compared with controls (see Box 13.1).[141,142]

COVID-19 and Cancer Therapy

As we begin our third year of the SARS-CoV-2 pandemic, much has been learned and more confidence exists today regarding the management of patients with cancer who, by the very nature of the COVID-19 pandemic, are exposed daily to the added risks of an aggressive respiratory virus.[5,143] Patients testing positive for SARS-CoV-2 infection may be totally asymptomatic or present as mildly symptomatic with flu-like symptoms, though many individuals become critically ill, requiring hospitalization, intubation for respiratory support, and intensive care. Today, those who do not survive COVID-19 infection are almost exclusively patients who are unvaccinated.

With its effects on the immune system, cancer is one of the confirmed risk factors for both an increased disease incidence and a greater severity of infection.[120] Thus, a critical question for oncologists and patients with cancer has been the effect of cancer therapy, especially immuno-therapy, on both an increased risk of COVID-19 infection and the clinical course of an infection. Previous reports, including the UK Coronavirus Cancer Monitoring Project (UKCCMP), indi-cated that COVID-19 mortality in patients with cancer was primarily associated with patient age, sex, comorbidities, and tumor subtype and not with the recent administration of systemic anticancer therapies.[120,144,145] In a UKCCMP multicenter study of 2515 unvaccinated patients with cancer between March 18 and August 1, 2020, the authors were able to draw several clini-cally relevant conclusions despite a short period of follow-up. First, patients with cancer had a poorer overall outcome when infected with COVID-19, but their analysis of these patients sug-gested that the poor outcome could be related to associated comorbidities and tumor subtype rather than anticancer treatment. Recent systemic chemotherapy, for example, was not associated with all-cause mortality. Interestingly, recent immunotherapy (principally ICIs) was found to be associated with less severe COVID-19 symptoms and a lower mortality rate from infection. The authors proposed that the association between recent ICI treatment and improved COVID-19 outcomes might be explained by enhanced anti-COVID-19 T-cell immunity.[145]

Anticancer hormonal therapy, targeted therapy, radiation therapy, and surgery within 4 weeks of COVID-19 infection were also not found to be associated with a higher COVID-19 mortality rate. The authors did find an association with higher COVID-19 mortality in patients with myeloma who received immunomodulatory therapy.[108] From this analysis and others, it would seem reasonable to conclude that fully vaccinated patients with cancer undergoing treatment would have similar or even better results if they were optimally vaccinated but contracted a "breakthrough" COVID-19 infection.[146]

Nevertheless, treatment decisions need to consider level of community viral transmission and to regularly test patients with cancer involved in all active therapies. This is especially critical for patients undergoing highly immunosuppressive systemic therapies such as oxaliplatin plus irino-tecan and infusional fluorouracil and leucovorin (FOLFIRINOX) for advanced colon cancer. Hematologic malignancies treated with anti-CD20 monoclonal antibodies are associated with B-cell depletion. These therapies are noted as a reminder of their potential association with an increased risk of COVID-19 infection and a suboptimal response to vaccination. Frequently updated websites hosted by the National Cancer Institute, the American Society of Clinical Oncology (ASCO), the National Comprehensive Cancer Network (NCCN), and the Centers for Disease Control and Prevention (CDC) are reliable sources for physicians to obtain up-to-date information and guidance for the care of the cancer patient during this pandemic.

Immunotherapies currently in use, whether as part of a clinical trial or as approved cancer thera-pies, include hematopoietic stem cell transplantation, cell-based therapies (CAR-T), bispecifics (BiTEs), and immune checkpoint inhibitors (ICIs). Of these immunotherapies, ICIs have gained considerable promise and use in the cancer population. PD-1-based ICI anticancer therapy acts through $CD8^+$ and $CD4^+$ T lymphocytes to effectively release the downregulation of the antitumor immune response caused by the increased PD-1 activity occurring in the patient with a progressing cancer. ICI therapy therefore acts to generate a more effective anticancer immune response.

$CD8^+$ and $CD4^+$ T cells, as noted previously, are also essential to the development of a robust immune response after the administration of a protective vaccine. Though it is certainly possible that ICI therapy could provide protection against the development of more severe COVID-19 infection, immune-related adverse events (irAEs) are a common complication of ICI therapy, with a reported incidence of between 54% and 76%.[147] The therapies used to manage ICI-induced irAEs make it difficult to interpret the role played by active ICI therapy in patients either exposed to COVID-19 or experiencing a breakthrough infection.

A look at the clinical effect of becoming infected with COVID-19 while being treated with an ICI must, of course, be examined in the two phases of COVID-19: prevaccination and post complete vaccination. An early multicenter study reported in December 2020 (prevaccine) involved

110 ICI-treated patients with cancer with a variety of cancer types who had laboratory-confirmed SARS-CoV-2 infection.[148] Approximately 40% were essentially asymptomatic, and the clinical presentation of those who became symptomatic did not appear different than expected despite being ICI treated. Thirty-five required hospitalization (32%), a slightly lower rate than that reported for patients with cancer. In this study, 18 patients died (16%). It was noted, however, that all deaths were in patients with advanced cancer and only eight deaths could be directly attributed to COVID-19. Though there are many limitations to interpreting the results of this study, it does suggest for the patient with cancer and the treating oncologist that ICI treatment does not appear to be an added risk factor for developing severe COVID-19 disease (Box 13.2).[147,148]

In summarizing where we are today as we plan going forward, several points seem important. As cancer physicians, we recognize that for our patients with cancer there are many tumor and health variables that each patient uniquely brings to their anti-cancer therapy. Each patient requires careful attention/monitoring regarding the details of their disease; their immune response to their cancer; their frailty, if present; and the known risks of therapy being provided. Immune system integrity is an important variable for all interventions, and all therapies, including surgery and radiation. All therapies can be considered to be immune altering, at least transiently. All patients with cancer, therefore, have the added risk of infectious disease complications. The COVID-19 pandemic has provided a stark reminder of the need to thoughtfully plan how to first optimize the patient with cancer against COVID-19 as well as against other serious infections and to carefully

---

BOX 13.2 ■ COVID-19 Emergent Use Authorized

Monoclonal Antibodies:

- Tixagevimab with cigavimab (Evusheld): antispike protein mAbs; blocks viral entry
- Casirivimab with imdevimab (Regen-CoV): antispike protein mAbs; blocks viral entry
- Sotrovimab (Xevudy): antispike protein mAb; blocks viral entry
- Bebtelovimab: antispike protein mAb; blocks viral attachment
- Bamlanivimab with etesevimab: antispike protein mAbs; blocks viral entry

Antivirals:

- Remdesivir (Veklury): nucleotide analog ribonucleic acid inhibitor; disrupts viral replication; intravenous
- Nirmatrelvir with ritonavir (Paxlovid): viral protease inhibitor; blocks replication; oral $\times$ 5 days to prevent hospitalization
- Molnupiravir (Lagevirio): nucleoside analog; causes mutagenesis to inhibit replication; oral medication

Immunomodulators:

- Dexamethasone: antiinflammatory for hospitalized patients requiring respiratory support
- Baricitinib (Olumiant): COVID-19-positive patients requiring respiratory support; oral medication; can be used with remdesivir; selective Janus kinases (JAK1/JAK2) inhibitor
- Tocilizumab: mAb that blocks IL-6 receptor (needs more study)

Notes: This table is meant to provide some historical perspective regarding efforts to modify the course of COVID-19 infection, especially to prevent hospitalization and mortality. It is important to consider that although having received FDA-EUA emergent use approval, whereever possible, therapies such as listed in this table should be used in the setting of a clinical trial. Other antivirals and immunomodulators are under development and clinical study. COVID-19 websites hosted by state medical boards, the FDA, CDC, and the Department of Health and Human Services (HHS) are useful resources to get up-to-date information on anti-COVID-19 therapies available and use guidelines for high-risk individuals such as patients with cancer and immunosuppression.
mAb, Monoclonal antibody.

consider how to best balance anticancer treatment, protective vaccination, and actual breakthrough infection on a highly individual basis. The opportunity for robust vaccination against COVID-19 will be the key for our patients with cancer as we move forward. There is much we will learn in the coming years, emphasizing the importance of our participation in COVID-19 research.

Effect of COVID-19 Pandemic on Clinical Cancer Care and Cancer Clinical Trials Research

The initial wave of SARS-CoV-2 infections was recognized in the United States in January 2020. By March it was obvious that COVID-19 was a greater health crisis than originally thought as it began rapidly spreading globally and within the United States.[1,2,4] The United States and many other countries essentially shut down their communities, enforcing stay-at-home orders and community business lockdowns in an unprecedented effort to moderate the scale of spread of a highly contagious respiratory coronavirus. Hospitals quickly filled to capacity with COVID-19-infected patients. Health care systems were forced to stop the care of nonemergent patients, all elective surgeries were halted, and many health care workers were redeployed to care for the multitude of seriously ill virus-infected patients.[149] Oncologists went to extreme efforts to continue the care of their patients with cancer, switching whereever possible from intravenous therapy to oral anticancer medications and to virtual patient visits. Much of cancer care attempted to avoid the need to use in-patient resources and personal protective equipment (PPE), which at the time was in extremely short supply.[150,151]

Patients with cancer worried about an increased risk of a serious outcome if they were to become infected with COVID-19. This caused many patients with cancer to interrupt their cancer treatment.[111,152,153] There was a documented break from routinely scheduled cancer screening during this time as routine nonessential health care was placed on hold.[154] Even today as the country begins to return to a more confident state in terms of COVID-19, appointments for routine health care and cancer screening are difficult to schedule and certainly not available within the timelines of what was available prepandemic.[155,156] The delays in scheduling are the result of ongoing efforts to maintain social distancing in office and clinic waiting rooms to optimally protect patients with cancer.

The majority of research activities, including clinical trials, were significantly reduced or even halted as the scientific community shifted to address research directly related to COVID-19 and to finding new antiviral therapies and vaccines. Cancer scientists and their laboratories proved to be valuable assets to address the rapidly spreading COVID-19 pandemic. They had experience in laboratory immunology procedures, in the technologies of monoclonal antibodies, and in the development and testing of targeted therapies.

However, many university laboratories essentially closed and laboratory experimental work was placed on hold as universities closed and shifted to virtual classrooms. Laboratory scientists, translational scientists, and clinical trialists were further affected by the cancellation of all in-person scientific meetings. With time, the organizers of these meetings began to adapt to the reality of the pandemic and worked to set in place what proved to be exceptional and critical virtual meetings.[157]

There was a significant effect on cancer translational research during the pandemic. Clinical trials support staff such as research nurses and data managers were forced by the pandemic and institutional policies to work off-site. Some research nurses and physicians were called upon for reassignment to assist in direct care of patients with COVID-19. Many early-phase clinical trials were halted, and new phase 1 trials were postponed, with priority given to maintaining ongoing phase 2 and 3 trials. In addition to the workforce effect of the COVID-19 pandemic in our major academic research-oriented health care systems, these institutions experienced major financial losses. In addition, many patients were reluctant to continue their participation in trials because of concerns about their own risks during the peak of the pandemic.[158]

The pandemic effect on clinical research was not limited to cancer trials. In a study of randomized controlled trials (RCTs), Audisio and colleagues queried the Clinical Trials.gov database in February 2020.[159] For their analysis, eligible trials included all non-COVID-19 RCTs with a start date after January 1, 2010, that were listed as active during the period January 1, 2015, through December 31, 2020. They used March 11, 2020, as the start date of the pandemic. The analysis endpoints were (1) early trial stoppage, (2) normal trial completion, and (3) new trial activation. The database contained 161,377 trials for analysis. They found that the number of active trials increased annually through 2019 but decreased significantly in 2020. They found that trial completion was not adversely affected by the pandemic ($P = .56$) but trial stoppage was significantly increased ($P = .001$). They found a sharp decline in new RCTs in 2020 at the beginning of the pandemic, with a gradual recovery.[159] Others have reported clinical research reductions of >50% during early 2020.[160]

As noted previously, beginning in 2021 with the availability of highly efficacious vaccines, the clinical care of patients with cancer and the clinical trials research that is so critical to optimizing their care began the slow progression back toward a degree of normalcy. This recovery will certainly be a gradual process because major shifts in the clinical trials support staff occurred during the pandemic. Major university cancer research centers uniformly reported a significant shortage of clinical research nurses, data managers, and other staff essential to the return to pre-COVID-19 levels of activity. Similar staffing needs also exist for the regular delivery of in-patient and ambulatory care of our patients with cancer.[161] Perhaps a positive effect of the COVID-19 pandemic on clinical investigation will be the transformation of how we conduct clinical trials going forward. The pandemic has caused us to generate new trial designs, with protocols adapted to virtual visits, in-home electronic monitoring, remote delivery of study drugs/interventions, and with fewer requirements for blood sampling and imaging. An approach to cancer clinical trials based on what we have learned from navigating the pandemic may result in greater participation by our patients.

Though the availability of highly efficacious vaccines has certainly changed the trajectory of the pandemic and our socioeconomic recovery appears underway, we must continue to be prudent in planning our return. We must take every opportunity to carefully research the effects of the COVID-19 pandemic on not only our patients with cancer, but most importantly on the way in which the pandemic effected our delivery of cancer care and the ability to conduct clinical cancer research in order to be better prepared for the next pandemic.

Mutations, which are prominent in viruses with RNA as their genetic material, are expected in the genetic code of the COVID-19 virus.[162] Though there has been a high rate of mutations occurring in COVID-19, the United States has experienced only two additional major variant waves: the second, or Delta, wave, which peaked in early September 2021, and the third wave, the Omicron BA.1 variant, which peaked in January 2022. It is not clear what we should expect from a second Omicron variant BA.2 that is currently spreading in the United States (https://coronavirus.jhu.edu/map.html, accessed March 10, 2022).[13] Despite these second and third waves, the general acceptance of masking and the rapid availability of highly efficacious mRNA vaccines and vaccination has provided new hope and expectations. Mask mandates are being set aside, schools have been open during the 2021–2022 school year, and schools and businesses have been able to test for infection, contact tracet, and as a result to stay open. Our health care systems may not yet be back to prepandemic functioning, but they are progressing to a new state of accessibility and function. Despite the significant setbacks to clinical trials research, it appears that the continuation of accrual to trials has returned to prior levels and the level of new trial starts is approaching an expected normal level.

Post-Acute SARS-CoV-2 Syndrome and Its Effect on the Patient With Cancer

It is perhaps much too early in the study of the COVID-19 viral pathogen for us to understand either the potential long-term health effects of even the subacute (nonhospitalized) infections of

---

BOX 13.3 ■ Post-Acute COVID-19 Organ-Specific Sequelae

- Fatigue, muscle weakness, joint symptoms, hair loss (20%), and declining quality of life
- Anxiety, depression, sleep disturbances, posttraumatic stress disorder, cognition disturbances, and chronic headache (30%–40%)
- Dyspnea on exertion, persistent dry cough, nasal oxygen requirement
- Irregular heart rhythms, chest pain, thrombosis, and thromboembolism
- Decrease in kidney function

COVID-19 or the long-term effects that severe infection requiring intensive hospitalized care may have on multiple organ systems. "Postacute COVID-19 syndrome" is characterized by persistence of symptoms of the acute disease or of the subsequent onset of a wide range of organ-specific sequelae. Many patients post-COVID-19 infection identify themselves as "long-haulers," and in many cases the severity of the sequelae is severely debilitating. There were similar reports associated with severe infections of SARS and MERS, but the sheer magnitude of the COVID-19 pandemic and the unprecedented scale of global morbidity and mortality have generated a much larger population of patients with chronic post-COVID-19 morbidities and therefore much greater awareness of these debilitating post-COVID-19 illnesses.

To date there is very little information concerning the incidence of prolonged COVID-19 symptoms in patients with cancer and the effect of complete vaccination on mitigating the incidence of the postacute COVID-19 morbidities. The relationships of cancer and complete vaccination to prolonged postacute COVID-19 morbidities remain to be studied (Box 13.3).[163]

A study of 1250 patients using medical records and telephone surveys of patients discharged and alive 60 days postacute COVID-19 hospitalization was conducted in Michigan.[164] Of the original 1250 study subjects, 488 completed the telephone survey; 32.6% reported persistent symptoms, including 18.9% with new or worsened symptoms. Dyspnea on exertion was reported in 22.9%, persistent dry cough in 15.4%, and persistent loss of taste and/or smell in 13.1%.[163,164] Similar findings have been reported in Europe, the United Kingdom, and Asia.[163-166]

Given the scale and global nature of this unprecedented viral pandemic, it is imperative that oncologists understand the history of their patients with regard to prior acute COVID-19 infection and be more clinically attuned to symptoms that may suggest occult organ damage secondary to the infection. It will, at times, be necessary to separate symptoms associated with a history of COVID-19 infection from those commonly recognized as related to cancer treatment and cancer progression. Documented post-COVID-19 illness may have relevance to planned immunotherapies and to the nature of clinical follow-up and cancer management to avoid compounding unnecessary toxicities. Oncologists should be aware of ongoing studies and encourage their patients to participate where possible to further our understanding of the true long-term pathophysiology of COVID-19. There is much to learn going forward.

Some Concluding Thoughts

During the first quarter of the 21st century, scientists and clinicians worldwide became increasingly aware of the complete globalization and interactivity of the world's populations. The result is the ease of rapid global transmission of human infectious pathogens. Recent epidemics of Ebola, Zika, SARS, MERS, and COVID-19 have focused our attention on this new reality of the 21st century in terms of the challenges that lie ahead in the management of global infectious diseases. There is a recognition that these pandemics will continue to be a threat and that they will always need to be considered in the context of our management of patients with other chronic diseases such as cancer. Cancer and viral infections have an intimate immune system interaction and a somewhat similar relationship with the host adaptive immune system, as described in this chapter and in Chapters 4, 5, 6, and 7 of this text. The SARS-CoV-2 pandemic continues and has underscored our vulnerability as a society and the importance of continuing our laboratory-based and clinical research to find new ways to use the immune system to better treat our patients.

Key References

4. Lai C-C, Shih T-P, Ko W-C, Tang H-J, Hsueh P-R. Severe acute respiratory syndrome coronavirus 2 (SARS-CoV-2) and coronavirus disease-2019 (COVID-19): the epidemic and the challenges. *Int J Antimicrob Agents*. 2020;55(3):105924. doi:10.1016/j.ijantimicag.2020.105924.

5. Bora VR, Patel BM. The deadly duo of COVID-19 and cancer! *Front Mol Biosci*. 2021;8:643004. doi:10.3389/fmolb.2021.643004.

7. Lou E, Teoh D, Brown K, et al. Perspectives of cancer patients and their health during the COVID-19 pandemic. *PLoS ONE*. 2020;15(10):e0241741. doi:10.1371/journal.pone.0241741.

22. Rana R, Tripathi A, Kumar N, Ganguly NK. A comprehensive overview on COVID-19: future perspectives. *Front Cell Infect Microbiol*. 2021;11:744903. doi:10.3389/fcimb.2021.744903.

36. Abdool Karim SS, de Oliveira T. New SARS-CoV-2 variants – clinical, public health, and vaccine implications. *N Engl J Med*. 2021;384:1866-1868. doi:10.1056/NEJMc2100362.

40. Gralton J, Tovey E, Mclaws M-L, Rawlinson WD. The role of particle size in aerosolized pathogen transmission: a review. *J Infect*. 2011;62:1-13. doi:10.1016/j.jinf.2010.11.010.

43. Wang Q, Zhang Y, Wu L, et al. Structural and functional basis of SARS-CoV-2 entry by using human ACE2. *Cell*. 2020;181:894-904.e9. doi:10.1016/j.cell.2020.03.045.

54. Diamond MS, Kanneganti T-D. Innate immunity: the first line of defense against SARS-CoV-2. *Nat Immunol*. 2022;23(2):165-176. doi:10.1038/s41590-021-01091-0.

58. Li Y, Wang X, Wang W. The impact of COVID-19 on cancer. *Infect Drug Resist*. 2021;14:3809-3816.

59. Ren P, Gong C, Ma S. Evaluation of COVID-19 based on ACE2 expression in normal and cancer patients. *Open Med*. 2020;15:613-622.

69. Zindel J, Kubes P. DAMPs, PAMPs and LAMPs in immunity and sterile inflammation. *Annu Rev Pathol*. 2020;15:493-518. doi:10.1146/annurev-pathmechdis-012419-032847.

85. Kleinnijenhuis J, Quintin J, Preijers F, et al. BCG-induced trained immunity in NK cells: role for non-specific protection to infection. *Clin Immunol*. 2014;155(2):213-219. doi:10.1016/j.clim.2014.10.005.

87. Kleinnijenhuis J, Quintin J, Preijers F, et al. Bacille Calmette-Guerin induces NOD2-dependent non-specific protection from reinfection via epigenetic reprogramming of monocytes. *Proc Natl Acad Sci U S A*. 2012;109(43):17537-17542. doi:10.1073/pnas.1202870109.

89. Mogensen TH. Pathogen recognition and inflammatory signaling in innate immune defenses. *Clin Microbiol Rev*. 2009;22(2):240-272.

94. Sette A, Crotty S. Adaptive immunity to SARS-CoV-2 and COVID-19. *Cell*. 2021;184:861-880.

102. Israel A, Shenhar Y, Green I, et al. Large scale study of antibody titer decay following BNT162b2 mRNA vaccine or SARS-CoV-2 infection. *Vaccines (Basel)*. 2021;10(1):64. doi:10.3390/vaccines10010064.

106. Shrotri M, van Schalkwyk MC, Post N, et al. T cell response to SARS-CoV-2 infection in humans: a systematic review. *PLOS ONE*. 2021;16(1):e0245532. doi:10.1371/journal.pone.0245532.

119. Di Lorenzo G, Di Trolio R, Kozlakidis Z, et al. COVID-19 therapies and anti-cancer drugs: a systematic review of recent literature. *Crit Rev Oncol Hematol*. 2020;152:102991. doi:10.1016/j.critrevonc.2020.102991.

121. Westblade LF, Brar G, Pinheiro LC, et al. SARS-CoV-2 viral load predicts mortality in patients with and without cancer who are hospitalized with COVID-19. *Cancer Cell*. 2020;38(5):661-671.e2. doi:10.1016/j.ccell.2020.09.007.

122. Jee J, Foote MB, Lumish M, et al. Chemotherapy and COVID-19 outcomes in patients with cancer. *J Clin Oncol*. 2020;38:3538-3546. doi:10.1200/JCO.20.01307.

126. Shroff RT, Chalasani P, Wei R, et al. Immune responses to two and three doses of the BNT162b2 mRNA vaccine in adults with solid tumors. *Nat Med*. 2021;27:2002-2011. doi:10.1038/s41591-021-01542-z.

130. Fendler A, Shepherd STC, Au L, et al. Omicron neutralizing antibodies after third COVID-19 vaccine dose in patients with cancer. *Lancet*. 2022;399(10328):905-907. doi:10.1016/S0140-6736(22)00147-7.
161. Lamont EB, Diamond SS, Katriel RG, et al. Trends in oncology clinical trials launched before and during the COVID-19 pandemic. *JAMA Netw Open*. 2021;4:e2036353.
166. Halpin SJ, McIvor C, Whyatt G, et al. Postdischarge symptoms and rehabilitation needs in survivors of COVID-19 infection: a cross-sectional evaluation. *J Med Virol*. 2021;93(2):1013-1022. doi:10.1002/jmv.26368.

Visit Elsevier eBooks + (eBooks.Health.Elsevier.com) for complete set of references.

Page numbers followed by "*f*" indicate figures, "*t*" indicate tables, and "*b*" indicate boxes.